P9-CMT-177

Nursing Leadership, Management, and Professional Practice for the LPN/LVN

SIXTH EDITION

Tamara R. Dahlkemper, MSN, RN, CNE
Associate Professor
Weber State University School of Nursing
Ogden, Utah

F.A. Davis Company • Philadelphia

F.A. Davis Company
1915 Arch Street
Philadelphia, PA 19103
www.fadavis.com

Copyright © 2018 by F.A. Davis Company

Copyright © 2013, 2009, 2005, 2001, 1997 by F.A. Davis Company. All rights reserved. This book is protected by copyright. No part of it may be reproduced, stored in a retrieval system, or transmitted in any form or by any means, electronic, mechanical, photocopying, recording, or otherwise, without written permission from the publisher.

Printed in the United States of America

Last digit indicates print number: 10 9 8 7 6 5 4 3 2 1

Publisher, Nursing: Terri W. Allen
Content Project Manager II: Amy M. Romano
Design and Illustration Manager: Carolyn O'Brien

As new scientific information becomes available through basic and clinical research, recommended treatments and drug therapies undergo changes. The author(s) and publisher have done everything possible to make this book accurate, up to date, and in accord with accepted standards at the time of publication. The author(s), editors, and publisher are not responsible for errors or omissions or for consequences from application of the book, and make no warranty, expressed or implied, in regard to the contents of the book. Any practice described in this book should be applied by the reader in accordance with professional standards of care used in regard to the unique circumstances that may apply in each situation. The reader is advised always to check product information (package inserts) for changes and new information regarding dose and contraindications before administering any drug. Caution is especially urged when using new or infrequently ordered drugs.

Library of Congress Cataloging-in-Publication Data

Names: Dahlkemper, Tamara R., author.
Title: Nursing leadership, management, and professional practice for the LPN/LVN / Tamara Dahlkemper.
Other titles: Anderson's nursing leadership, management, and professional practice for the LPN/LVN
Description: Sixth edition. | Philadelphia, PA : F.A. Davis Company, [2018] | Preceded by Anderson's nursing leadership, management, and professional practice for the LPN/LVN / Tamara R. Dahlkemper. 5th ed. c2013. | Includes bibliographical references and index.
Identifiers: LCCN 2017014423 | ISBN 9780803660854 (alk. paper)
Subjects: | MESH: Nursing, Practical—organization & administration | Nursing Services—organization & administration | Nurse Administrators | Licensed Practical Nurses | Leadership | Vocational Guidance
Classification: LCC RT62 | NLM WY 195 | DDC 610.7306/93—dc23
LC record available at https://lccn.loc.gov/2017014423

Authorization to photocopy items for internal or personal use, or the internal or personal use of specific clients, is granted by F. A. Davis Company for users registered with the Copyright Clearance Center (CCC) Transactional Reporting Service, provided that the fee of $.10 per copy is paid directly to CCC, 222 Rosewood Drive, Danvers, MA 01923. For those organizations that have been granted a photocopy license by CCC, a separate system of payment has been arranged. The fee code for users of the Transactional Reporting Service is: 978-8036-6085-4/18 0 + $.25.

Foreword

Nursing at all levels is a field that is changing in its roles and functions to respond better to the changing health needs of the public. Licensed practical nurses (LPNs) and licensed vocational nurses (LVNs) are caught up in these ever-demanding changes and challenges. As they seek new solutions, they too are in need of new models, new theories, and new paradigms to accommodate to and address their work requirements amidst the increasing complexities of the systems in which they work.

This leadership-management text for LPNs and LVNs comes at an important time—a time when nurses at all levels are being reduced in number, and quality patient care is being challenged by the public at large. During such turmoil, LPNs and LVNs are being expected to rise to new challenges of patient care and new system role relationships. They are being thrust into a new environment that expects and requires team building, an ethic of accountability, relationship skills, and leadership that stretches their current scope of practice, transcending established educational-clinical role boundaries for better or for worse. It is in the midst of such dramas that these nurses need the most sophisticated education and professional preparation they can possibly obtain, formally or informally.

It is here, in the midst of this need for education and practice reform, that this book on leadership and management provides some much-needed answers and educational material not generally available. This work not only offers "how tos" but, more important, it also offers some "whys" within the context of broader paradigm changes. As a result of this broader context, the text helps the student better understand the nature of change and leadership within the framework of caring and relationships and within the realities of conflict, employment processes, motivation, and use of power.

Such a broad framework for leadership and management places the issues within an even more fundamental structure related to ethics, teamwork, and the benefits of change and growth. In addition, this text provides an assessment guide for how to critique oneself and one's assignment and how to engage in making assignments for others and to engage in counseling and performance assessment. All of these are basic essentials and fundamentals for improving clinical care and practice in the arena of teamwork and assuming leadership roles.

In a field that is often replete with intellectual tools and professional development in areas that affect one's daily work life, this book fills a critical gap. It instructs, it informs, it coaches, and it inspires. In a field that is searching for new approaches to old problems, in a field that is seeking new questions for old answers that no longer hold true, this work holds out a glimmer of light and solid ground by which LPNs and LVNs can enter the 21st century for reformed health-care nursing practices.

Dr. Jean Watson
Distinguished Professor Emerita
University of Colorado Health Sciences Center
Denver, Colorado
and
Founder and Director
Watson Caring Science Institute
Boulder, Colorado

Preface

Licensed practical nurses (LPNs) and licensed vocational nurses (LVNs) are a vital element in health care today. They assume responsibility in multiple arenas of care that go far beyond the traditional hospital setting. Demands on the health-care system have expanded the role of the LPN and LVN to include, among other responsibilities, that of leadership in the profession and management of complex situations and groups of people who also give care.

Traditionally, LPNs and LVNs have assumed leadership and management roles in nursing homes and have validated that they are capable in that position. The demands are now more diverse, however, and it is appropriate for nursing education to respect the changes that have occurred in the role of these caregivers by providing them with the theoretical background they need to fulfill successfully the positions they are being asked to assume.

The purpose of this book is to provide LPNs and LVNs with the knowledge they need to assume the current leadership-management roles asked of them. It was written in response to LPN and LVN nursing educators asking for a text clarifying and supporting the leadership-management role of their students. This book is designed to give the learner the information needed to make the transition successfully from student to LPN and LVN. In a clear and concise manner, it presents basic information on the skills and knowledge needed to fulfill leadership and management role requirements. It covers multiple practice settings and presents the information with sound and practical theory. Clinical application examples of the content complement current LPN and LVN roles, and case studies at the end of each chapter call on the student to make personal applications of the information.

Although this text was written specifically for the expanded role of the LPN and LVN, its content also is relevant to registered nurses (RNs) seeking basic information. It can be used as a required or supplemental text in various leadership-management courses for RNs, LPN, and LVN career-ladder courses and courses for other health-care workers for whom leadership-management roles are expanding.

The book is written with an emphasis on the humanistic aspects of caring and is based on Dr. Jean Watson's nursing theory, *Nursing: human science and human care.* This approach provides students with leadership and management theories grounded in a meaningful nursing theoretical framework.

The content in this edition has been enhanced with updated information on current trends and issues such as bioethics, genetics, and substance use disorders in nursing. The informatics content has been enhanced to include information about electronic health records, telemedicine, meaningful use, HIPAA concerns when using health-care technology, and evidence-based practice that requires students to think critically. The chapter on culture includes new information that addresses hiring and managing diverse employees as well as developing and maintaining a culturally sensitive staff and recognizing its impact on patient outcomes. The chapter on delegation has been updated to include the principles of delegation from the nurse manager's perspective.

In an effort to enhance the learning process for students reading this textbook, new features have been added to each chapter in this edition. A list of key terms has been added at the beginning of each chapter to introduce the important terms covered. Additional tables and boxes have been added to a number of chapters to better highlight information in the chapter. Key points have been added at the end of each chapter to summarize important information discussed in the chapter. A list of chapter concepts has been added at the beginning of each chapter to facilitate use of this book in programs that teach conceptually. In addition, the textbook now includes five NCLEX-style review questions at the end of each chapter to help students review what they have learned.

Student Resources

To further the student learning experience, supplemental learning materials are available on Davis*Plus*. They include NCLEX-style quiz questions for each chapter, unfolding case studies that build on concepts as students progress through the textbook, and the ability to complete online the reflective thinking activities from each chapter and submit them to an instructor. The supplemental materials are designed to reinforce the student's comprehension of concepts introduced in each chapter.

Instructor Resources

Instructor resources for this edition include active classroom lesson plans mapped to content addressed in chapter PowerPoint slides. Lesson plans include integrated discussion questions and activities. The instructor resources also include a test bank with NCLEX-style questions for each chapter.

I hope you enjoy reading this textbook. Best of luck in your future nursing career!

TAMARA DAHLKEMPER

Contributors

Sally Cantwell, PhD, RN
Associate Chair of School of Nursing
Director, Associate Degree Program
School of Nursing
Weber State University
Ogden, Utah
Chapter 13 Understanding Benefits of Change,
* Chapter 21 Delegating, Coaching, and*
* Evaluating Performance*

Richard Dahlkemper, PhD
Faculty Emeritus
Health Administrative Services
Dumke College of Health Professions
Weber State University
Ogden, Utah
Chapter 4 Health-Care Environment

Carolyn Anita Jones, MS, RN
Dean of School of Nursing (Retired)
Oklahoma City Community College
Oklahoma City, Oklahoma
Chapter 12 Considering Culture

Diane Leggett-Fife, PhD, RN
Associate Professor
School of Nursing
Weber State University
Ogden, Utah
Chapter 5 Nursing and Informatics

Cory Moss, DHA, MBA, NHA
Assistant Professor
Health Administrative Services
Dumke College of Health Professions
Weber State University
Ogden, Utah
Chapter 12 Considering Culture

Melissa NeVille, DNP, APRN, CPNP-PC
Associate Professor
Director, MSN Program
School of Nursing
Weber State University
Ogden, Utah
Chapter 15 Handling Conflict in the Nursing
* Profession*

Julie Rhodes, MSN, RN
Nursing Instructor
School of Nursing
Weber State University
Ogden, Utah
Chapter 15 Handling Conflict in the Nursing
* Profession*

Holli Sowerby, EdD, MSN, RN, CNE
Assistant Professor
School of Nursing
Weber State University
Ogden, Utah
Chapter 2 Caring as a Person and Professional
* Behavior, Chapter 3 Understanding the*
* Changing Roles in Nursing, Chapter 4*
* Health-Care Environment*

Amy Stegen, MSN, RN
Assistant Professor
Director, RN-BSN Program
School of Nursing
Weber State University
Ogden, Utah
Chapter 6 Fulfill Your Role as a Student

LPN/LVN Advisory Board

Deborah D. Brabham, PhDc, RN, CNE
Instructional Program Manager
Scholar in Residence
Frisch Institute for Senior Care
Associate Degree and Practical Nursing
    Programs
Florida State College at Jacksonville
Jacksonville, Florida

Mark Donoghue, MS, RN
Faculty
Isabella Graham Hart School of Practical
    Nursing
Rochester, New York

Shelley Eckvahl, MSN, BSN
Lead Instructor
Chaffey College
Chino Hills, California

Marie Hedgpeth, MSN, MHA, RN
Practical Nursing Instructor
Robeson Community College
Lumberton, North Carolina

Kaye Henry, BSN
Program Director
School of Practical Nursing
Georgia Piedmont Technical College
Covington, Georgia

Dawn Johnson, DNP, RN, Ed
Practical Nurse Program Director
Great Lakes Institute of Technology
Erie, Pennsylvania

Paula K. Mundell, MSN, RN
Coordinator, Nursing Program
Delaware Technical Community College
Dover, Delaware

Sonia Rudolph, APRN, FNP-BC
Nursing Division Chair
Jefferson Community & Technical College
Louisville, Kentucky

Patricia Taylor, MSN-Ed, RN
Practical Nursing Coordinator
Kapi'olani Community College
University of Hawaii
Honolulu, Hawaii

Reviewers

Ruth Fee Blackmore, MSN, RN, CNOR
Faculty of Nursing
Isabella Graham Hart School of Practical
    Nursing
Rochester, New York

Pauletta Brady, RN, BSN
Practical Nursing Instructor
Tennessee College of Applied Technology
Livingston, Tennessee

Kelly Claycomb, RN, MSN
Nurse Educator/Program Coordinator
North Central Missouri College
Trenton, Missouri

Michele A. Dickson, DNP, RN, CNE
Professor of Nursing
Prince George's Community College
Largo, Maryland

Diane Duffy, RN, BSN, M.Ed.
Practical Nursing Director
Northwest Technology Center
Alva, Oklahoma

Alisha Edmunds, BSN, RN
Vocational Nursing Instructor
South Plains College
Plainview, Texas

Crystal Higgins, MS, RN, CNE
Program Chair Practical Nursing
Southeast Community College
Beatrice, Nebraska

Monica Iaquinta, RN, MSN, MS
Coordinator, Practical Nursing
United Technical Center
Clarksburg, West Virginia

Thirty H. Lacy, BSN, RN
Instructor, Vocational Nursing
Alvin Community College
Alvin, Texas

Belinda Rogers, RN, BSN, WHNP-BC
Director Practical Nursing
Ozarks Technical Community College
Lebanon, Missouri

Elizabeth Stingo, MSN, RN
LPN Instructor
Fred Eberle School of Practical Nursing
Buckhannon, West Virginia

Nancy Wiseman, RN, MSN
PN Instructor
Saline County Career Center
Marshall, Missouri

Amy Young, MSN, RN
Assistant Professor
Community College of Baltimore County
Dundalk, Maryland

STRESSED ABOUT THE
NCLEX®?

LATEST TEST PLAN!

Turn to Davis Edge NCLEX-PN®

- An online experience that prepares you for the exam

- 6,000+ questions, including 20% alternate format like "select-all-that-apply" (SATA), video, and audio questions

- Identifying weak areas and creating quizzes by client needs category, concept, or content area

- Exam-builder that generates 75-150 question simulated experience

- Test-taking tips to help reduce anxiety

Over **6,000** QUESTIONS

All with comprehensive rationales so you know exactly why your answer is correct or incorrect.

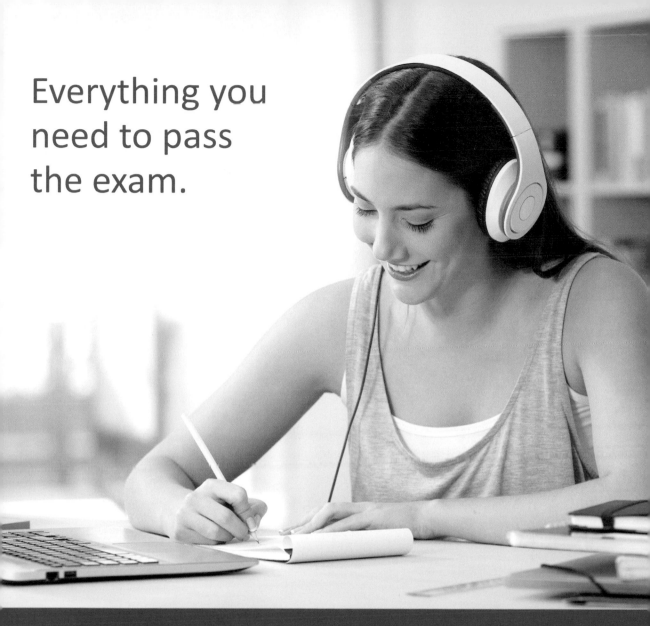

Everything you
need to pass
the exam.

SAVE 20%
Use Promo Code: NCLEXREADY

Order today on www.FADavis.com

Promotion subject to change without notice. Offer valid for purchases by individuals from www.FADavis.com in the US only.

Acknowledgments

I would like to thank all of the individuals, past and present, who have contributed their expertise and knowledge to this book. I also would like to thank Terri Allen and Amy Romano at F.A. Davis for their assistance and guidance in completing this edition. I would especially like to thank Developmental Editor Julie Scardiglia for her suggestions to improve the textbook and her words of encouragement that helped see me through the many hours of editing.

Most of all I would like to thank my husband and family for their constant support in all of my endeavors. I would not be who I am today without them.

Table of Contents

unit ONE

The Nursing Profession in Today's Health-Care Environment

1

Historical Perspective and Current Trends

KEY TERMS

Healthcare-associated
  infections (HAIs)
Impaired nurse
Medical model
Nursing model
Quality and Safety Education
  for Nurses (QSEN)

CHAPTER CONCEPTS

Addiction and Behaviors
Health-Care System
Professionalism

LEARNING OUTCOMES

1. Verbalize the importance of understanding the
   history of nursing.
2. Identify the accomplishments of nurses during
   ancient times, the Dark Ages, and modern times.
3. List four modern nurses who significantly contributed to the history of nursing and identify a
   major contribution of each.
4. Discuss the role of the LPN and the evolution of
   the role historically.
5. Name two official membership organizations for
   LPNs concerned with practical nursing education
   and nursing practice.
6. Discuss three current trends and issues that affect
   the practice of LPNs.

[F]orward-looking nurses endeavor to perfect their abilities to work effectively across organizational boundaries and pull together all the forces that must converge to create high-quality, cost-effective care. Moreover, such nurses also continually seek to understand the past, present, and future of the volatile environment in which nurses work.

—Philip A. Kalisch and Beatrice J. Kalisch

History is one class that is always required in educational curricula because examining historical evidence of a profession, a country, or a specific group of people establishes pride and knowledge in the mind of the learner. This chapter focuses on the history of nursing, with an emphasis on the evolution of the role of the licensed practical nurse (LPN) and the demands of current trends and issues in modern health care. One historical fact about this role is that it has more than one legally recognized title. LPNs and licensed vocational nurses (LVNs) are legally recognized and practice in diverse health-care settings today. LVN education predominantly takes place in California and Texas, whereas LPN education is common in other geographic areas of the United States. Throughout this book, both categories of licensure and nurse are referred to as LPN; this is not done to devalue LVNs but rather for the purpose of ease in reading.

This chapter establishes a historical perspective of your profession. Nursing is in a period of change, as are all health-care disciplines. Hospitals and other health-care delivery systems in the United States increasingly have been assaulted with major financial and quality concerns. The profession of nursing is changing in response to the powerful economic, ethical, and technological forces affecting health care. This is the state of the profession you are preparing to enter. It will be exciting and challenging! This chapter focuses on how history evolved to bring the profession to this point. This chapter also gives you the opportunity to write your own history. As a beginning nurse, you are at the perfect place in your career to consider what you want your history to be. In what type of nursing do you want to become an expert? Do you anticipate continuing school after completing your LPN education? Do you plan on moving to another geographic area? Because of the many people, predominantly women, who have written the profession's history to date, you will be able to make many informed decisions about your career. It may be too early in your career to answer

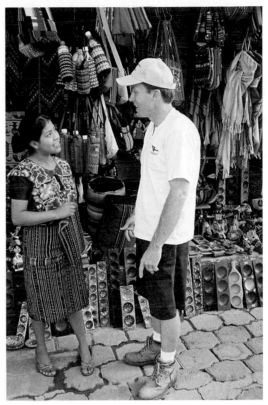

The history of nursing extends back to ancient times. Currently nurses in developing countries provide health care in situations that resemble the conditions in ancient times. This nurse in Guatemala is following up on a newborn visit. He had to find the mother and make an appointment to see her at home to examine the baby.

all of your questions; however, because of the people you will read about in this chapter, you will have choices.

By reviewing this chapter, you will be able to identify some aspects of nursing that have allowed it to be different for you. Many opportunities exist because nurses and others had the vision and did the work needed for nursing to evolve as we currently know it. So have fun. Read about the history of nursing and try to imagine what you would have done in situations similar to those described. Then consider what you will contribute to the historical pages of nursing that are still blank and waiting for what you have to offer.

THE BEGINNING OF NURSING

All historical writings have a beginning point and for nursing that was the dawn of civilization. Nursing is as old as humanity itself. The word *nursing* comes from the Latin word *nutricitus,* which means "nourishing." People have always needed and desired nurturing people in their lives. New babies and sick, deformed, injured, or dying individuals have always needed someone to give them care.

In ancient times, alterations in health were believed to have been caused by the presence of evil spirits. The shaman was sought to improve a person's health with masks, herbs, and noise sticks designed to ward off evil spirits. Eventually this ancient version of health care became more focused on the actual person, and care was entrusted to the priests who served as physicians. Women and nursing were not recognized as actual entities except for the brave women who practiced midwifery. (I applaud their courage.) Try to imagine delivering babies without knowledge of the germ theory, clean sheets, medications, incubators, or radiant warmers. The mortality rates had to have been discouraging. Many women died from puerperal fever caused by cross contamination (no hand washing or clean linens). Yet those women persisted, giving the best care they had to offer to anyone who needed it.

Except for the midwives, the primitive health care that was available was provided by men and was promoted by a belief in Apollo, the mythical Greek healer. From this beginning, temples were built, and men were recruited as priests to serve the sick. This allowed the priests not only to give nursing care but also to intercede for the ill person with God.

From this ancient beginning, the medical model, following the physician's approach to disease, has dominated the delivery of health care. You may have heard that doctors study disease, whereas nurses study human responses to disease. It is sometimes referred to as cure (medical model) versus care (nursing model). This is an interesting thread for you to follow through the history of nursing, identifying the strengths it has added and the hurdles it has created. The reality of health care being dominated by men from early times should clarify for each of us the strength it took for modern nurses to advance the position of nursing in society. All social, political, educational, and economic gains for women throughout the world's history also brought parallel gains for the nursing profession.

Some interesting bits of information have been preserved for your review regarding the ancient era. Hammurabi, an ancient Babylonian king

(about 2000 B.C.), wrote a code of laws designed to protect individuals who were ill. It defined the legal limitations placed on caregivers. This concept has been carried through history and into the current licensing laws. Such laws were written to protect the public from unsafe practitioners and to elevate the status of nursing by ensuring standards of knowledge, skill, and accountability. References in the Old Testament indicate that women performed nursing care at home and Hebrew priests worked as public health officers. People always have had the motivation to change their lives through improved health, and, fortunately for society, there have been people available and willing to assist in the process.

During the 5th century B.C., the Greek scholar Hippocrates translated the work of the priests who had been administering to the sick into a textbook of medicine. Hippocrates is referred to as the father of medicine, and his ethical oath is still taken today by physicians as they enter medical practice. The great contributions of Hippocrates were (1) to make a written record of the health-care practices being used and (2) to remove the mythical aspects of health care (based on the belief that Apollo controlled people's health and other such superstitions) at the time and replace them with the underpinnings of science as it was developed at that point. (Contemporaries of Hippocrates were the great philosophers Socrates, Plato, and Aristotle.) During the ancient Greek era, women nursed their own children at home. They were not allowed to work beyond the health needs of their family. Because it was an oppressive time for women, their contributions to nursing were minimal.

DARK AGES AND INTRODUCTION OF CHRISTIANITY

Beginning at the fall of the Roman Empire, the Dark Ages represented a period of about 500 years when learning in all disciplines disintegrated. People essentially lost the ability to read, which rendered the work of Hippocrates useless. Nursing care was practiced by friends and relatives. There was no scientific basis for the care given, and medical theory disintegrated along with the level of civilization.

Society recovered from this bleak period at the end of A.D. 1000. Scientific medicine survived the Dark Ages because of the Jewish scholars who maintained the written work of others and served as translators. The revival of medicine occurred in Italy at the famous school of Salerno. Medicine was once again taught and women were admitted to the school to study nursing and midwifery. The school became famous for its midwifery graduates; some of them published treatises on the care of women. Another positive aspect for nursing in this era was the growth of Christianity. As this religion spread, convents were established where women administered health care to the sick and the poor. The first public health nurses were the deaconesses from this historical period.

In that era, it was not easy to break new ground and promote women's issues through study or publication. Those heroines of the profession deserve our praise. We do not know their names, but they had courage and strength much like what you may be asked to contribute in the ever-changing dynamics of nursing today.

One of the realities of health care during the Middle Ages was the absence of ways of meeting basic health needs. The windows in the hospitals were too high to open, so little fresh air was available. Plumbing, heating, and lighting were essentially nonexistent. Linens were washed at the river, but contagious elements seldom were washed away. As modern nurses in the United States, we cannot imagine working without fresh air or plumbing. Yet many developing countries have similar circumstances for their health-care delivery. In many countries, medications are given to patients in hospitals only if the families fill the prescriptions and bring the drugs to the patient. The same is true of special foods or devices such as braces or crutches. To be responsible in the nursing profession today, it is important to recognize the reality of global health and health care and the problems that exist on that scale.

RENAISSANCE PERIOD

Nursing during the Renaissance period was not forward moving or powerful. The Renaissance was an era of musical and artistic development for societies, and an increased interest in scientific method and medicine allowed many basic principles of medicine to be established and supported. Martin Luther, who opposed the teachings of the Catholic Church, led the fight for the decline of women's roles and nursing as a profession. Because of the rise of Protestantism, monasteries and convents were closed, religious orders were abolished, and nursing progress was halted.

ERA OF INDUSTRIALIZATION

This was the time in history when women began moving to hospitals for delivery of their babies. Because of the poor conditions in the hospitals, the spread of puerperal fever was rampant, as were infant–mother mortality rates. Hungarian obstetrician Ignaz Semmelweis (1818–1865) first identified and used antiseptic methods to assist in controlling the high maternal death rates. Unfortunately, Semmelweis died of an untreated postoperative infection at age 47.

EARLY HEALTH CARE IN THE UNITED STATES

Hospitals in the United States evolved from cities and communities needing to provide care primarily for the disabled and chronically ill. In the early nineteenth century, many individuals gave birth and endured extended illnesses at home. By the late 1800s, hospitals were staffed by trained physicians and nurses and became a key component in providing health care to communities. By the 1920s, hospitals became a place where illness could be treated and hopefully cured. Many hospitals began affiliating with educational institutions with the hope of attracting the upper middle class. The public hospitals continued to provide care to the poor (America's Essential Hospitals, n.d.).

THE BEGINNING OF MODERN NURSING

The beginning of modern nursing covers the 19th and early 20th centuries. It was a time when hospitals were places to go to die, and people with mental illness were warehoused in jails and county poorhouses. Living conditions were appalling, and the mortality rate was very high. Nursing was not a defined profession in the United States unless it was administered by Catholic orders of nuns and priests. These people emigrated from Europe with knowledge, skills, and a willingness to serve. The communities where they settled generally built hospitals, and the religious orders gave a higher level of care than in other places in the country. Generally there was no supervision of nursing care, and nurses did not work night shifts.

REFLECTIVE THINKING

The late industrialization era in the United States brought marvelous inventions, such as the cotton mill and the steam engine. At the same time, child labor laws were nonexistent. In addition, large waves of immigrants came to the United States. In your class notebook, list three health-care issues you sense would be critical to address if you were a nurse in an urban community hospital during that time. How would you attempt to improve the problems that were clearly a part of the industrial era?

The purpose of this assignment and others like it that occur throughout this book is to stimulate your thinking about an issue at hand. It is hoped that you will discuss possible answers for this assignment with other people so that your concept of the industrial era and the demands of nurses who worked in it will be clearer to you.

I will not usually share possible answers here, but because this is the first assignment, it seems reasonable to do so. Although nurses in the United States did not have to deal with the bubonic plague, they did have to deal with bacteria and viruses before there was a clear understanding of germ theory. One of your responses could be a comment about that issue. As machinery became a major part of the industrial era, an increasing number of accidents related to machinery began to occur. What would some of those accidents be, and how could a nurse conduct teaching that would prevent some of those accidents? The large number of immigrants who were coming to the United States brought with them extreme poverty and infectious diseases that had not been seen in this country previously. What role could you take as a nurse in controlling and treating such diseases?

In the United States and Europe, society openly disapproved of educated upper-class women doing manual labor. Such activities were left to the poor and the newly emerging middle class. In addition, families with money kept their sick loved ones at home during this period because it was considered a disgrace to send a family member to a hospital.

Nursing Education

The first school of nursing, located in Kaiserworth, Germany, was established in 1836 by the German pastor Theodor Fliedner. The purpose of this hospital training was far-reaching. Students, always women, would come to the school for 2 or 3 years. When their educational experience was complete, these women were referred to as Kaiserworth deaconesses and were sent to various places in the world to educate other women to be nurses. Much of the education was focused on scrubbing floors and cleaning and changing bed linen. Florence Nightingale received her 3-month education at Kaiserworth. Her appearance into the profession marks the beginning of modern nursing.

Florence Nightingale

Florence Nightingale was exactly the type of person that society did not expect to become a nurse. Nursing was considered a disreputable job, and because Florence was from a wealthy family, it was never thought that she would take a job and go to work!

Florence benefited from the education and social experiences of wealthy British society. She had the opportunity to travel to Egypt for a year, spend time in Paris, and receive an education that most people of her era could not have because of the time and money it required. She had an excellent mind and found that her learning needs exceeded counting linen, studying French, and enjoying theater arts. She insisted on taking classes with a science background, was proficient in accounting, and quickly mastered statistical analysis of data. These were nontraditional educational experiences for a young woman of her position and resulted in many disagreements with her mother and younger sister. Her quiet and understanding father tried hard to support her interests while maintaining the standards of the society in which the family lived.

Florence's behavior was always a point of controversy between her parents. The Nightingales had a winter home in London and a summer home outside the city (a practice started by many wealthy people to provide them with a place to go to avoid the plague). Surrounding the country estate were small, one-room houses where poor people who worked for the estate manager lived. When Florence was old enough, she would take a servant with her and visit these homes, bringing fresh fruits and vegetables. Often she would bandage the festering wounds of the workers, and eventually she assisted a local midwife who attended to the needs of the women who lived there. These behaviors upset Florence's mother because they did not conform to what a wealthy young lady should be doing with her time. Florence made it clear to her mother that needlework was not what she wanted to do!

Florence eventually arranged to attend the Kaiserworth Deaconess Institution in 1851 to receive her nursing education; she was 31 at the time. She also spent time studying with the Sisters of Charity in Paris. Her first position was superintendent of a small hospital in London called the Establishment for Gentle Women. Florence was successful in this position and implemented changes in nursing practice that greatly enhanced the health of the women there. She strongly believed that promoting good health and treating the ill were the priorities of nursing. Florence performed her job without pay.

The Crimean War, which involved England, Russia, and France, gave Florence the opportunity to show what nursing could do for a vulnerable population—wounded soldiers. Russia and France had nuns to care for their wounded and sick. England, however, had only untrained men.

REFLECTIVE THINKING

I have a book in my office that was published in 1897. In the book, there is a comment that states, "Nurses are born, not made." This definitely is a statement against nursing education. You, as an LPN student, obviously do not believe in that statement or you would not be making the sacrifices you will be making in nursing school. Ponder the question. Why are you in school?

The first LPN class to graduate went to school for only 3 months. That is also the length of time Florence Nightingale spent at Kaiserworth. Linda Richards was the first "trained" registered nurse (RN) in the United States, and her education took only 1 year. Why do you believe it is important to make the time and financial commitment to attend school for 9 to 12 months to be an LPN? Write your response in your class notebook.

In Chapter 2, you will have the opportunity to read more about the work Florence Nightingale did during the Crimean War. Briefly, she saved thousands of lives with the help of the 38 women she took with her, she earned the respect of the entire country, and she learned the value of recording statistical data and sharing them with government heads as a step toward making change. Florence often worked on her data through the night so she could send critical reports to the Secretary of War. The work she did in the Crimea changed the face of nursing forever. Her work reflected the first effort at using evidence-based practice in nursing.

In 1862, Nightingale assisted in establishing a home nursing service in London where nurses were made available for private duty, hospital coverage, and home visits. Nightingale's establishment is seen as the beginning of the modern visiting nursing service. She continued to use her knowledge, skill, and influence to establish formal nursing education programs, improving women's place in society, impacting the care given in hospitals, and introducing the philosophy of "treating the patient rather than the disease." Nightingale published many bulletins and reports; her two books, *Notes on Nursing* and *Notes on Hospitals* (both published in 1859), are still used in educational programs today. If you have the opportunity to look through her *Notes on Nursing* text, you will find it practical and meaningful. Florence Nightingale was a very focused woman, and her work is still valuable to the profession.

The first three hospital schools of nursing in the United States, which focused on overall nursing education as opposed to just midwifery or medicine, were Florence Nightingale schools that followed her traditions. The hospitals were located in Boston, New York, and New Haven, Connecticut. The programs were modeled after the famous Nightingale school at St. Thomas in London. The introduction of these nursing programs brought nursing to the forefront of health care and differentiated between classes for medical students, which nurses attended but could not participate in, and classes specifically for nursing students.

Florence Nightingale died at age 90 in 1910. Her contributions to the profession of nursing can never be replicated or discounted. She willingly gave her fortune, her health, and 60 years of her life to the establishment of nursing as a creditable and enduring profession.

Other Modern Nursing Leaders

Once the barriers to modern nursing were recognized and broken, opportunities arose for other nurses to contribute to the structure of the profession, and many nurses took advantage of these opportunities. The developments and principles that have been established by these women deserve to be recognized and appreciated. Through the work of these people, nursing grew from a job to a profession; every nurse should be grateful for their contributions. Because of these people of courage and foresight, we nurses can eagerly embrace our profession and work toward the resolution of today's concerns in nursing. These leaders developed a pathway and process for change and acceptance to occur, which should inspire pride in every nurse. As you review the following summaries of some of these leaders in nursing, consider what made their history possible. It required a level of strength and vision that is admirable. Consider the obstacles they identified and overcame. Ponder the sacrifices they made in their personal lives to accomplish what they did. Not everyone will have a page in a history book because of his or her contributions to nursing. Another aspect for you to consider, however, as you continue your reading of this chapter is how you can write your own page of history. For most of you, your contribution to history will not be something related to the national or international agenda, but it could make a profound difference where you work. It could be an idea that you follow through to completion that affects daily care or the quality of caring that you give your clients each day. Each page—yours, mine, and Nightingale's—is crucial for the overall history to be complete. As you review the accomplishments of the following history makers, don't forget to consider your own historical contributions now and in the future.

Clara Barton

Clara Barton was a schoolteacher who became a Civil War nurse. She also worked tirelessly for the American Red Cross. She based her work during the Civil War on the work Nightingale did during the Crimean War. While she was volunteering her nursing skills during the war, she was known for giving care to soldiers on both sides of the conflict. She was referred to as the "Angel of the Battlefield." Barton was the first president of the Red Cross Association, which

Clara Barton was known as the "Angel of the Battlefield" for her heroic work during the Civil War. She eventually became the first president of the American Red Cross. (Source: *http://www.redcross.org/hec/pre1900/_bartonimg.html*)

today meets the needs of people both nationally and internationally.

Dorothea Dix

Dorothea Dix was a retired schoolteacher; however, her impact on nursing was profound. She first encountered mentally ill people who were warehoused in jails and treated brutally. She championed the development of psychiatric hospitals, and her work brought about improvement for prisoners in jails. Dix was appointed the U.S. Army's Superintendent of Female Nurses in 1861. She did not have a nursing background or military rank, yet she organized army hospitals and their equipment and staffed them with qualified nurses.

Linda Richards

Linda Richards graduated from the New England Hospital for Women and Children in Boston in 1872 as the first trained nurse. Her educational program lasted 1 year. About a year later, Richards was appointed as the superintendent of the school. In addition to her teaching duties, she maintained her love for people by continuing to care for the sick. When she worked as the night superintendent at Bellevue Hospital, she developed a system for recording details about patients, which served as the basis for modern nursing notes. She served a medical mission in Japan, and while there she established the first school of nursing in Japan.

Isabel Hampton Robb

Isabel Hampton Robb was a strong activist for nursing. She initiated reform for nurses and students. Some of her changes were a 12-hour workday (as opposed to a 24-hour workday), breaks for meals, and time for rest and recreation. She also initiated the 3-year educational program for nursing and fought for licensing examinations and registration to protect patients from incompetent nurses and to raise the standards of the profession. She was the first principal at the Johns Hopkins School of Nursing and one of the founders and original stockholders of the American Journal of Nursing Company.

Mary Adelaide Nutting

Mary Adelaide Nutting graduated with the first class of the Johns Hopkins School of Nursing and, as a friend of Robb, continued Robb's reform issues. She was the first nurse to receive the title of First Professor of Nursing and created the Nursing and Teachers College of Columbia University. Nutting was instrumental in the formation of the International Council of Nursing.

Lavinia L. Dock

Lavinia L. Dock worked as an assistant to Isabel Hampton Robb. She established an organization for nursing school superintendents, known today as the National League for Nursing (NLN). This organization is responsible for accrediting schools of nursing in the United States. Dock wrote *History of Nursing,* which is a classic text on the topic.

Mary Eliza Mahoney

Mary Eliza Mahoney was the first African American nurse in the United States. She graduated from the New England Hospital for Women and Children. She spent her life working for acceptance of African Americans in the nursing profession. Mahoney was the organizer and first president of the National Association for Colored Graduate Nurses (NACGN).

Lillian D. Wald

Lillian D. Wald is known for opening the Henry Street Settlement in New York City; she is recognized as the first community health nurse in the United States. She served as the first president of the National Organization of Public Health Nursing. Wald and her work in the Henry Street Settlement are discussed in detail in Chapter 10.

Annie Goodrich

Annie Goodrich was an advocate of nursing education and worked tirelessly to promote nursing as a profession. Goodrich developed the Army School of Nursing, which earned her the Distinguished Service Award. She also served as Dean of Nursing at Yale University, President of the American Nurses Association, President of the International Council of Nursing, and Director of the Visiting Nursing Service at the Henry Street Settlement.

Goodrich, Wald, and Nutting are known as the "Great Trio" because of the developments in nursing attributed to them.

HISTORY OF THE LICENSED PRACTICAL AND VOCATIONAL NURSE

Early in the modern history of nursing, society and nursing leaders recognized a need for nurses who were excellent in delivering care at the bedside of individuals who were ill. That person was the LPN. The first training for practical nurses was offered in 1892 at the Young Women's Christian Association (YWCA) in New York City. The first official school for LPN education was established in 1893 at the Ballard School in New York; the program was 3 months long. The curriculum

As these retired LPNs reminisce about their school and working days, they recall the rich tradition and hard work of being among the first LPNs in their hospital.

Risk Takers and Role Breakers in Nursing

FLORENCE NIGHTINGALE
Went to school for 3 months at age 31.
Mother of modern nursing.
Famous for her work during the Crimean War, including her use of statistics.
Decreased death rates by 70% by using nurses.
Established the first formal schools of nursing including the first three hospital schools in the United States.

CLARA BARTON
No formal education.
"Angel of the Battlefield" during the Civil War. Treated wounded on both sides.
First president of the American Red Cross.

DOROTHEA DIX
Retired schoolteacher.
Championed the development of psychiatric hospitals. Also improved health care in prisons.
Appointed U.S. Army's Superintendent of Nurses; organized, equipped, and staffed army hospitals.

LINDA RICHARDS
First trained nurse to graduate after 1 year of school.
Was appointed superintendent of school 1 year after graduation.
Served a medical mission in Japan and established the first school of nursing there.
Developed the first format for patient charting.

ISABELLE HAMPTON ROBB
Graduate nurse.
Strong activist; changed shifts from 24 hours to 12 hours.
Developed 3-year educational program for nursing.
Fought for licensing examinations and registration.
First principal of Johns Hopkins School of Nursing.
One of the founders of the *American Journal of Nursing*.

MARY ADELAIDE NUTTING
Graduated from the first class at Johns Hopkins.
Worked with Robb on nursing reform issues.
First professor of nursing in the United States.
Created the Teachers and Nursing College of Columbia University in New York.
Instrumental in the formation of the International Council of Nursing.

LAVINIA DOCK
Assistant to Robb in nursing activist work.
Established the National League for Nursing (NLN), the organization that certifies schools of nursing.

MARY ELIZA MAHONEY
First African American nurse in the United States.
Spent her life working for the acceptance of African Americans.
Organizer and first president of the National Association for Colored Graduate Nurses (NACGN).

LILLIAN WALD
Opened the Henry Street Settlement.
Recognized as the first community health nurse in the United States.
First president of the National Organization of Public Health Nursing.

ANNIE GOODRICH
Dean of Nursing at Yale University.
Tireless advocate for nursing education and promoted nursing as a profession.
President of the American Nurses Association.
President of the International Council of Nursing.
Director of Visiting Nurse Service at the Henry Street Settlement.
Goodrich, Wald, and Nutting are known as the "Great Trio" because of their major contributions to nursing.

consisted of various homemaking skills in addition to techniques of caring for sick people. Students were sought who "had a special way with the sick," which often was referred to as a mothering quality. During this historical era, much of the care of the ill was done at home, which immediately made the LPN a home health or visiting nurse. The role of the LPN has a rich history, which is based on excellence in the actual person-to-person delivery of care.

LPNs have their own licensure but work under the direct supervision of a registered nurse, advanced practice nurse, or physician. Current educational programs are 9 to 12 months long, and passing the National Council Licensure Examination for Practical Nurses (NCLEX-PN) is required for licensure. As an LPN, you have the opportunity to work directly with people, sick or well (as in health promotion). Although LPNs are sought after to attend planning meetings because of their clinical expertise, they generally are required to do that less than other licensed health-care workers. This gives LPNs the opportunity to perform the duties for which they sought education—the direct care of other people. What an opportunity it is to enhance the philosophy of Nightingale—to "treat the patient rather than the illness." What a privilege it is to be entrusted with the health care of society in such a direct manner. After the turn of the 20th century, LPN education and licensure became more formalized in the nursing profession. The National League for Nursing (NLN) developed a system for standardization of requirements for the LPN. However, all states did not pass LPN licensure laws until 1955. World War II brought with it the need for additional nurses, which focused attention on the contributions of LPNs to health care. At this time, the role of the LPN expanded from home and visiting nursing to industrial and hospital nursing.

The National Association for Practical Nurse Education and Service (NAPNES) was formed in 1941. This was the first national organization with a focus on LPNs. NAPNES accredited LPN educational programs from 1945 through 1984. The NLN established the Council for Practical Nursing Programs in 1961, which assumed the responsibility for promoting LPN interests within the NLN.

In 1949, the National Federation of Licensed Practical Nurses (NFLPN) was founded. This organization is considered the official membership organization for LPNs and LVNs, and only people

with that licensure can join. Both of these organizations have continuing education opportunities and publications of interest to LPNs.

The role of the LPN is ever changing. With the future demands on the health-care system, the LPN will fulfill a critical role in providing care to patients in multiple care settings. According to the Bureau of Labor Statistics (2016b), the demand for the LPN is projected to increase 16% by 2024. As the population ages, there will continue to be a need to provide care to individuals with chronic conditions in long-term care and assisted living facilities. As health care focuses on providing more community-based care, LPNs will continue to provide care in community-based settings such as home care and hospice. There will also be an increased need for LPNs to work in outpatient and ambulatory care centers that provide primary and preventive care. The National League for Nursing (2014) has identified a definite role for the LPN in providing quality health care for our nation and encourages the nursing profession to provide support for the LPN in fulfilling this role.

As health-care providers, LPNs can work in any health-care arena and be effective. With health care being redesigned at such a rapid pace, LPNs today need to be alert to all that is happening and to proceed with confidence to write histories for themselves and for the profession. One way to do that is to stay alert to current trends and issues in nursing.

CURRENT TRENDS AND ISSUES

This section addresses current trends and issues that you need to recognize in your education and practice. Many of these current issues focus on the concern for patient safety in the health-care environment.

Healthcare-Associated Infections

Healthcare-associated infections (HAIs) are infections individuals acquire while receiving care for other conditions in a health-care setting. These settings include acute inpatient hospitals, outpatient surgery centers and clinics, dialysis centers, and the various long-term care settings such as assisted living facilities, nursing homes, and rehabilitation centers. Health care–associated infections are associated with high mortality and morbidity rates and increased health-care costs. Unless appropriately managed, HAIs can be transmitted between health-care settings. HAIs affect about 1 in 25 patients in inpatient settings. Patients who acquire an HAI can experience emotional, financial, and medical consequences (Health.gov, 2016). Many HAIs are preventable.

Risk factors for acquiring HAIs are indwelling urinary catheters and other medical devices, the overuse of antibiotics, surgical procedures, unsanitary environments, and the transmission of infections from health-care employees to patients. The most common HAIs include urinary tract infections, pneumonia, surgical site infections, and bloodstream infections, and these can be caused by bacteria, fungus, viruses, and other less common pathogens. The most difficult HAIs to treat are those caused by antibiotic-resistant bacteria. The most common antibiotic-resistant bacteria include methicillin-resistant *Staphylococcus aureus,* multidrug-resistant *Pseudomonas aeruginosa,* and multidrug-resistant *Acinetobacter* (Brooks, 2016).

Although health-care professionals have made progress in preventing HAIs, there is still work to be done. Healthy People 2020 has established a goal to reduce and ultimately eliminate HAIs in health-care settings (Healthy People 2020, 2016). Research indicates that by practicing current prevention protocols such as hand hygiene and isolation, the occurrence of HAIs can be reduced. Educating health-care employees about the importance of maintaining strict hand-washing and isolation procedures will go a long way in the prevention of HAIs.

Disaster Nursing

The occurrence of natural and man-made disasters has made disaster preparedness a priority for individuals, communities, and health-care facilities throughout the United States. Have you or a family member been affected by a disaster? Are you prepared to respond to a disaster? Many of you may remember Hurricane Katrina. Katrina was a level 5 hurricane that devastated the Gulf region in August 2005. This hurricane was considered one of the five deadliest hurricanes ever to affect the United States. Individuals who survived lost their homes and places of employment. Although there has been much rehabilitation in the past several years, to date many homes and businesses have not been rebuilt. One long-term care facility was unable to evacuate the residents, and they all drowned in the rising waters. One hospital was completely destroyed by the winds and rising water. Fortunately, the hospital was able to evacuate most of the patients before the storm hit. The patients who could not be evacuated were cared for by hospital employees over several days in a building with no electricity or running water. In more recent years, other parts of the United States have been devastated by tornados and hurricanes.

Most nurses have not had the education or training necessary to respond to a disaster. However, with more than 2 million nurses throughout the United States as well as millions more worldwide, the nursing profession is in a unique position to provide leadership and support during disaster response.

To be prepared for the next disaster, nurses need to understand emergency response planning and the role nurses will play in critical decision-making situations during and after disasters. It will be important for you to participate on the disaster committee at your place of employment. This would include planning and participating in disaster activities and drills. You will need the ability to identify patients who would receive priority care during a disaster. Deciding which patient will be placed on the limited number of available ventilators is a likely decision that would need to be made. Nurses will be involved in making these decisions while also providing safe quality care to their patients. In the most recent update of the NCLEX-PN exam, questions regarding disaster management were added, so nursing programs are adding disaster management concepts to their curriculums.

Cultural Diversity

The society of the United States weaves a beautiful fabric of diversity. Although 75% of the United States is Caucasian, the country has double-digit percentages of Hispanic/Latinos, African Americans, and foreign-born residents.

One obvious barrier to health-care delivery is language. To give effective care to people who are not fluent in English, nurses need to know a foreign language or have access to qualified interpreters. Some health-care facilities use interactive technology to provide access to interpreters.

Although the focus of diversity is primarily on our patient populations, we need to consider the increasing diversity of health-care professionals. More foreign nurses and physicians are coming to the United States to practice. In order to collaborate well with diverse health-care providers, we need to understand and respect the differences they bring to the health-care setting. For more information about cultural issues in health-care settings, refer to Chapter 12.

Technology

The use of technology in health care has increased dramatically over the past several years. Nurses now use electronic charting to document the care they are providing to their patients. The information they record can be accessed by the rest of the health-care team to make decisions regarding care. Having the ability to access patient information at any point of care improves communication among providers and allows for care to be provided in a more timely manner. Telehealth is a sophisticated way to use technology to improve diagnosis and treatment of health conditions. It allows individuals to receive medical and nursing services from distant geographic regions. Telehealth providers can remotely interview a patient, review an x-ray or laboratory tests, or suggest treatments and procedures. This technology includes devices to remind patients to take medications, provides Web-based video office calls, and provides equipment that can monitor a person's vital signs at home and send electronic results to the doctor's office.

This type of health care is cost effective and convenient and conserves resources. Telehealth is widely used around the world and allows for greater flexibility in accessing services, more options for consultation, and a reduction in service costs. Technology is now being used in nursing education to provide simulated clinical practice for nursing students. High-tech mannequins can be programmed to present physical signs and symptoms that mimic those of an actual patient. These simulations give students the opportunity to learn in a closely monitored, low stress environment. Chapter 5 discusses additional ways technology is used in nursing.

Nursing Shortages

Nursing shortages continue to exist in various geographic areas and tend to fluctuate. It is predicted that by 2024 the demand for nurses will increase by 16% (Bureau of Labor Statistics, U.S. Department of Labor, 2015). This increased demand is due to the aging population with increased medical and health needs as well as current health-care reforms that are increasing the number of health-care consumers and putting a strain on the health-care

system (American Nurses Association, 2016). These issues will definitely have an impact on the nursing shortage.

One reality of the nursing shortage is that the 21st-century woman has more employment options than women had previously. Now women can become astronauts, chief executive officers of companies, doctors, and dentists. These options have not always been available. Because 90% of nurses are women (Bureau of Labor Statistics, U.S. Department of Labor, 2015), this change has a definite impact.

The nursing shortage itself is a contributing factor because the shortage creates staffing problems, mandatory overtime, and constant calls for additional shift work. These issues contribute to nurses becoming disillusioned with the nursing profession.

Another reality is the shortage of nursing faculty, which limits the enrollment of students. Most schools of nursing require faculty to be doctorally prepared nurses and there is currently a shortage of nurses with doctoral degrees. In most states, faculty salaries do not compete with clinical practice salaries. In addition, as with the general nursing workforce, nursing faculty are also aging and looking forward to retirement.

National nursing organizations are making strong efforts at reversing the shortage by mandating better nurse-to-patient ratios, eliminating mandatory overtime, and increasing salaries and benefits for nurses. Change will take time, but adjustments to the health-care arena will happen. In the meantime, you as an LPN need to ensure your place on the team. When you graduate, take advantage of ongoing educational programs at your place of employment or online. Be an eager learner on the unit and in the education department's classroom. Take care of yourself so that you don't get tired and make mistakes or become less communicative. Be alert and work to become better at the art and the science of nursing. That is the way to ensure your role in the new arena of health care.

Substance Use Disorders in Nurses

The American Nurses Association (ANA) estimated that 6% to 8% of nurses use substances to such an extent that patient safety is jeopardized (Leverence, 2015). Impaired nurses may come to the workplace with a long-term substance abuse disorder or may begin using a substance as a coping mechanism for stress in their lives or in the workplace.

Signs of impairment include offering to give pain medications for other nurses, questionable behaviors related to medication counts and waste, giving more pain medications than other nurses, having more drug-tolerant patients, coming into the work setting on days off, and frequently staying after shifts to help with drug counts (Leverence, 2015). If diverting drugs, the nurse may substitute saline for injectable medications or may dilute medications after using some of it. The nurse abusing alcohol may drink during breaks and meals, hiding the smell of alcohol with toothpaste, gum, or mouthwash. If actively using at work, the nurse may have slowed speech and poor coordination. By the time the impairment is noticed by others, the nurse may be in advanced stages of the addiction.

Many nurses are not sure what to do when a nurse colleague is suspected of being impaired. They are hesitant to confront the colleague, so they will often report their concern to the nurse manager. In some cases, nurses do not report their peers. This is can lead to potential harm to patients and delays in treatment for the nurse (Kunyk, 2015). Nurses should be taught the signs of impairment and how to report a colleague. The legal aspects regarding reporting an impaired nurse vary from state to state. To find the requirements for reporting an impaired nurse in your state, contact your state board of nursing.

Studies have shown that nurses need treatment and follow-up support for a full recovery. The length of treatment and the willingness of the nurse are good indicators for success but recovery will need to last a lifetime. Many organizations offer alternative treatment programs instead of termination. In the early 1980s, the American Nurses Association called for non-disciplinary programs to address substance abuse in nurses. Several states offer programs in which nurses are directed to treatment options and long-term monitoring, including drug testing, until the nurse is determined safe to return to practice. Most employers have established after-care programs to support long-term recovery and potential relapse. Nursing managers play a significant role in addressing substance abuse concerns among their staff. Developing a workplace environment that supports the reporting and educating of staff in identifying impaired colleagues will provide earlier intervention for the nurse and increased patient safety.

Aging U.S. Population

Currently in the United States there are more than 40 million persons 65 years old or older. This represents almost 14% of the U.S. population. This number is expected to increase to 21% by 2040 (Administration on Aging, 2015). As mentioned previously, as the population ages, the increased numbers will put a strain on the health-care system, requiring more nurses to provide care. A person aged 65 or older will be likely to develop one to five chronic illnesses, such as arthritis, diabetes mellitus, congestive heart disease, and dementia. These illnesses cause an increase in hospitalizations and admissions to long-term care facilities. Chronic conditions are a leading cause of death for older adults.

At this point you may be thinking to yourself, I am not planning to take care of the elderly when I am a nurse. As LPNs, many of you will work in long-term care facilities taking care of 7% of the elderly population that currently reside in long-term care facilities. Ninety percent of the elderly population lives in the community either independently or with assistance of some kind. These individuals represent 60% of the patient population on adult care units such as general medical-surgical units, intensive care units, and emergency departments. For home care and hospice agencies, that number is much higher. As the older adult population increases, these percentages will also increase. So, the truth is that most of you will take care of the elderly at some point in your nursing career.

Quality and Safety Education for Nurses

Throughout the past 40 years of my nursing career, I have seen many changes in nursing. Many are mentioned in the prior section. One of the most dramatic changes has been in how patients are managed related to their level of sickness. A patient having minor abdominal surgery 40 years ago would stay in the hospital for a minimum of 5 days. Today most patients having a similar surgery go home the same day or stay for 24 to 48 hours. Patients on the general medical-surgical floors have more complex needs, similar to patients in the intensive care unit (ICU) 40 years ago. As you move into your practice, it will not be uncommon for you to take care of a patient on a ventilator in a skilled care facility. With the increase

An older adult receives care from an LPN.

in patient medical needs, there is increased concern about patient safety.

To address this concern, the Quality and Safety Education for Nurses (QSEN) project was developed. The focus of the QSEN project is to prepare future nurses with the knowledge, skills, and attitudes needed to provide safe quality care to their patients. Six quality and safety competencies were identified (QSEN). These competencies are being integrated into nursing program curricula throughout the United States. To read more about the QSEN competencies, go to www.qsen.org.

Providing safe care means not only that you perform the procedure correctly but also that you understand why you are doing the procedure and how it will affect your patient.

REFLECTIVE THINKING

As you continue with your nursing education, how will you incorporate the six QSEN competencies into your practice? How will you ensure that the care you give to your patients will be safe?

REAL-WORLD CASE STUDY

■ In each of the following chapters, you are asked to respond to a specific situation relating to the content of the chapter. Most of the case studies are based on actual clinical situations and ask you to work through a resolution of the problems presented. This case study is unique, however. Explore it and complete it in a manner that is meaningful to you. For this assignment, there is no right or wrong response. Spend some time considering what you are asked to write and then write it. Sharing this assignment with your faculty person should prove to be beneficial to your future plans.

My Contribution to Nursing History

■ Record your thoughts about the contributions you are interested in making to nursing history. You may present some grand dreams and ideas as well as more immediate or less complex ideas. Whatever you write will be valued by the faculty person reading this assignment. Please record thoughts about what you believe you, as a future LPN, can contribute to nursing overall. You may wish to refer to a specialty area in nursing in which you have a particular interest, or you may focus on being the best day-to-day caregiver in your place of employment. Perhaps you have been discriminated against because of a learning disability, body size, skin color, or opinions. This could be a focus to explore as you write your page in the nursing history book. Feel free to make this magical like a fairy tale or clear and formal like a report. It is your history page, and whatever you choose to record on it is important and needs to be shared. Best wishes!

Key Points

■ Understanding the history of the nursing profession gives today's nurses a sense of pride in knowing how far the profession has come. Many opportunities exist in nursing today because nurses and others had the vision and did the work needed for nursing to evolve as we know the profession today. Because of the accomplishments of other nurses, you are able to make better decisions about the direction your

career will take and what you want to contribute to nursing history.

■ Primitive health care was performed by men and was promoted by a belief in Apollo, the mythical Greek healer. The initial approach to health care focused on the disease and curing the disease and not on the human response to disease. The medical model for today's health care still focuses on curing the disease and the nursing model's focus is on the human response to disease.

- Hippocrates is referred to as the father of medicine and his ethical oath is still taken by physicians today. His contributions were to make a written record of health-care practices, remove the mythical aspects of health care, and replace them with the underpinnings of science. During this time, women were not allowed to provide nursing care beyond the health needs of their families.

- Scientific medicine survived the Dark Ages and medical schools were started during that time. Women were admitted to these schools to study nursing and midwifery. During the rise of Christianity, nursing care was given to the sick and poor by the deaconesses of the churches. The Renaissance period saw a rise in the interest of medicine and many basic health-care principles were established.

- During the industrial era, women began using hospitals to deliver their babies. A Hungarian obstetrician, Ignaz Semmelweis, identified and used antiseptic methods to control high maternal death rates. By the 1920s, hospitals became a place where illness could be treated and cured.

- The first nursing school was established in Germany by Theodor Fliedner. The graduates of this school were sent to various places in the world to educate other women to be nurses. Florence Nightingale was a graduate of the school.

- Florence Nightingale is considered the mother of modern nursing and was the first nurse to use evidence-based practice. She used statistical data obtained by observing her patients to make changes to patient care. She established the first formal schools of nursing, including the first three hospital schools in the United States.

- Other women also contributed to modern nursing. They include Clara Barton, who was the first president of the Red Cross; Dorothea Dix, who championed the development of psychiatric hospitals; Lavinia Dock, who established the National League for Nursing; Linda Richards, who developed the early version of documenting patient care; Isabel Hampton Robb, who improved working conditions for nurses and fought for licensure for nurses; Mary Adelaide Nutting, who created the International Council for Nursing; Mary Eliza Mahoney, who was the first African American nurse in the United States; Lillian Wald, who is recognized as the first community health nurse; and Annie Goodrich, who developed the Army School of Nursing.

- LPNs have a rich history of providing excellent primary patient care. LPNs play a critical role in providing care to patients in multiple health-care settings, and the demand for LPNs is projected to grow in the next several years. There are two organizations that focus on the LPN: the National Association for Practical Nurse Education and Services (NAPNES) and the National Association of Licensed Practical Nurses (NALPN).

- The population is becoming more diverse. Language and other cultural needs can create a barrier to providing quality patient care. In addition, the population continues to age and nurses need to know how to take care of patients with multiple chronic conditions. Currently about 60% of the patients on adult care units are 65 years or older.

- The use of technology in health care has increased over the past several years. Documentation of patient records is now done electronically in most health-care organizations. Telehealth uses computers and other electronic devices to assist physicians and nurses in providing care to patients remotely. This type of health care is cost effective and convenient, especially for patients living in rural areas.

- Health care–associated infections (HAIs) are infections acquired while accessing care in a health-care setting. They are attributed to high mortality and morbidity rates in the United States. Most can be prevented by following strict hand-washing and infection control procedures.

- Nurses need to understand disaster management. They need to know how to develop an emergency response plan and understand the critical role nurses play in disaster response.

- The demand for nurses by 2024 will increase by 16%. As the population ages, the United States will need more nurses to care for their elderly. In addition, older nurses are preparing for retirement, which will increase the need for nurses.

- According to the American Nurses Association, 6% to 8% of nurses are dealing with a substance abuse disorder. Impaired nurses can impact patient care and safety. An impaired nurse should be reported to avoid patient harm and so that treatment for the impaired nurse can be provided.

■ Quality and Safety Education for Nurses (QSEN) is a national initiative to prepare nurses with the knowledge, skills, and attitudes needed to provide safe, quality care to patients. The six competencies include patient-centered care, teamwork and collaboration, quality improvement, informatics, safety, and evidence-based practice.

ANSWERS TO REAL-WORLD CASE STUDY

Although this case study is designed to focus on you, I will share my response to this activity.

For my application to nursing I was asked to write an essay. One of the questions asked what I wanted to do in the future with my nursing degree. I remember writing that I wanted to teach at a nursing school. As it turned out, several years later I ended up teaching at the same nursing school at which I earned my associate nursing degree. I love teaching because I enjoy the positive interactions with my students and watching them learn new things. I think my contribution to nursing history will be the education I have provided to the many nursing students I have taught over the past 16 years and will continue to teach during the next several years. I have been fortunate to work with students who have studied and worked hard to earn their nursing degree and are now positively contributing to the nursing profession.

REVIEW QUESTIONS

1. Florence Nightingale:
   1. Became the first president of the American Red Cross.
   2. Championed the development of psychiatric hospitals.
   3. Used evidence-based practice to improve patient outcomes.
   4. Established the National League for Nursing.

2. Dorthea Dix:
   1. Established the National League for Nursing.
   2. Used evidence-based practice to improve patient outcomes.
   3. Fought for licensing examinations and registration.
   4. Championed the development of psychiatric hospitals.

3. Risk factors for acquiring health-care associated infections include:
   1. The use of urinary catheters.
   2. Improper hand-washing technique.
   3. The overuse of antibiotics.
   4. Undergoing surgical procedures.
   5. All of the above.

4. What organization is considered the official membership organization for LPNs and LVNs?
   1. National League for Nursing
   2. National Association of Licensed Practical Nurses
   3. National Association for Practical Nurse Education and Services
   4. American Nurses Association

5. Signs that a nurse might be impaired include:
   1. Frequently staying after her or his shift to help with drug counts.
   2. Suspicious activity related to drug counts.
   3. Coming to the work setting on days off.
   4. Offering to give pain medications for other nurses.
   5. All of the above.

References

Administration on Aging. (2015). Aging statistics. Retrieved from http://www.aoa.acl.gov/Aging

American Nurses Association. (2016). Nursing shortage. Received from http://www.nursingworld.org/MainMenuCategories/ThePracticeofProfessionalNursing/workforce/NursingShortage

America's Essential Hospitals. (n.d.). Emergence of public hospitals: 1860–1930. Retrieved from http://essentialhospitals.org/about-americas-essential-hospitals/history-of-public-hospitals-in-the-united-states/emergence-of-public-hospitals-1860-1930/

Brooks, M. (2016). "Chilling" data on antibiotic-resistant infections in US hospital patients. Retrieved from http://www.medscape.com/viewarticle/859829

Bureau of Labor Statistics, U.S. Department of Labor. (2015). Labor force statistics from the current population survey. Retrieved from http://www.bls.gov/cps/cpsaat11.htm

Bureau of Labor Statistics, U.S. Department of Labor. (2016a). Registered nurses. *Occupational Outlook Handbook, 2016-17 Edition*. Retrieved from http://www.bls.gov/ooh/healthcare/registered-nurses.htm

Bureau of Labor Statistics, U.S. Department of Labor. (2016b). Licensed practical and licensed vocational nurses. Retrieved from http://www.bls.gov/ooh/healthcare/licensed-practical-and-licensed-vocational-nurses.htm

Health.gov. (2016). Healthcare-associated infections. Retrieved from http://health.gov/hcq/prevent-hai.asp

Healthy People 2020. (2016). Retrieved from https://www.healthypeople.gov/2020/topics-objectives/topic/healthcare-associated-infections

Kunyk, D. (2015). Substance use disorders among registered nurses: Prevalence, risks and perceptions in a disciplinary jurisdiction. *Journal of Nursing Management, 23*(1), 54–64.

Leverence, K. (2015). Tackling the taboo of substance abuse among nurses. *ONS Connect, 30*(4), 64–64.

National League for Nursing. (2014). A vision for recognition of the role of licensed practical/vocational nurses in advancing the nation's health. Retrieved from http://www.nln.org/docs/default-source/about/nln-vision-series-(position-statements)/nlnvision_7.pdf?sfvrsn=4

Nightingale, F. (1859a). *Notes on hospitals*. London: Harrison.

Nightingale, F. (1859b). *Notes on nursing*. Philadelphia: J. B. Lippincott.

Quality and Safety Education for Nurses (QSEN). (n.d.). http://www.qsen.org/

Web Resources

American Association for the History of Nursing (AAHN) www.aahn.org

American Nurses Association (ANA) www.nursingworld.org

National Association for Practical Nurse Education and Services (NAPNES) www.napnes.org

National Association of Licensed Practical Nurses (NALPN) www.nalpn.org

National League for Nursing (NLN) www.nln.org

Quality and Safety Education for Nurses (QSEN) www.qsen.org

2 Caring as a Personal and Professional Behavior

HOLLI SOWERBY

KEY TERMS

Caritas
High-touch nursing care
Holistic nursing
Paradigm
Transpersonal caring

CHAPTER CONCEPTS

Evidence-Based Practice
Patient-Centered Care
Collaboration

LEARNING OUTCOMES

1. Discuss the basic principles of caring practiced by Florence Nightingale.
2. Discuss the differences between medical models and nursing models of care.
3. Define transpersonal caring and holistic nursing within the framework of Dr. Jean Watson's theory of human caring.
4. Apply Watson's theory to the classroom.
5. Apply Watson's theory to colleagues in a nursing setting.
6. Apply Watson's theory to patient care.
7. Define what motivation is and express concepts of personal motivation.

*Let us each and all realize the importance of
our influence on others—stand shoulder to
shoulder—and not alone in a good cause.*

—Florence Nightingale

Throughout history, caring has been the hallmark
of nursing. Florence Nightingale, a British philan-
thropist who is considered the first nurse in the
modern era of nursing and the founder of nursing
as a profession, spent her career serving others.
When she went to help during the Crimean War,
she tied a bag of gold coins to her slip where no
one could see it. Florence did not know how she
would use those coins, but she knew they might
be needed to keep her and her nurses safe.

When Florence Nightingale and her 38 uneducated but committed women reached the Crimea,
the conditions were appalling. The surgeons did not
want nurses and put all 38 of them in quarters so
small they lacked privacy and had to sleep in shifts
because of the lack of space. They had to walk in
raw sewage to reach and treat their patients, and
they developed strategies to avoid rats.

Florence Nightingale began modern nursing
with a strong tradition of caring. Would you like
to know how she spent her bag of gold? She used
it to buy fresh fruit and vegetables so the soldiers
could have better nutrition.

Florence Nightingale. (Source: *Anderson, M. A.
[2000]. To be a nurse [p. 66]. Philadelphia:
F. A. Davis.)*

WHAT IS CARING?

Because most students and even practicing nurses
do not have bags of gold to ensure better care for
their patients, it is important to look at caring from
several different perspectives. Metaphorically, caring could be seen as the bag of gold that would help
you give the best care to your patients. I like the following definition of *caring:* Caring means responding to others as unique individuals, sensing their
emotions, and accepting them as they are unconditionally. Caring makes a connection with another
human being and breaks down the alienation that
not caring creates.

One of the foundational concepts of caring as a
science is "caring for the whole person," also
known as *transpersonal caring* or *holistic nursing.*
If I were to ask you what these terms mean, how
would you answer? The following list of definitions should help clarify these important concepts:

• Transpersonal caring is a human-to-human
  caring (e.g., the patient and the nurse or the

patient, nurse, and family) with an acceptance
of the uniqueness of the other person(s)
(Watson, 2012).
• Caring for the whole person is paying attention to
  and caring for a person's body, mind, and spirit.
• Holistic nursing is caring for the whole person
  and all ramifications of that person (e.g., family,
  significant other, pet).

Now that you have read the definitions, you can
see that I am talking about essentially the same
thing with each concept. The terms *transpersonal
caring* and *holistic nursing* are used interchangeably throughout this book. It is important for you
to understand these terms and to be able to use
them. It is crucial, however, for you to be able to
use the knowledge and skills that constitute the
overall principle of caring.

REFLECTIVE THINKING

How do the concepts of transpersonal caring and
holistic nursing relate to the QSEN competency
"patient-centered care"? Write your response in
your class notebook.

Dr. Jean Watson

Dr. Jean Watson, a nurse, distinguished professor, and nurse theorist, has devoted her life to understanding and teaching nurses about the science of human caring and the "high-touch" aspect of nursing that is needed in nursing today. Watson refers to high-touch nursing care as transpersonal caring in which the nurse respects the whole person and his or her existence in the world (Watson, 2012).

Watson believes that nursing has long neglected the development of the art of nursing, and her theory is a strong support for revaluing that aspect of care (Box 2.1). Watson (2012) believes that it is important to incorporate more than just the hard scientific facts into nursing. She proposes that we need to include the beauty and art of human caring into the science of nursing. My idea is that the art of nursing is the reason many people are nurses. I believe that the human-to-human caring process is what attracted many people as they made the decision to become a nurse.

In her writings, Watson shares examples of what a nurse practicing in a caring paradigm looks like. Such a person has a deep human regard for the lives of others. When giving care, the nurse practices as a coparticipant. This means that the nurse is not the "boss" or the only one with knowledge; instead, the nurse and the patient work together to achieve the best outcomes possible for the patient receiving care. Watson talks about the caring moment, when the nurse and the patient share something personal while nursing care is being given. That "something personal" is the ability of the nurse to focus knowledge, skills, and wisdom completely on one person for the moments they are together.

Another basic premise of Watson's theory is the intentionality of the nurse. The nurse should enter every interaction and caring moment with the intention of giving nursing care in a personalized, human, and scientific manner; this means that the focus of care is beyond the cellular needs of the patient and extends to the entire person and his or her needs.

Direct caregivers, in my experience, are masters of practicing the art of nursing, and they generally do it without knowing anything about nursing theory. I'm sharing Watson's theory in this book because it supports licensed practical nurses (LPNs) in their daily practice. I want you to recognize your foundation as you "stretch and grow" into the sometimes new, always challenging role of a nurse manager. Please don't lose the caring basis for your practice; just add to it as you read and study this book and in your future management experiences. In Chapter 3, you will be introduced to Dr. Abraham Maslow's theory of human motivation, referred to as his "hierarchy of needs." Throughout this book, Watson's theory is integrated with Maslow's as a framework for understanding the work of the nurse manager.

Let's go back to the phrase *transpersonal caring moment*. Can you recall the last time you experienced one? It would have involved seeing people giving up thinking about themselves and putting their focus and energy on someone else. If you are a parent, it is possible that you often use transpersonal caring with your children. People who are newly in love also seem to use transpersonal caring more often. However, what about your real day-to-day world? Does transpersonal caring exist there? It would be meaningful for you to stop and consider where the transpersonal caring moments are in your daily life. Is there someone who gives you such caring moments? Is there someone special that you give transpersonal caring to regularly?

Watson's theory also discusses caritas (caring) versus curative nursing measures. Caritas measures are described as transpersonal caring or "high touch." Curative nursing care is high-tech, or nursing care that is based on the medical model of care, which often is based on the use of technology. Watson has written an entire book about the caritas versus curative features of nursing care (Watson, 2012). One of the most profound examples of high-touch nursing is the "pneumonia nurse."

Box 2.1 Examples of Nurses Practicing in a Caring Paradigm

1. A deep human regard for the lives of others
2. Work together with patient to meet best outcomes
3. Complete focus on the person receiving care
4. Enter every caring moment with intention to give personalized care

In the history of nursing and before antibiotics were invented, nurses predominantly had to rely on their high-touch skills to assist them in healing people. A classic example is the "pneumonia nurse." People with pneumonia generally were cared for in their homes by a nurse who specialized in caring for people with that infection. I cannot imagine the problems that a nurse would have encountered while giving pneumonia care without antibiotics. Massive lung congestions and long bouts with high fever would have been common. Nurses didn't administer intravenous therapy in those days, so every sip of fluid into the patient would have been carefully monitored and valued. I think the healing hands of the pneumonia nurses were the best they had to offer their patients. They gave exquisite care to people who had little chance of survival—24 hours a day, 7 days a week. Their hands and hearts gently served, fed, and bathed patients who were critically ill. The nurses turned their patients and "clapped" their chests to help the mucus move out. The work of the pneumonia nurses was heroic. They definitely were high-touch nurses because they had little else to use in their healing art.

REFLECTIVE THINKING

Take some quiet time and record in your class notebook responses to the questions listed in the text. Seriously consider when and with whom you have genuine, transpersonal caring moments. Do you observe transpersonal caring in your work or clinical setting? Be prepared to discuss this concept in class.

High-tech nurses are nurses who use the complex and sophisticated equipment that is currently available for health-care workers. I think of intensive care nurses when I think of high-tech care. Other examples are nurses in emergency departments, burn units, shock/trauma units, and oncology units. Telemetry is another example of a high-tech arena. Nurses who work in high-tech arenas spend approximately as much time with the technology that is saving the patient's life as they do with the patient. They work long and hard to master the complexity of the technology and manage it effectively. Think what the simplest of modern nursing equipment would have done to assist the pneumonia nurse.

Ideally, a nurse can work equally well in high-tech and high-touch arenas of care. To be able to do so is a challenge, but it is one well worth focusing on as you go through your educational experience.

As a student LPN and future nurse, you need to begin to develop transpersonal caring characteristics. If you focus on developing the awareness and skill of transpersonal caring as a student, you will be more successful as a nurse. There are some prejudices and negative thinking, however, about transpersonal caring.

Some professionals with excellent high-tech skills and behaviors—expert intensive care, emergency department, or transplant nurses and physicians—are critical of the high-touch concept of transpersonal caring. Patients in these areas often have acute conditions (seriously demanding urgent attention), which forces their caregivers to focus on what is happening with the body; these caregivers may not appear to care about what is happening to the mind or spirit of the patient. I can understand their viewpoint. If a patient or visitor were suddenly to have a heart attack, it is preferable for a high-tech expert to focus on saving the person's life. Once the patient was stable, however, I would hope someone would hold his or her hand because I know the person would be afraid. That would be high-touch care. Skill is required in both arenas to give truly holistic nursing care to people.

Holding a patient's hand to offer strength and consolation is characteristic of transpersonal caring. Another act that incorporates the principles of transpersonal caring is contacting the patient's religious advisor to have someone to pray with or for the person, depending on the situation. If the patient dies, you should still care about the individual and treat his or her body with gentleness and love. There is no way to avoid being caring if you want to be successful at the art of nursing.

The spiritual aspect of caring is sometimes uncomfortable for nurses. Some people express offense at the mention of "spirit" because of its religious connotation, and some nurses do not accept the validity of organized religion or do not believe in God. Nurses need to respect and support the religious or spiritual needs of patients, however, because that is caring for the spirit, an integral aspect of transpersonal caring. Think of it as nursing care for the spiritual aspect of a person. Your beliefs do not enter in, but your quality of nursing does. If you are a caring person, you accept people unconditionally. That

Spirituality is a crucial aspect of holistic nursing.

means you accept people's needs and behaviors as being real for them. You do not have to convert to Judaism, Islam, or Christianity to be a caring nurse. But it is essential that you respect those beliefs in others.

Watson says, "A nurse may perform actions toward a patient out of a sense of duty or moral obligation, and would be an ethical nurse. Yet it may be false to say he or she cared about the patient. The value of human care and caring involves a higher sense of self. Caring calls for a philosophy of moral commitment toward protecting human dignity and preserving humanity" (Watson, 2012, p. 41).

REFLECTIVE THINKING

What does Watson's quote mean to you? Can you think of an example in your life when someone has met his or her ethical responsibility but has not cared about you in the process? Take a moment and think about such an event that you experienced and record it in your class notebook.

Your teacher may ask you to discuss your example or story in class.

You may want to share your example with a classmate and get feedback about it. It also would be interesting to read another person's example. I won't ask you to write it, but think of a time when you were noncaring. The example probably comes from your personal life. I wonder if it is a behavior you feel sorry about now or even felt that way soon after you did it? Do you know how to avoid such a behavior again? Talking to others about such a situation can be helpful.

APPLYING CARING THEORY IN YOUR PERSONAL LIFE

Is there someone you care about in your personal life, such as a classmate or a friend, who drives you crazy at times? As a caring person or someone who wants to be a caring nurse, you have given the relationship some thought, I hope. When I say you care about someone, I am not referring to love or even a close friendship. I am talking about caring that is transpersonal and as such can be shared with any human being anywhere. You do not have to know the person and develop a strong relationship; it does not have to be intimate caring or the caring that exists in most families. All of those situations count, but transpersonal caring is the caring you give another person—a stranger—because you both are human and your lives have crossed paths. This type of caring is seen by philosophers as a human trait or as a moral imperative. There are other ways to examine caring, but they are not discussed in this chapter.

A classic example of caring for a stranger is your response when another driver cuts you off in traffic. Justified or not, is your response based on caring principles?

What about the irritating person in class who talks too much, or knocked your books off your desk and didn't apologize or pick them up? Or the neighbor who keeps watering his lawn so the water spots your front windows every time? Or the friend who is consistently late in picking you up to drive to school? Or the mother who constantly yells at you to help her with the housework and the younger children despite the amount of homework you have to do? Do these people deserve your transpersonal caring? Yes, they do because they are human beings, and true caring does not discriminate based on race, religion, age, behavior, or any other characteristic. This is one of the challenges of being a professional nurse.

As a class, you could begin a project to practice transpersonal caring. Ask your instructor for some time to discuss caring in the classroom, then talk about how transpersonal caring could be implemented. There are some simple ways. Begin by learning everyone's name. I know LPN classes vary in size, and you already may know everyone's name. I have taught classes, however, where students graduated without knowing the names of their classmates. Caring is getting to know each other. You will find the power in names once you learn them. Being able to address a person by name allows barriers to a relationship to be removed so that caring can occur.

Another thing you could discuss as a class is how the class should be conducted. This is not the process of setting up rules for class. Instead, it is a discussion in which everyone gets to voice his or her opinion. Because I am hoping for an empowering environment for this discussion, every comment and idea should be treated with respect. The topics listed in Box 2.2 might be discussed in such a forum.

By thinking about and implementing transpersonal caring concepts in your personal life, you are making a change within yourself. I sense that most nurses struggle with transpersonal caring principles because of nursing's long history of being obedient to physicians. Obedience in itself is not

a bad thing, unless it keeps you from thinking independently. But it does place a nurse directly within the medical model, whereas I think nurses should be practicing within a nursing model such as Watson's.

UNDERSTANDING NURSING MODELS

The profession of modern nursing is approximately 100 years old. As a new profession, nurses had to concede to physicians, just as Florence Nightingale did to make and keep peace, or she and her nurses would not have been allowed to visit and treat the soldiers in the Crimea. Obedience was a matter of necessity if nursing care was to be administered. Another reason nurses were subservient to physicians is that white men with money traditionally have had the power in our culture; women have not. Because of the power structure and social constraints, female nurses were subservient to male physicians.

Subservience is one of the characteristics nursing inherited. If the profession of nursing is going to overcome that inheritance, there is a need for empowerment and caring. Why caring? It is the overwhelming characteristic that differentiates nursing from medicine. I am not saying physicians are not caring people. I am saying they do not learn how to practice transpersonal caring because it is a nursing model of practice. There are several nursing models of care, and caring is a basic part of many of them.

To understand medical and nursing models of practice better, let's look at the case of a 17-year-old girl named Sarah who is an outstanding cellist. She plays in the high school orchestra and in a statewide youth orchestra. The youth orchestra requires travel to the capital city (1 hour each way) twice a week for rehearsal as well as hours of practice. Sarah recently was admitted to the hospital in a diabetic coma. The physician did an excellent job of saving Sarah's life, stabilizing her condition, and planning for her future health. This was accomplished by following the medical model, which states that physicians treat the cells in the human body. The physician ordered the diet, medication, and exercise that would stabilize Sarah's diabetes and allow her to live. If Sarah experiences complications with her diabetes, the physician will take tests that will indicate what the cells are doing and write orders accordingly. The physician will keep Sarah alive and functioning.

Box 2.2 The Caring Classroom

1. The respectful caring that is shown when people come to class on time
2. The higher quality of class discussion that occurs when people come well prepared
3. The importance of allowing others to finish what they were saying before starting your comment
4. Being watchful about not taking more than your share of the time so that others can share their ideas too
5. General rules of courtesy to be used with each other
6. Accepting and valuing others' comments that are new or foreign to you (e.g., religious or cultural comments)

What is the nurse's role? The nurse follows the physician's orders, ensuring that Sarah gets the medication and diet that have been ordered in the right way and at the right time. In addition, the nurse practices within the nursing model of transpersonal caring. This means that when Sarah is found crying late at night because she thinks she cannot stay with the statewide orchestra, the nurse stays with her while she cries, reassures her that with good management she can work out a healthy schedule, and does not leave until Sarah is feeling better informed about her disease. All of this happens even if the nurse thinks cello music is unpleasant and "scratchy." The nurse does not share her feelings but instead values the patient and her dreams and concerns without judging them. That is a nursing model. The same nurse will patiently teach Sarah and repeat the lesson to the family members who are interested but who arrive late for every teaching session. The nurse is the person who will "sneak in" Sarah's orchestra friends for an afternoon mini-concert and chat.

Nursing goes beyond the body's cellular response. Let physicians do what they do so well—treat patients on the cellular level. Nurses should do what they do so well—treat the patient holistically using transpersonal caring.

APPLYING CARING THEORY IN YOUR PROFESSIONAL LIFE

I was educated more than 40 years ago to practice nursing within the medical model of thinking. It is only because I have continued to go to school that I learned about nursing models of care. At the time

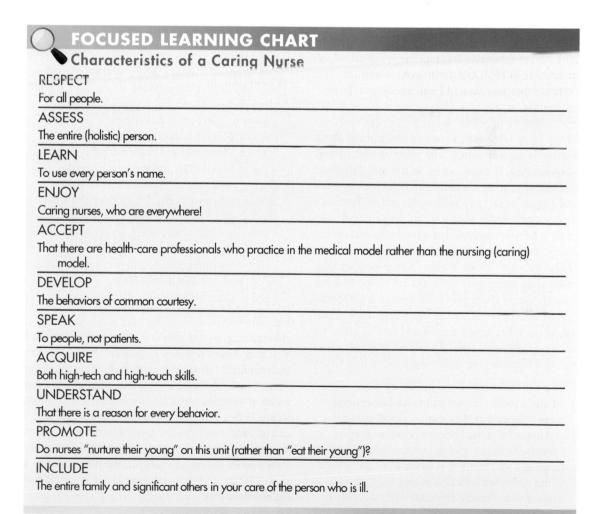

FOCUSED LEARNING CHART
Characteristics of a Caring Nurse

RESPECT
For all people.

ASSESS
The entire (holistic) person.

LEARN
To use every person's name.

ENJOY
Caring nurses, who are everywhere!

ACCEPT
That there are health-care professionals who practice in the medical model rather than the nursing (caring) model.

DEVELOP
The behaviors of common courtesy.

SPEAK
To people, not patients.

ACQUIRE
Both high-tech and high-touch skills.

UNDERSTAND
That there is a reason for every behavior.

PROMOTE
Do nurses "nurture their young" on this unit (rather than "eat their young")?

INCLUDE
The entire family and significant others in your care of the person who is ill.

I earned my registered nurse (RN) degree, the focus was on learning to take blood pressures (the physicians had just recently given that up and were allowing nurses to take them!) and starting intravenous (IV) fluids. Rapid response teams were just being organized, and the first intensive care unit, in the large city where I went to school, opened soon after I graduated. Nurses were working hard to prove they had the technical competence to practice alongside physicians. During this time, the nurse practitioner (NP) role was identified, and nurses went to school to learn to practice as "personal care providers." NPs from the first schools were taught to practice in the medical model, not the nursing model. I see the current trend for NPs to practice independent of physicians and within nursing frameworks as a positive part of nursing's evolution.

As a new student in the profession, you do not have to unlearn medical model approaches to care as I did. Instead, you can learn nursing models of care from the beginning of your career. You also will learn the high-tech information necessary for you to do your job effectively. Don't worry; no one will let you graduate without knowing all of the technical skills so crucial to your licensure. The bonus is that you also will learn caring theories.

Caring as It Relates to Colleagues

When I first went back to school and learned about Watson's nursing model and other models, I was very excited. It made sense to me and felt good emotionally. In my excitement, I went back to work and began to tell my colleagues about Watson's theory and what it meant to nursing overall. The most common response I received was that nurses always had been caring, and "they" didn't need to study to learn about caring. Some people who made such comments were unkind to me because I was bringing them new information. An RN who taught the paramedics (a very high-tech field) asked me what caring meant and how it could be done on ambulance runs. These responses surprised me, but I learned the following lessons that I now share with you to make your life easier:

1. Medical model nurses still exist. Older nurses were educated in the medical model paradigm. If a nurse has never been exposed to nursing models, he or she will not understand when first hearing about them. It is much like taking third-year French without first taking the first and second year French. If we are truly working on

being transpersonal caring nurses, we need to acknowledge and respect medical model nurses and teach them if they are interested. We should not be judgmental or critical, just caring.

2. Despite all of the good that people such as Watson have done to change the focus of nursing from medical to nursing models, nurses can still be unkind to each other. This is a terrible reality, but one many nurses attest to regularly. Not all nurses are caring. If it suits them and generally if they were hurt as they progressed through the profession, they will hurt you as a less experienced nurse. A newly graduated nurse remembers feeling embarrassed when an experienced nurse criticized her in front of a patient and a physician. She also clearly recalls being unable to find help in learning the responsibilities of being a new charge nurse. Without understanding transpersonal caring, nurses often subject new graduates to the same negative things they experienced. The phrase "nurses eat their young" really portrays a nightmare scenario. I wonder if the phrase would go out of vogue if nurses quit using it? You are the generation of nurses who can do that by refusing to use such a negative phrase. You could replace it with the question, "Do nurses nurture their young on this unit?" Such a question would refocus the listener's thinking and share with the listener what your priorities are regarding people.

3. Caring nurses are everywhere. Find those nurses and enjoy them. Learn from them and share your ideas with them. The nursing profession is filled with caring, compassionate people who work the continuum from emergency departments to health promotion clinics. Seek them out and do not let the few who still need to learn about caring theories interfere with your career.

As you begin your clinical practice, look around you and observe nurses in general. Watch for the techniques (high-tech) and the behaviors of caring (high-touch) that you want to incorporate into your nursing practice. Work toward developing such skills. When you are a more experienced nurse, go out of your way to be the type of nurse you admire by sharing your knowledge with others, especially new nurses. Being an example and role model is a powerful thing. Find such people for yourself and be one for others.

Caring for Patients

Being a caring person enhances your personal life and your professional skills and ability. When I was a young nurse, I was with a patient who was near death, homeless, and without family. My role model in nursing was with me. It was a busy day on a 40-bed surgical floor, but another nurse and I stayed with that man for more than 3 hours as he was dying and while waiting for the mortuary to come for his body. He received precious care and the gift of our time. The other nurses on the floor knew what we were doing and picked up our workload. It was a cherished time in which the other nurse and I gave the best of ourselves to that patient, and the other nurses on the unit showed supportive caring for us by doing our other work. How could something like that happen? It is because nurses, by their nature, are caring people.

The concept of transpersonal caring makes sense when applied to patients. Watson would encourage us not to call people who are sick *patients*. We all do, but in a theoretical sense, it is better to recognize them as individuals rather than label them as patients. You already may have discovered, however, that most people who are in hospitals and nursing homes are referred to by their diagnosis (e.g., "the fractured hip in 113" or "the knee replacement down the hall"). Such language is uncaring. Remember when I told you about the power in knowing a person's name? This is an important application of that principle. Motivate yourself to learn the names of the people for whom you provide care. Write them down or refer to your assignment sheet. If you need to, pull out the sheet and refresh your memory before walking into the room. If you are dashing into the room to respond to an emergency, the priority is to get into the room and attend to the crisis at hand. When the emergency has been managed, you can check on the name.

SETTING PRIORITIES USING TRANSPERSONAL CARING

In this chapter, you are learning about holistic care within the framework of a caring theory. As an LPN, you will need to apply the skills and knowledge you have learned and set priorities for patients' care. As you read the following case study, evaluate the two approaches to the care presented. Which approach is most effective?

In a report, you are told about Mrs. Lopez, who had abdominal surgery that was more extensive than expected. Mrs. Lopez is receiving IV fluids and blood transfusions, and her dressing has been saturated and changed every 2 to 3 hours. (Although an uncommon practice, in some states LPNs are taught to manage IVs in their basic program. In all states, the RN is responsible for the blood transfusion. Whatever your education, if you are assigned to Mrs. Lopez, you need to be aware of the blood and the IV and know your legal responsibilities.) The pain medication Mrs. Lopez is taking does not relieve her discomfort. She is divorced and has no family nearby, so she is alone. Mrs. Lopez is the most ill person you have been assigned, and as you walk to the room to evaluate her, you are planning how to prioritize her needs. You decide the following:

1. Survival is the most important need, so checking the dressing is the first priority.
2. It is sad that Mrs. Lopez has no one to be with her while she is so sick, but there are other needs to consider first.

Efficient approach. As you enter Mrs. Lopez's room, you notice she is pale. You remember her name and greet her while you put on your gloves. Then you proceed to check her dressing, which is saturated. You quickly and efficiently remove the dressing, examine the wound, and reapply a stronger dressing while thinking that the RN needs to know about the seepage on the dressing right away. Then you check the IV and blood to see that they are still running and leave the room to inform the nurse about Mrs. Lopez's saturated dressing.

If you were the nurse just described, you were very efficient, but not very caring. Let's reenact the same scenario using a caring approach.

Caring approach. As you walk into Mrs. Lopez's room, you notice she is pale and apparently has been crying. Because you practice holistic nursing, you take 2 to 3 minutes and introduce yourself to her, pull up a chair, and hold her hand while you look directly into her eyes and ask her how she is. She may cry because she is lonely and in pain. Perhaps she is afraid she is dying and has just spent the night worrying alone. She is afraid to move because she thinks it will cause more bleeding, and her arm is numb at the IV site because she is terrified to move it.

By actually talking to Mrs. Lopez, rather than around her, you have demonstrated one of the strongest points of caring for another person. You know the dressing needs to be checked and probably changed immediately; yet by speaking to Mrs. Lopez, you have discovered other needs that cannot be ignored. What do you do? (This dilemma is why some nurses do not talk to patients.) You should explain to Mrs. Lopez that you care about her and her feelings and let her know that there are some things you need to teach her about her postoperative healing. But for the moment you need to look at and change the dressing and check her IV lines. She will want you to do that because she is very worried herself. While you are checking her dressing, you can explain that moving will not cause her incision to bleed more. Then make a note to teach her about moving and coughing as part of her postoperative healing plan.

After you have changed the dressing, you should explain to Mrs. Lopez that you would like the RN to know what you saw, then excuse yourself and go find the RN. Mrs. Lopez obviously has concerns, so it would be thoughtful to let her know when you will be back: "I will be back within the next 10 minutes, Mrs. Lopez. Here is your call light if you need me before then."

The difference between these two scenarios is caring. In the first situation, the LPN was focused on the wound and dressing and hardly spoke to Mrs. Lopez. It was as if Mrs. Lopez were a surgical incision rather than a person. This is a depersonalized approach to Mrs. Lopez's needs, yet the LPN performed the technical skills well. The first LPN would keep Mrs. Lopez alive, but the nurse failed to recognize many needs because the total person (holistic care) was not addressed.

In the second scenario, the LPN recognized and acknowledged Mrs. Lopez as a whole human being. The nurse immediately recognized the fear on Mrs. Lopez's face and addressed it. The nurse neglected neither the wound nor the personhood of Mrs. Lopez. The nurse showed transpersonal caring by being holistic in approach and informing Mrs. Lopez about what was being done and why.

CARING FOR FAMILY AND SIGNIFICANT OTHERS

As a holistic nurse who practices transpersonal caring, you have a responsibility to family members and to the person who is ill. Working with the family is always time-consuming and generally challenging. However, holism means the whole person. Most of us do not live in isolation but have family or significant others who are important in our lives. If the nurse can engage the family or significant others in the healing process of the patient, the healing process generally is enhanced. Patient stress is reduced, and patient support is increased because others know and understand current happenings and plans for the future. What follows is an example of how including the family can be done with everyone benefiting.

Mrs. Romer is a widowed, 80-year-old, alert mother of six adult daughters. Two of her six daughters are nurses. All six of her daughters are strongly independent women accustomed to being in charge. Mrs. Romer was admitted to the emergency department of the local hospital for a pathological fracture of her left femur. A pathological fracture means the injury did not occur because of a fall; instead, the fracture resulted from a disease process—in this case, osteoporosis. Two months before she fractured her femur, Mrs. Romer had fallen and fractured the neck of her femur. The fracture was repaired with a pinning procedure, and she went home and did well with a walker until the femur itself fractured.

An LPN provides high-touch care.

Mrs. Romer's surgery to repair her fracture was 7 hours long because it necessitated repinning the hip, doing a bone graft, and placing a steel rod in her femur. She was very ill and at risk of dying when she left the recovery room. Mrs. Romer spent 8 weeks in the hospital, had three surgeries, and spent time on five different nursing units. With aggressive rehabilitation, she was able to transfer from the hospital to a rehabilitation center. After 2 months there, she was discharged to live with one of her daughters.

During the acute phase, Mrs. Romer's situation, including her family, posed many challenges. Each daughter wanted to know exactly what was happening at all times and wanted to be a part of all decisions made. Can you see how these six strong women, all with different opinions, could drive the physician and the nursing staff crazy? It took approximately 48 hours for everyone to recognize what was happening—the nursing staff received calls from a different daughter about every hour, and the physician received six calls a day about Mrs. Romer's condition.

To solve this problem and to meet the family's needs, the daughters and the case manager designed a plan. The daughter who lived the closest was selected to be the information person. The physician would call that daughter every morning after he had made rounds. (It was worth his time because it saved him from the six calls he would have had to manage otherwise.) Then the informant would visit her mother every morning after the day shift was on duty, gather first-hand information from her mother and the nurse, and call the other sisters.

The plan worked beautifully. Mrs. Romer did not have to deal with "daughter stress." The nurses had to deal with only one daughter once a day (instead of all six of them throughout the day), and the physician was glad to report to only one person. The important point from the nurses' standpoint was that the daughters could relax and allow their mother to heal instead of adding to her stress.

Talk to families, teach them, care about their concerns, and respect them. Include them in the information loop, unless they tell you they just don't want to know. Allow them to be with their family member and assist them in the healing process. I want to clarify two important points: (1) When I say family, I mean all significant others. (2) When I say healing, I also mean dying well if that is the case.

 ## CARING INCLUDES EVERYONE

Although it may be difficult to value and respect all patients, you need to show caring to everyone. In one of my classes, a student RN, who is practicing as an LPN, said that he had no respect for patients who brought on their own diseases. I jokingly told him I was writing this chapter on caring and he may need to read it. His response was that some people are not worth caring about! I told him I didn't agree with him and then went on with class. I didn't want to embarrass him in front of his peers, but I am going to give him a copy of this chapter.

The student was referring to a quadriplegic (paralyzed in all four extremities) patient who had been in a car accident after trying to elude the police. He was a known heroin user. Because of this man's behavior before his paralysis, the student felt the patient deserved his resulting quadriplegia.

I say it unequivocally and with conviction: Every single human being deserves your respect and the highest level of nursing care possible—everyone!

Some people are homophobic, which means they have an aversion to homosexuals. Homophobia should not be expressed, either verbally or nonverbally, while you are practicing as a nurse. Some people feel disdain for feminists; others, for minorities. When you go home, you may say or think what you wish, but when you are on duty, you are obligated to practice professional nursing, which does not allow for discriminatory practices. One of my favorite phrases is "there is a reason for every behavior." You may not always know the reason for a patient's behavior, but your responsibility is not to criticize but rather to give holistic care to every person in your care. To give holistic care, you must recognize there is a reason for whatever behavior the patient exhibits; you just may not know what it is.

Some people work in prisons and jails where murderers, pedophiles (child molesters), and rapists need nursing care. If you work in such an institution, you need to work through any negative feelings you may have against such people and give them the same level of holistic care that you would give Mother Teresa, if she were still alive, or your own loved ones. Meeting the challenge of holistic nursing care is what makes nursing a profession. To be a nurse is difficult, demanding, and challenging.

The ability to give holistic, transpersonal care in all nursing care situations is how that challenge is met.

PERSONAL MOTIVATION

You may agree with the caring information shared in this chapter, but you will not use it unless you are motivated to do so. Just what is motivation, and what will motivate you personally to apply the principles you are taught?

What Is Motivation?

Motivation is defined by some as a caused behavior or a psychological process that gives behavior purpose and direction. As you begin your educational process to become an LPN, I am sure you have a strong motivation for what you are doing. Having purpose and direction as you go through school and eventually your nursing career is crucial.

Maureen O'Hara, a nurse I respect very highly, is a nationally recognized nursing leader in oncology (care of persons with cancer). In an interview discussing high-tech nursing care and high-touch nursing, she was asked what she considered the essence of nursing to be. She stated:

> *Clinical excellence coupled with heart and compassion. It's important to think, "What if this was my mother, my sister, or my daughter or son?" Our patients are somebody's mother or child and their families have entrusted their loved ones' lives to us. All patients and families deserve clinical excellence combined with compassion, kindness, dignity, and respect because that's how all human beings ought to be treated, whether they are prisoners or Silicon Valley executives. (O'Hara & de Ruiter, 2015, p. 229)*

I think such a positive statement from a nationally recognized nurse such as Maureen O'Hara is motivating for you. I share it with you as information for building your own understanding of what may have motivated you to become an LPN. Does it cause you to have good feelings about being an LPN?

I am interested in knowing why you chose to be an LPN. There are likely several reasons why you chose nursing overall and licensed practical nursing in particular. Although I may never know what they are, your reasons need to be clear to you.

As human beings, we do things based on our motivation to accomplish certain tasks. When I think of the people who have climbed Mount Everest or competed in the Iron Man Triathlon, I wonder why they do it! Those activities are of no interest to me. I would never train to compete in an athletic event. How about you? Are you motivated by sports, music, reading, or children?

To complete this textbook, I will spend many hours sitting in front of my computer with reference books stacked around me while I write. I do this day and night. I love weekends and holidays because I can sit and write uninterrupted. I am as excited about finishing this book or other scholarly projects as an athlete is about finishing a race or a tough climb. We are different people with different things motivating us to perform. I respect the motivation and success of any athlete and expect the same respect for my motivation and accomplishments. One of the richest aspects of living as human beings is the diversity of people. It is something I have learned to appreciate sincerely. Think about the people you know well and consider what motivates them. What gets them excited? More important, what gets *you* excited?

Why are you wearing the clothes you have on right now? Is the outfit you are wearing the last one clean? Is it something new you got for school, so you chose to wear it today? Are you curled up somewhere comfortably studying and chose to wear something comfortable as well? There is a reason for everything you do, and the reason behind your behavior is your personal motivation.

REFLECTIVE THINKING

Write in your class notebook the top three reasons you are in this class at this moment in your life.

Some students have been motivated to be nurses from childhood.

You may need to take a moment to think about it. Did you just graduate from high school and are fortunate enough to be able to go directly to nursing school? Have you recently been able to obtain enough money to go to school? Were you in the hospital as a patient and learned about the role of the LPN? Or have you wanted to be a nurse for your entire life and see LPN education as the way for you to achieve that dream? Whatever reasons you identify, record them to share in class. The thoughts you record should have something to do with your motivation to be an LPN.

There Is a Reason for Every Behavior

The critical concept of "there is a reason for every behavior" requires each of us to understand human nature and ourselves. It is a challenging concept to learn. One may say there is no good reason to take illegal drugs. That may be true, but I am not talking about good reasons. I am simply talking about reasons for what we do. Those reasons are based on personal motivation.

What did you eat for breakfast this morning? Perhaps you were motivated to stay up late last night studying, and you slept in this morning. You can honestly say you were not motivated to skip breakfast, but look at how your decision of last night (based on the motivation to study late) impacted the decision you made today. There is a reason for everything you do, and it is important that as you develop professionally, you learn to understand the impact motivation has on your behavior. By understanding motivation, you will learn to understand that there is a reason for every behavior and begin to look for the reason for a person's actions (such as taking drugs) rather than being confused or judgmental. Understanding is part of the professional behavior you want to develop as you venture through school.

Have you ever experienced conflict based on differing personal motivations? Perhaps you are motivated to study, but your family wants dinner. Such situations are difficult, but it is important to understand that people are working from what motivates them rather than being insensitive or unkind. As part of your educational process, I encourage you to examine your life and see whether you can determine the motivation of the people with whom you spend a great deal of time.

I recall rather shamefacedly a classic example of two people with different motivations. My 2-year-old granddaughter was crying and fussy on a day when I was very busy trying to meet a deadline. Finally, I looked at her in exasperation and asked, "Why are you crying?" Once she told me why she was crying, it was clear to me that I should have known. She simply stated that she was hungry. She was crying because she wanted food, and I wanted to meet my deadline. Fortunately, I was more than willing to stop what I was doing and feed her whatever she wanted! I was embarrassed at my insensitivity.

Has something like this happened to you in your personal life? Being aware of this type of behavior on a personal level should help you avoid the same behavior when you are caring for patients and residents. A nursing example that should never happen, but could, might involve an LPN keeping to a time schedule. Perhaps, as an LPN, you are passing medications, and you are motivated to do it on time (that is a good thing!). As you proceed, however, you find that many of the nursing home residents want to talk to you, perhaps asking you questions or simply enjoying your company. You need to decide whether you are going to keep your schedule or meet the emotional needs of others. What motivates you is the bottom-line question. You will have to keep within an appropriate time frame for passing the medications, which will allow for some visiting but not as much as you want. You may return to the residents who needed you and talk to them after medications are dispensed.

As you continue through school, you will experience many things that will change your motivational focus. Motivation is a dynamic process, one that changes over time because of experiences and the influence of others. When I went to school more than 40 years ago, there were only 11 women in my class. There were no men because they simply were not admitted to hospital schools of nursing. During one of my clinical rotations, there were only three students and one faculty person for the entire quarter. I was very motivated in that class because I received so much time and attention from the teacher.

When I went to a local university to take classes for my baccalaureate degree, there were 90 students in my first class. I was overwhelmed and just plain shocked. How could I be expected to learn, let alone understand the content? I had to stand in line to talk to the instructor, and there was never enough time to get to the front of the line before my next class. I had to learn a different form of motivation to complete that and other classes successfully. I wanted a baccalaureate degree in nursing, and attending a class with 90 students in it was the way to meet my goal. So I adapted; that is another way of saying I changed my motivational approach.

Have you ever had to adapt to achieve what motivates you? I am sure you made sacrifices to come to school. Did any of them require motivational adaptation? It is a common occurrence in the lives of most people. If you can identify motivational adaptation in yourself, you should be able to understand it in the people to whom you give nursing care.

There are ways to learn how to identify your personal motivation and to understand the motivation of others. The ways to understanding are called theories of motivation. In Chapter 3, you will learn about Maslow's theory of motivation and how to apply it to your clinical practice as well as to yourself.

Florence Nightingale stated: "It may seem a strange principle to enunciate as the very first requirement in a hospital that it should do the sick no harm" (Nightingale, 1863). When a nurse uses holistic practices within the framework of transpersonal caring, "no harm" is done to the person who is sick. Modern nurses have the opportunity to begin their practice without the constraints of the previously used medical model style of nursing. They are learning the knowledge and skills that allow a nurse to practice holistically in today's modern educational systems. This is knowledge that will have an impact on the nursing profession forever.

Learning and applying the principles of caring require LPNs to define and understand their personal motivation to learning and nursing practice. When you understand motivation for yourself, you will understand it better for the people to whom you give care.

REAL-WORLD CASE STUDY

■ Trish, a new employee at the Wasatch Gardens Skilled Nursing Facility, made the following comment: "I found it really easy to practice transpersonal caring while I was an LPN in the newborn nursery. But, I find that it is too hard to care about the residents because they are confused, smelly, and, well, just aren't pleasant."

Trish was a new LPN who had recently moved to the area and had been working at the long-term care center for the past 3 weeks. She made the previous comment while meeting with her nurse manager to discuss getting help or terminating her employment. Trish had excellent basic skills and was able to work with the certified nursing assistants (CNAs) effectively. Joe, the nurse manager, had been excited when he interviewed Trish because she knew about transpersonal caring and holistic nursing concepts. He believed the skilled nursing facility was the perfect place to practice caring theories in nursing. Based on the employment interview, the nurse manager was surprised to hear of Trish's dissatisfaction with her job.

After consulting with Trish and the staff development nurse, Joe gave Trish two weeks of education and orientation time to work with Mercy, the staff development coordinator. This act in itself was a caring one. If you were the LPN staff developer, what plan would you design to teach Trish how to apply caring theory in the long-term care setting?

Write the solution to the case study on a separate piece of paper to submit to your instructor.

Key Points

- ■ Florence Nightingale used her resources to provide for the basic needs of the sick and injured she cared for. She overcame the lack of education of her nurses, the attitudes of physicians, and basic health and sanitation issues to provide holistic care for her patients.
- ■ The nursing model has traditionally been a subservient one. Nurses need to become more empowered and caring while focusing on holistic transpersonal care. Traditionally, the medical model has been focused on the diagnosis and treatment of illness.
- ■ Dr. Jean Watson teaches that transpersonal caring has been neglected in nursing education. She values the nurse–patient relationship and says that they should work together to achieve the best outcomes. Caring should be the intent of every interaction with the patient.

- Caring includes everyone. Nurses care for patients but they also provide care and education to families and other significant people in their patients' lives. In addition, they must demonstrate caring for their colleagues, other members of the health-care team, and themselves.
- Watson's theories can be applied in personal life and in the classroom by showing care and concern for those people with whom we interact. We demonstrate this concern when we value and respect the comments and opinions of others.
- Nurses are not always welcoming of new graduates and may not show the caring that is important to successful transition into the profession. Application of Watson's theories in the workplace includes finding good role

models and then being a good role model. In this way, new nurses can help to improve this unfortunate part of nursing culture.
- Watson's theories should be applied to patient care. By referring to patients by name and carefully prioritizing their needs, nurses can demonstrate caring. It is important to consider all of the patient's needs, both those concerned with health and those concerned with emotional well-being, and develop a holistic plan of care.
- Understanding what motivates you is an important part of personal success and satisfaction in a nursing career. People are motivated by different things. Spending some time thinking about why you want to be an LPN and what things motivate you to complete your goals will help you succeed.

ANSWERS TO REAL-WORLD CASE STUDY

As the staff developer in a long-term care setting, you have seen other employees who have had to struggle either learning caring theory or applying it to the long-term care environment. You have a plan as to what to do to help Trish. You know to keep it simple but meaningful so that Trish won't be frustrated or overwhelmed. Here is one possible educational plan for Trish. You may have other ideas. If so, be sure to share them.

Mercy assigned Trish to work an entire week with the facility's most outstanding CNA to provide Trish the orientation she needs to make the transition from newborn nursery care to long-term care nursing. Trish should not feel devalued because she is working with a CNA. CNAs know how to give "caring" care, which is what Trish needs to learn. Mercy picked the most caring and efficient CNA in the skilled nursing facility to work with Trish and encouraged them to develop their own caring relationship.

During her first week, Trish spent the afternoons sitting and talking with the residents. Her objective was to learn residents' names and personal aspects of their lives. In this way, Trish learned to relate to the residents as human beings with individual personalities, needs, and desires. Trish was encouraged to talk to the CNAs about the information she learned from the residents and to observe how the CNAs, especially

the outstanding one she was assigned to work with, gave transpersonal care to the residents.

When a nurse has been used to working in a newborn nursery where the RN gives most of the medications, the large number of medications that need to be given in a skilled facility can be overwhelming. So, during the second week, Mercy assigned Trish to work with the medication nurse so that by the end of the week Trish had gradually taken over the administration of all medication. This task was made easier for Trish because now she knew the CNAs and the residents as individuals.

■ *Results*

Trish decided to stay at the skilled facility because she learned to care about the residents. She saw the CNAs as role models who cared about the residents and knew about them personally. She was the recipient of transpersonal caring from her nurse manager and Mercy who had given her two extra weeks (a big budget item) to learn her role in the nursing home. The staff members were caring toward her as well.

You may have designed a different solution to Trish's problem. If so, go through it and identify the caring aspects. This case study gives you the opportunity to consider residents, staff, and colleagues in the solution.

REVIEW QUESTIONS

1. Sarah is a 17-year-old newly diagnosed diabetic. Which statement reflects the medical model of care?
   1. Sarah will need a consultation with a dietician.
   2. Sarah will need support from her family and friends.
   3. Sarah will need time to accept her diagnosis.
   4. Sarah will need reassurance that she can continue favorite activities.

2. What is the main idea of holistic care?
   1. Providing access to spiritual advisors
   2. Listening to patients and using reassuring touch
   3. Allowing family and friends to visit patient
   4. Caring for the mind, body, and spirit

3. Which statement is an example of transpersonal caring?
   1. Care is transferred to another person.
   2. The person giving care is feeling mind, body, and soul.
   3. Each person feels a connection at a deeper level.
   4. The person receiving care feels unity of mind, body, and spirit.

4. Which of the following is not part of a holistic, caring method of healing?
   1. Dieting
   2. Music
   3. Aromatherapy
   4. Meditation

5. Which statement is true about motivation?
   1. People are motivated by the same things in the same career field.
   2. Motivation is caused by indecision and turmoil.
   3. Motivation usually begins in childhood and it remains constant.
   4. Motivation is a caused behavior that gives actions purpose and direction.

References

Dahlkemper, T. R. (2016). *Caring for the elderly client holistically.* Philadelphia: F. A. Davis.

Nightingale, F. (1863). *Notes on hospitals* (3rd ed.). London: Longman, Green, Longman, Roberts, and Green.

O'Hara, M., & de Ruiter, H. P. (2015). From high touch to high tech: A conversation with Maureen O'Hara, BSN, RN, OCN. *Creative Nursing, 21*(4), 228–233

Watson, J. (2012). *Nursing: Human science and human care: A theory of nursing* (2nd ed.). Sudbury, MA: Jones & Bartlett.

Web Resource

Watson Caring Science Institute www.watsoncaringscience.org

3

Understanding the Changing Roles in Nursing

HOLLI SOWERBY

KEY TERMS

Ageism
Caring intentionality
Clinical judgment
Clinical reasoning
Critical thinking
Hierarchy
Institutional review board (IRB)
Patient advocacy

CHAPTER CONCEPTS

Evidence-Based Practice
Patient-Centered Care
Collaboration

LEARNING OUTCOMES

1. Define the word *paradigm* and its current meaning in nursing education.
2. List three paradigm shifts that have had an impact on modern nursing.
3. Share three examples of how to use critical thinking in nursing practice.
4. Discuss the four critical thinking themes presented in the text.
5. Describe how Dr. Abraham Maslow's theory, "a hierarchy of human needs: a theory of motivation and development," relates to being an effective nurse manager.
6. Discuss Dr. Jean Watson's theory, "nursing: human science and human care," and its impact on the management role of the LPN.
7. Define the principle of advocacy as used in contemporary nursing.
8. Describe four components of a person's identity for which nurses should be advocates.

The significant problems we face cannot be solved at the same level of thinking we were at when we created them.

— Albert Einstein

The purpose of this chapter is to introduce some basic concepts that will be used throughout the rest of the book. They are the foundations for the knowledge you will develop as a nurse manager.

The future history of the licensed practical nurse (LPN) is still to be written. Future chapters will be scripted and lived by individuals such as you and by the profession as a group. With the tidal waves of change that are occurring throughout health care, the LPN needs to develop the ability to observe those changes and define a personal role that fits in with what is happening. Basic to understanding one's professional role in modern health-care settings is the concept of paradigm thinking. Supporting that concept is the development of the ability to shift one's paradigm to accommodate the demands of the industry.

PARADIGM THINKING DEFINED

The word *paradigm* comes from ancient Greek. It originally was a scientific term but is used more commonly today to mean a model, theory, perception, assumption, or frame of reference. In a general sense, it is the way a person "views" the world. It does not refer to visual ability but rather to one's perception, assumption, or frame of mind. In the 17th century, Galileo was imprisoned because he told the scientific and religious communities that the sun was the center of the universe and all planets, including Earth, revolved around it. Before his revelation, the scientific community believed that Earth was the center of the universe and all else revolved around it. It was not until the 20th century that the Catholic Church officially forgave Galileo for his "false teachings." Galileo shifted the paradigm thinking of the universe with his discovery.

Do you remember stories from the 17th and 18th centuries in which midwives went from woman to woman assisting with deliveries without washing their hands? The disease that resulted from this unknowing cross contamination was puerperal fever, and most women who contracted it died, as did their infants. The work of those midwives was done in the paradigm of care that existed before the germ theory was described. The midwives did not understand what caused the deaths and had absolutely no concept of germs or cross contamination.

In today's world of labor and delivery care, it is unthinkable for health-care personnel to move from person to person or room to room without washing their hands. In addition, rooms and linen are cleaned between deliveries, and sterile instruments are always used. Modern care given to women in labor is based on knowledge of germs and their potential for harm. This is a monumental paradigm shift for nursing.

Do you require yourself to make your bed every morning before going to school, or do you feel that making the bed only on weekends is more realistic? These ideas represent different paradigms. As an LPN, you should be able to identify the paradigms that govern your personal and professional thinking. Another paradigm that is individualized in the practice setting is the use of touch in clinical practice. Some nurses believe it is inappropriate to touch patients unless doing a procedure. This type of touch is referred to as task touch. Others feel comfortable touching patients except when the patients indicate they don't want the physical contact. Another touch paradigm is that of using therapeutic touch as a healing modality. What is your touch paradigm? Your way of "viewing" how touch is used in your clinical practice is individualized and generally based on your personal and professional experiences.

Most nursing paradigms are based on learning through theoretical or clinical experiences. Most students model their behavior after an admired instructor or clinical nurse; others read and critically evaluate their readings to define their paradigms. Some use a mix of both approaches to determine their way of "viewing" nursing practice.

Other paradigms that have an impact on nursing are based on cultural differences and personal biases. Most nurses bring their cultural belief systems with them to school and work. These paradigms generally enrich the environment and add the needed component of diversity to a setting. The same is true of personal biases. I personally value the elderly person with dementia as my favorite client. That is a personal bias that has developed into my paradigm of care. Some people are offended when I share that with them; that response represents their paradigm. The purpose of exploring paradigm thinking is to be able to recognize existing paradigms and work within their different frameworks as a nurse.

Your paradigm is the accumulation of experience and reason that determines your thinking about all aspects of the care you deliver. This concept is similar to the accumulation of information that is condensed into a map. Consider this for a moment. If a paradigm is compared to a map, what happens if the map is the wrong one for the environment? As an example, consider what might occur if you used a map of Paris while you were exploring New York City. The paradigm (map) would not be helpful to your exploration. It would cause you to become lost and feel frustrated, and using it would be ineffective in reaching your objective of exploring New York. In this situation, you could change your behavior by working harder, being more diligent, or reading the map faster. These efforts would succeed only in getting you to the wrong place more quickly. You also could decide to work on your attitude in an effort to achieve your goal. This could result in thinking more positively. It wouldn't help you with your exploration, but perhaps you wouldn't care. Your attitude would be so positive that you'd be happy wherever you were!

Working harder or changing your attitude to achieve a goal works only if you are in the right paradigm or if you are able to shift your paradigm to fit the current environment. The shift has to be authentic in terms of understanding the rationale and purpose of making the shift. The purpose of this discussion on understanding paradigms is to encourage you to identify your work environment paradigm and to learn how to shift it or yourself, if necessary.

Paradigm Shift

The term *paradigm shift* was introduced by Kuhn (1962) in his influential book *The Structure of Scientific Revolutions*. Kuhn shows how almost every significant breakthrough in science is first a break with tradition, a shift away from old ways of thinking and old paradigms. The government of the United States is an example of a profound paradigm shift. For centuries before 1776, the traditional concept of governments was that of imperial rule—the divine right of kings. It was a powerful shift for the early colonists to determine the rule of their country to be "by the people, for the people, and of the people." When the Constitution was written, democracy was born and a centuries-old paradigm was altered.

Whether the shift is positive or negative, a paradigm shift changes the world of the person experiencing it. Paradigm shifts are powerful. Correct or incorrect, they are the sources of attitude and behavior and ultimately the basis for relationships with others. See Box 3.1 for the difference between *paradigm* and *paradigm shift.*

Several years ago, I was the clinical instructor in a busy emergency department. After I had assigned the students to various nurses and situations, I noticed three small children in the TV room and visitors' lounge. The children were unkempt and rowdy. They were hitting each other and crying while moving constantly around the small room. The TV was on at an irritatingly high volume, and junk-food wrappers were scattered throughout the room. The scene was upsetting to me, and in my paradigm of a low noise level and minimal disruption in an emergency department waiting room, I was ready to change the situation. As I walked into the room, I saw the person I assumed to be the mother of the children. She also was disheveled and sat in a corner of the room with her head down, ignoring the children. I was really irritated when I saw her indifference to the chaos. I thought, "She should at least keep them quiet or call a family member to get them." In that frame of reference, I was ready with a list of suggestions as I approached the mother. I was surprised when she didn't notice me standing in front of her, so I sat down beside her. Because the couch was small, I was forced to sit near her and I later realized that she assumed this to be a caring act. When she looked up at me, I realized she had been crying for a long time. By acknowledging me, she also acknowledged the behavior of her children and immediately spoke to them in a tender way. With her quiet approach, she quickly brought them

---

Box 3.1 The Difference Between a Paradigm and a Paradigm Shift

Paradigm: One's assumptions or perception of the world

Paradigm shift: A break with old ways of thinking or traditions under control. When they were quiet, she apologized to me for their behavior and with fresh tears explained that her husband had just been killed in an automobile accident and she simply didn't know what to do. I quickly shifted my paradigm and began to assist her in calling family members, and I played with the children to keep them happy. (Notice that my objective was not to keep them quiet, as it was previously.) This was a humbling example of how information can shift one's paradigm of thinking.

Shifting Paradigm of Nursing Practice

A more recent paradigm shift in nursing is that of placing LPNs into more and varied management positions. Many nurse practice acts allow LPNs to assume charge nurse positions if they are working under the supervision of a registered nurse (RN). Long-term care facilities throughout the United States have a successful history of using LPNs in such positions, and now opportunities for management positions have moved beyond the nursing home. LPNs work in home health agencies, where they manage patients under the supervision of an RN; they work in hospitals as dyad members as they give care; and they fulfill management roles in nursing homes, subacute care units, and physicians' offices.

This LPN is working hard to learn the concepts of the latest paradigm shift on her unit.

REFLECTIVE THINKING

Take some time and determine your paradigm of thinking as an LPN. What is it that you value most? What, if anything, would you find intolerable in nursing practice? What is your strongest emotion regarding the nursing profession? What experiences have you had that helped define your nursing paradigm? Write your thoughts in your class notebook and share your thinking with others.

Paradigms dictate how a nurse thinks and approaches patient care needs. The LPN manager needs to acknowledge existing paradigms in patients, staff members, physicians, and nursing supervisors. Understanding and acknowledging the paradigms of all these people can result in more effective and meaningful care.

LPNs are being asked to assume management responsibilities that have never been asked for previously. In every situation, the LPN is the manager

of the patients who have been assigned; this is a strong management role. In addition, changes caused by downsizing or reorganizing have extended the management role for many LPNs to managing other personnel. This additional or extended role of the LPN may require a paradigm shift for the LPN, for the RN supervisor, or for the personnel being managed by the LPN. It is important for the LPN manager to recognize that not everyone may have made the current shift regarding the LPN role.

Recall my paradigm shift once I understood the situation of the mother and her children in the emergency department waiting room. The shift occurred quickly because I saw the situation differently, I felt differently, and I behaved differently. Not everyone is able to shift quickly. That is why it is so important for LPNs to understand the use of paradigm thinking and use that knowledge in their work with others.

It takes patience and tolerance to wait for people to go through the process of making a shift.

The keys to supporting the process in a timely manner are education and awareness. The responsibility of providing education to promote the awareness needed for the shift process often falls to the nurse manager.

It is important for the LPN to be aware of the paradigms that guide practice and management in the current work setting. Frequently paradigms change or are different from one health-care environment to another. This awareness is a significant key to success. The understanding that occurs with attention to personal and existing professional paradigms enhances the role of the LPN nurse manager in all settings.

CRITICAL THINKING CONCEPTS

To be a successful manager, it is crucial to identify the prevailing paradigm of a nursing unit, a new employee, or an RN supervisor. The LPN must develop the tools to assist in the identification of paradigm strategies. One tool is the ability to examine situations and issues critically.

Critical thinking is what allows you, the nurse, to identify the existing paradigms and devise the education or other strategies that are needed to shift paradigms of others or yourself. It also allows for broader decision making regarding treatment modalities, human interactions, and the split-second decision making that often is necessary to save a life.

Critical thinking is one of the most significant activities of adult life. It is a method of thinking that allows you to be skeptical of quick-fix solutions, single answers to problems, or claims of universal truth. It allows you to become open to alternative ways of looking at or behaving in society (or paradigm shifting) personally and professionally.

Do you remember the moment you realized that Santa Claus was a myth? That was possibly your first critical thinking activity. You had been told by people you trusted and loved that there was a Santa Claus. You also were told by another second grader that there was not a real Santa. Why did you believe the kid in second grade instead of your parents? It was because you critically examined all of the information you had on Santa Claus and found enough discrepancy to question the universal truth that your parents had given you.

People with critical thinking skills are able to question the assumptions underlying their customary, habitual ways of thinking and acting. They are able to think and act differently on the basis of their critical thinking ability. An example is a patient looking "just fine" but complaining of not feeling well. The nursing assistant has reported to you that the patient's vital signs are within normal limits and the dressing is dry. Yet somewhere in the LPN's knowledge there is a reason to feel concern over this patient's complaint. Instead of ignoring the feeling, the critically thinking LPN talks to the patient personally, retakes vital signs, and rechecks the surgical dressing. Even though the vital signs are normal, when the LPN touches the patient, the skin is cold and clammy. The dressing is dry, but there is a large, dark discoloration under the skin adjacent to the wound that is tender to the touch. The LPN who uses critical thinking in this situation is going to get help for the patient before a potential crisis occurs. The universal truth in this scenario is that normal vital signs and a dry dressing indicate there is not a problem despite the patient's complaints of not feeling well. Compare this with the critical thinker who questions the universal truth of stable vital signs and searches until a satisfactory explanation is identified.

Following is another example that is not as serious but makes the point. As a nursing instructor, I remember faculty meetings that focused on the three-cotton-ball and the five-cotton-ball technique for inserting a Foley catheter. Some faculty members held firm and non-negotiable positions about the number of cotton balls to use. Because of the unwavering commitment of the faculty to one procedure or another, it seemed that the number of cotton balls used to cleanse the perineum determined the life and death of the patient. Every licensed nurse knows that this is not true!

As an instructor, my objective was to teach the students excellent sterile technique, the purpose and insertion techniques of the catheter, and the way to relate to a patient who was experiencing catheter insertion. If a student knows excellent sterile technique, it doesn't matter how many cotton balls are used because the student uses enough to cleanse the area appropriately. This happens through the ability of the student to use critical thinking rather than to follow blindly the instructions given for a procedure.

Wilkinson and Treas (2015) state that critical thinkers are flexible, honest, inquisitive, and nonjudgmental and are interested in the truth. The

FOCUSED LEARNING CHART
Advantages of Being a Critical Thinker

CRITICAL THINKING:

Is one of the most significant activities of adult life.
Allows skepticism about "quick-fix" solutions.
Opens alternative ways of behaving in society, both personally and professionally.
Allows for broader decision making regarding critical issues.
Encourages people to question the personal assumptions that underlie their habitual ways of thinking.
Is a productive and positive activity.
Requires both emotional and rational thinking.

following are some common themes helpful in identifying just what critical thinking is:

- **Critical thinking is a productive and positive activity.** Critical thinkers are actively engaged in life. They value creativity and are innovative people. Critical thinkers are confident about themselves and their ability to contribute to a group process.
- **Critical thinking is a process, not an outcome.** No one is ever "done" if he or she is a critical thinker. Critical thinking suggests a continual assessment of the "certainties" of life. Common procedures and methodologies should be critically examined repeatedly because, by its nature, critical thinking can never be finished in some final, static manner.
- **Manifestations of critical thinking vary depending on the context in which they occur.** Critical thinking can be demonstrated quietly through writing or talking. It also can be more dramatic when it is a political change, a march for a particular cause, or a strike.
- **Critical thinking is triggered by both positive and negative events.** A common theme to many discussions of critical thinking is an activity resulting from a person's traumatic experience that prompts reexamining the situation that caused the trauma. Just as true is the occurrence of a joyful, pleasing, or fulfilling event—a hallmark life experience that alters one's view of how the world has previously functioned. Examples are having a baby, falling in love, or passing the NCLEX-PN® examination.

Clinical Judgment and Clinical Reasoning

I want to introduce you to two additional concepts related to critical thinking: clinical judgment and clinical reasoning. *Clinical judgment* is a nurse's ability to assess a patient's problems and needs and use the information gathered to address those needs as they pertain specifically to that patient. Clinical judgment is influenced by prior experiences of the nurse and what he or she may know about the current situation. It is also based on what the nurse knows about how the patient has responded to prior treatments and how well the nurse is engaged with the patient's concerns. *Clinical reasoning* addresses the processes used by nurses to make clinical judgments about patient care. The nursing process is one example of a process that may be used as a form of clinical reasoning (Bussard, 2015). See Box 3.2 for the difference between *clinical reasoning* and *clinical judgment*.

Box 3.2 The Difference Between Clinical Judgment and Clinical Reasoning

Clinical judgment: The ability to use gathered clinical information to address specific patient needs

Clinical reasoning: A way of thinking that addresses the processes used by nurses to make clinical judgements

Let us refer back to the patient described earlier. Despite the normal blood pressure and the fact that the dressing was dry, the LPN was still concerned there was something wrong with the patient. Without further assessment, on what was the LPN basing her concerns? Why did she decide to do a more thorough assessment? This LPN may have taken care of this patient enough times to know that if she states she doesn't feel well, then there is a problem. Or this LPN may have taken care of a prior surgical patient who presented in the same manner. Using clinical reasoning, the LPN used the first steps of the nursing process and further assessed the patient to find the skin discoloration and cold, clammy skin that are signs of a possible hemorrhage.

In conjunction with being a critical thinker and using clinical reasoning and judgment, the LPN needs to be aware of and follow the guidelines and laws found in the current state nurse practice act. These laws generally state that the LPN is to follow orders from the physician and the RN. It is essential to know the laws for your state and practice within them; the guidelines are in place to ensure nurses are effective in clinical practice. Thinking about and knowing what is being asked of you is critical. Don't do things blindly; think about them and talk about them with the physician, RN, or other nurses. Do all you can to assure patients, residents, and personnel who depend on you that you are participating in reasonable and safe care, which is the highest quality care possible.

THEORETICAL FRAMEWORKS FOR MANAGEMENT

Another important aspect of management is that of understanding people, both care recipients and caregivers, within an acceptable framework of thinking. This discussion covers two theories of human understanding. One is Maslow's (1963) "hierarchy of needs: a theory of human motivation and development," and the second is Watson's (2012) caring theory.

Dr. Abraham Maslow

Maslow's theory is familiar to most LPNs and LPN students. It is a basic source of information in academic settings and is considered fundamental to understanding human behavior. The basis of Maslow's theory is that people have to meet their lower level needs (e.g., food and oxygen) before they can move up Maslow's pyramidal structure to higher order needs. Continuing up the pyramid, a person must feel safe before that individual can meet social needs and must meet social needs before self-esteem can be developed. Maslow indicates that self-actualization is the ultimate achievement for a person and cannot be achieved without the other needs being met. The hierarchy of needs, from top to bottom, is as follows:

- Self-actualization
- Esteem
- Love and belongingness
- Safety
- Physiological

How does an understanding of these levels of need assist you in being a more effective manager? The answer is that the pyramid is the key to understanding human behavior.

If an employee has recently been hired but has been too shy to make friends with the other staff members, and the other staff members do not make an effort to include the new person, what happens? According to Maslow's theory, the new employee does not meet his or her belonging needs and is unable to develop self-esteem at work. Does this have an impact on the quality and amount of work the person does? Generally it does. Is it important for the

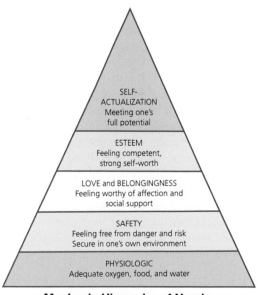

Maslow's Hierarchy of Needs

Maslow's hierarchy of needs. (Source: Maslow, A. [1963]. Toward a psychology of being. *New York: Van Nostrand Reinhold.*)

LPN manager to understand what is going on so that a successful intervention can be made? Yes, it is.

I often try to clarify this concept with the fantasy of being chased down the street of your hometown by a pride of saber-toothed tigers. If you were running for your life from such creatures (the first two levels of hierarchy—survival and safety), you definitely would not be concerned about whether your boyfriend is going to call you tonight (third level of hierarchy—love and belonging)! Stopping to visit someone watching the event (level four—esteem) or the meditation time (level five—self-actualization) you were missing because of being chased by the tigers would not be a priority. I find Maslow's leveling of needs meaningful as a basic method for understanding human behavior.

Consider this application example: When a patient is having pain and you as the LPN try to do patient teaching, minimal learning will occur. The reason is that people generally cannot move to a higher level, such as learning, when they do not feel safe because of the threat of physiological discomfort. Another practical example is an employee who is having marital problems at home that are causing feelings of fear for personal safety or the inability to feed and house her children. Because basic needs are not being met, that employee will not be effective in the work setting. It is important to understand the employee's behavior and what is causing it.

The reason for introducing Maslow's hierarchy of needs in this text is based on the essential quality of a manager to be able to understand human behavior rather than judge it. It is so simple for people to judge, criticize, or reject the behavior of other people and not have to deal with the behavior and its consequences. A nurse manager cannot afford to have those attitudes. Instead, it is essential that there be an understanding of human behavior so that every aspect of an employee's or patient's behavior can be enhanced. Subsequent chapters identify direct application of Maslow's theory in management situations. For now, this information is shared in an effort to stimulate thinking and reinforce previous learning on the theory.

The following are two thoughts for successfully working with people:

1. It is better to understand people than to judge them.
2. There is a reason for every behavior. (It is the nurse manager's responsibility to identify the reason and work with it.)

Dr. Jean Watson

Watson's nursing theory, "nursing: human science and human care," is an internationally recognized nursing theory that has deep meaning for the art of nursing practice. This is important because the LPN manager needs to preserve and enhance the art and the science of nursing. This theory has been discussed in the previous chapter, but to understand Watson's theory the reader may need to make a paradigm shift.

Watson's theory addresses the art of nursing. The art of nursing moves beyond the cellular response of the human body and goes to the overall response of the human being and that person's total life values and experiences. Watson believes that nursing has neglected the development of the art of nursing, and her theory strongly supports revaluing that aspect of care. Watson (2012) states, ". . . if we view nursing as a human science, we get to cocreate, combine, integrate, and transform our views of science, restoring unitary notions of beauty, art, ethics, and aesthetics of the human-to-human care process, and even love back into nursing." My idea is that the art of nursing is the reason many people are nurses. I believe that the human-to-human care process was the attraction for many people as they made the decision to become licensed nurses. I also think it is a good reason to make that decision.

In her writings, Watson shares examples of what a nurse practicing in a caring paradigm looks like. Such a person has a deep human regard for the lives of others. When giving care, the nurse practices in a coparticipating manner. Watson also talks about the caring moment, called *transpersonal caring,* when the nurse and the patient share a personal connection while nursing care is being given.

Another basic premise of Watson's theory is the *intentionality* (or the intentions) of the nurse. The nurse enters every interaction and caring moment with the intention of giving nursing care in a personalized, human science manner; this means that the focus of the care is beyond the cellular needs of the patient and extends to the entire person and his or her needs.

REFLECTIVE THINKING

List three experiences in which you have participated in the caring-healing moment of coparticipating with another person, as described by

Watson. After you have described the moment, share the paradigm shifting or critical thinking skills that were involved in the experience. Write these experiences in your class notebook and be prepared to share them in class.

The new vocabulary that accompanies Watson's theory should become part of your conversation as a nurse. There were three new phrases from Chapter 2. Do you remember them? If not, go back to the beginning of Chapter 2 and review them. There is one more phrase to add to your "Watson List." It is *caring intentionality.*

 ## BASIC PRINCIPLE OF PATIENT ADVOCACY

Another essential skill nurses need to develop is that of *patient advocacy.* This ability requires skill and caring and a clearly defined concept of who you are. In a patient advocacy situation, the nurse's thinking needs to be at its best. It requires critical thinking and the ability to shift one's paradigm

The needs of people in the health-care system are diverse and complex. This situation is not expected to change. Because of the complexity of health care and the health-care system, people need a guide to assist them in achieving the level of health they desire. This role most often belongs to the nurse and is that of *patient advocate.*

The term *patient,* as it is used in the term *patient advocate,* refers to people in all arenas of health-care delivery. Some people are referred to as clients and others as residents. For this concept, however, the term *patient* refers to all persons who seek out health care wherever the health-care delivery site is located. It could be a homeless center, clinic for birth control, or the Mayo Clinic. A patient advocate fulfills the role of guide and support at the bedside, chair side, and curbside. It is a serious responsibility for every nurse. Box 3.3 provides some principles basic to patient advocacy.

As the head of the nursing team, the RN often takes an active role in being the patient advocate; however, the role of advocate also belongs to the LPN. Often the LPN gives more personal care and is able to spend more time with the patient. You often learn of issues that need to be advocated for when you are alone with a patient or the patient's family. Take seriously what you learn from patients

---

Box 3.3 Principles of Patient Advocacy

- Guiding patients to achieve the level of health they desire
- Protecting patients from the infringement of their rights
- Informing and supporting patients to make the best decisions for their personal health

---

about their needs and wants, share them with the RN, and follow up in the role as advocate.

The fundamental principle of patient advocacy is protecting people from infringement on their rights as patients and human beings. Gazarian, Fernberg, and Sheehan (2016) define patient advocacy as the primary role of advocacy [for nurses] and go on to define the concept as the protection of patients' rights and interests. Advocacy is the act of informing and supporting a person (the patient) so that the person can make the best decisions for personal health.

Protecting the Rights of Patients

Licensed nurses are educated to recognize the need to protect the rights of people as human beings and as patients in the health-care system. I feel confident that as you grow in your role as an LPN, you will learn and act on your knowledge to protect patients from having their rights abused. Examples of nursing conduct that protects the basic rights of all people include the following:

1. Nurses do not hit or yell at patients.
2. Medications and treatments must be given correctly and in a timely fashion.
3. People are treated in a respectful and caring manner.
4. The principles of aseptic and sterile technique are not violated.

Research-Related Rights

The medical atrocities performed on Jewish concentration camp prisoners are an example of breaching patients' research-related rights. Some of the most horrific incidents of health-care research abuse in the history of the world occurred in Germany during World War II. Because health-care personnel performed such acts against unwilling human beings, the Nuremberg trials were held to prosecute the "medical researchers" and others as war criminals. One positive result of the Nuremberg trials was the development of the institutional review board (IRB), which is used to protect patients from inappropriate research. No one can perform research, even of an innocent nature such as an interview, without the research process being scrutinized by a committee (the IRB) and the patient being fully informed of the research being done. IRB committees in health-care organizations are designed to ensure safety to all patients. Patients involved in research projects can withdraw at any time. It is important for you to know this and remind the patient of it if the patient expresses any distress or concern. As the patient advocate, it is your responsibility to ensure that the patient's rights are not infringed on when participating in research.

Right to Refuse Treatment or Medication

A classic example of a patient's right is the right to refuse treatment or medication. I work with people with dementia. I respect their right to refuse a medication and encourage others also to be respectful of this right. I remember the days of my nursing youth when nurses (not me!) used syringes to force medication on an elderly person or, even worse, held the person's nose to get the individual to open his or her mouth and take the medication. Such actions are a violation of the person's rights.

Whatever the ailment or disease, every patient has the right to refuse treatments, including medications, surgery, or something as simple as a bath or the measurement of one's blood pressure. This right is stated in the Patient Care Partnership, a document listing all rights of any patient.

Additional examples of choices patients may make include the following: (1) A patient with

These young parents have the right to refuse the surgery suggested for their baby's medical condition.

cancer has the right to refuse chemotherapy, (2) a person needing a liver transplant can refuse to have the transplant, and (3) a patient with congestive heart failure has the right to eat French fries (although this is dangerous because of the salt on the fries). Part of the responsibility of being an advocate is to inform the patient fully of the consequences of all treatment choices. When you are sure the patient knows and understands all of the options, he or she has the right to make the personal choice about what will be done. As the patient advocate, it is your responsibility to support the person in the choice made and to facilitate other options that may be more acceptable for health's sake. The patient with congestive heart failure may be encouraged to use a salt substitute. This simple change may necessitate calling the dietary department or even for you to "run to the store" to get the important item. Don't just let things happen. Instead, work tirelessly to promote the best options possible.

Informed Consent

Another aspect of patient advocacy is informed consent for procedures such as surgery. It is the physician's responsibility to explain what will be done and all possible consequences of the operation. Physicians are responsible for medical aspects of care, and this is a prime example of their medical responsibility. It generally is the responsibility of the nurse, however, to have the signature on the consent form. If you are asked to have a consent form signed, and as you talk to the patient about the procedure you realize he or she neither understands it nor the possible consequences, you have a responsibility to ensure that the patient is informed before consent is given.

First, stop what you are doing and tell the patient you will be back. Then find the RN and inform him or her about the situation. The RN should assume responsibility from that point, but if not, the bottom line is that the patient should not go to surgery until there is full understanding and information has been shared. This patient needs an advocate.

Safe Care

Every patient has the right to safe care. Although the patient's right to safe care seems a simple concept, it can become complicated as the following example illustrates. You are working the 7 p.m. to 7 a.m. shift along with an RN, another LPN, and two certified nursing assistants (CNAs). It is a busy night and the shift is going fast, but you can't help noticing that the RN is slow in her work and seems confused by the questions you ask or the comments you make. By 3 a.m. you are quite sure you smell liquor on the RN's breath. What is your responsibility as a patient advocate?

As a licensed nurse, you are responsible for the safety of all patients on the unit, not just the patients assigned to you. If an RN is drinking on duty, he or she is endangering all patients on the unit, which places a tremendous responsibility on you. Protocol requires that you talk to the RN about your suspicions. You do not say, "I think you are drinking." Instead, start with something like, "Are you feeling OK?" Then point out some of the errors she has made during the shift. Offer to divide up her load between the LPNs if she needs to leave or identify some other solution.

If the RN refuses to leave and still seems impaired in her ability to do her work, let her know you are going to call the supervisor or nurse manager. Then make the call. Letting people continue to work when you have identified they are not functioning in a safe manner is a serious breach of the patient's right to safety. When you call the supervisor or manager, you do not say the nurse is drinking on duty unless you have actually seen her do so. Perhaps she has an illness that makes her behave as though she has been drinking. You do not want to destroy someone's reputation or be held accountable for slander. Simply report the facts and ask for help. The nurse is now the supervisor's responsibility, but you are still responsible for the safety of the patients on the unit. You have to provide that safety in any way that is feasible and responsible.

Nurses who abuse drugs and alcohol are often referred to as *impaired nurses*. Refer to Chapter 1 for information about impaired nurses.

Safety needs for patients also include ensuring the availability of proper and safe equipment and a safe standard of staffing. Many situations in nursing are unsafe, and only nurses with awareness of their responsibility are able to change such situations. These are not easy challenges, but they do come with the license you are striving to earn. Being a licensed nurse is a complex responsibility.

The most humbling and difficult example of patient advocacy in my practice occurred with a 70-year-old man. He lived alone and had been a widower for several years. His overall health was worsening. He had arthritis and heart disease. His diabetes was difficult for him to manage because his eyesight had diminished, and he found it challenging to buy food and medication on his limited retirement income. His children and grandchildren lived in distant communities and did not visit him often. His finances had forced him to discontinue his telephone service.

When this man was brought to the emergency department by a neighbor who had found him wandering outside, confused and without a coat, I was assigned to be his case manager. I immediately liked this man because of his sense of humor, which was readily apparent after he was stabilized, and his practical way of looking at life. I was fortunate to have the time to talk with him in a transpersonal, caring manner.

His physician ordered a pacemaker implant for him and did a good job of explaining to the patient the procedure and the consequences of having or not having it.

When the physician was finished, I stayed with the patient to see whether he had any questions. But before I could ask, he said to me, "I don't want the pacemaker. I am ready to die." He went on to explain to me his religious beliefs, which included an afterlife. He wanted to be reunited with his wife and strongly believed that would happen when he was dead. He wanted to go home after calling his children to meet with him individually for one last time, and then he wanted to die. He was ready.

I became quietly frantic. How could anyone choose not to have a pacemaker? It was a simple procedure with minimal risks and Medicare would pay for it. I began imparting what I thought was crucial information to the patient. He was very polite and listened to everything I said. When I was through, he quietly repeated his wishes and why they were his wishes. Then he asked me for the telephone so he could call his children.

Before this strong and independent man was discharged, I became his advocate. It was challenging to keep explaining to the physician, nurse manager, and the social worker, among others, why I was supporting him in his decision. The physician even called in a psychiatric consultation, but the man was declared sane and rational. I never wavered, despite the criticism I received, because I believed in the patient's right to make his life choices. His choice was much more serious than a patient refusing a bath or a medication. This man was rationally choosing not to live any longer.

Looked at in another way, he was allowing the natural course of his life to be lived out rather than being interfered with by others.

I arranged for home health and kept in contact with the patient until his death. I also attended his funeral. His children expressed their gratitude to me for helping him die as he wished. They each told me of the special times and memories they had built in the few weeks they had with their father after he was discharged from the hospital. It did seem to end as he had wished. I feel strongly that was my purpose for being involved in that man's life; it was to advocate for his death.

I recognize that you are still students, and you are not going to go out to your clinical assignment this week and participate in a situation like the one I just described. It may be years before you are prepared to perform such deeds of advocacy. I want you to know, however, that such responsibilities exist. In the meantime, work on the fundamental level of advocacy. Protect patients in all settings from having their rights infringed on by others. Take the risks necessary to keep them safe. Use transpersonal caring as part of your everyday care. If you are unsure of how to use transpersonal caring, refer to the section on Dr. Jean Watson presented earlier in this chapter.

REFLECTIVE THINKING

How will you use your critical thinking skills to provide safe patient care? Record your thoughts in your class notebook.

Other Aspects of Advocacy

In society, there are several components of identity that characterize and define each of us as individuals. To be an effective advocate for all patients, you need to understand your feelings and the patient's feelings regarding the following components of identity: spirituality, sexuality, ethnicity, and age.

Spirituality

Spirituality is a significant aspect of a person's identity. It often influences how the person manages loss, illness, and death. A person's spirituality generally is based on religious beliefs or the formal or informal belief in a higher power. Spiritual fulfillment provides meaning and purpose for

some people, and it is a source of strength and hope for others. Because of the powerful meaning religion has for many people, it is important for you, as a nurse, to understand the beliefs and customs related to the religion of the people to whom you give care.

Even in a major religion, such as Christianity, there are many different beliefs. Some Christians believe in deathbed repentance, and others believe in lifelong repentance for their "sins." Understanding what a dying patient believes is important in providing spiritual comfort. One person may want last rites, and another may simply want to talk with a clergy person. Fasting is another aspect of religion that is variable. In some religions, a person fasts for 24 hours once a month or more. In the Muslim faith, persons fast annually for 40 days, eating only in the evening. This observance is called Ramadan and is viewed as sacred. What are you going to do when you have a patient who is hospitalized during Ramadan? There are serious nutritional consequences for someone who is ill and fasting, even for part of a day, let alone for 40 days.

Some religious people express their spirituality by praying out loud, whereas others pray silently. Some people pray kneeling on the floor, and others pray facing east. To respect a patient's religious beliefs, you need to be aware of those beliefs and understand them.

REFLECTIVE THINKING

Spend some time talking to people of different religions and ask them about prayer, fasting, religious celebrations, and special care to be given when someone is ill or has died. This information is important to you as a holistic patient advocate. After you have talked to at least three people who have religious beliefs different from yours, record what you learned from them in your class notebook. Be prepared to share what you have learned in class.

Sexuality

Sexuality is a powerful aspect of every person's identity. We all are male, female, or transgender; homosexual or heterosexual; modest or casual in our sexuality. Every individual has definite feelings about how they express their sexuality. Some people are modest and easily embarrassed. Generally, a modest person would have difficulty discussing sexual matters even if they relate to the person's health. Others are comfortable with their sexuality and discuss it freely. You need to develop the skills to work with the sexuality of every person. It is a challenging assignment.

As the patient advocate, it is important for you to assess each person's sexual health and to support individuals in the right to express their own sexuality. Some people need privacy to be able to talk about their sexuality. However, you should not endanger yourself by being alone with someone who is sexually abusive or behaves inappropriately. Such people need to be referred to the proper authorities or to appropriate counseling. The RN and physician make this referral. They may need your assessment information and observations, however, to make the right treatment decision. Always report inappropriate sexual behavior to the RN.

If you are uncomfortable discussing factors that relate to sexuality, you need to start now, as a student, to overcome such feelings. You could consider trying to identify why you feel uncomfortable and work to understand your feelings. For some nurses, it is difficult to discuss sexual health issues because of their cultural background. For others, it may be because of personal experiences. Some people have an aversion to sexuality that is different from their own. Your responsibility as an LPN is to be an advocate for all patients in all aspects of their lives. Recognize the need to resolve

The sexuality of every patient needs to be respected; it must also be considered in the holistic plan of care.

any sexual issues you have that may interfere with your being a strong patient advocate. Another thing you can do, if you are uncomfortable with sexuality, is practice asking people questions related to their sexual health. Your physical assessment text should have information to assist you in determining questions you can use to practice. The most important concept to remember is to treat all people holistically and with caring. That way you cannot go wrong.

Ethnicity

Just as each person is unique in his or her religious beliefs and sexuality, each person is unique in his or her ethnicity. Unless you are Native American, you have ancestral roots that eventually can be traced beyond the shores of the United States. The ancestry we each have gives us our unique ethnic background. I am proud of my European background, and I hope you feel pride in your ancestors also.

My ancestors immigrated to the United States as poor farmers. Eventually they ended up in Utah, where they were still farmers with limited income. They worked hard to make the farm produce quality food. If they didn't, the family didn't eat. I do know how to work hard and be productive. I credit my ancestors with giving me these traits; they have been of great benefit to me throughout my career as a nurse.

What traits do you have that you can identify with your ancestors? Think about where they came from and the situations they had to manage when they came to the United States. Obviously they survived the trials of immigration because you were born. What were some of those survival traits, and which ones did you inherit or learn? They may help you to be successful in your nursing program.

The same is true of all people. Everyone has ancestors and receives gifts from their ancestors' gene pool. As a nurse, you need to recognize the differences among people who are part of the wide variety of people living in the United States. Along with recognizing the differences and the uniqueness of each person, you need to respect the diversity you find.

Individuals' cultural heritage brings the richness of diversity to the health-care setting. I strongly suggest all health-care professionals learn to embrace diversity and reject prejudice. Look forward to the differences in all people and the interest those differences can bring to a day or a care plan.

Ethnicity is a subcategory of culture. Some people travel the world to experience different cultural events, people, food, and history. For some nurses, similar cultural events can occur in the hospital emergency department or in any waiting room. Treasure what others can teach you about their lives. It is an education in itself. If you truly are a caring nurse, all you need to know about ethnicity is that it represents cultural experiences, so be prepared to learn and grow with the knowledge that a patient shares with you. Then apply the knowledge to giving culturally specific care to the person who has come to you for nursing care.

Age

Society has coined terms that relate to prejudicial and discriminatory behavior regarding three of the four components of identity that are being discussed here: sexism, racism, and ageism. Most people have an understanding of sexism and racism because they have been part of the prejudicial cycle for a long time. Unspeakable things have been done to women and people of color because of prejudice. Society is slowly dealing with these issues, but in many environments they still exist. You may be called on to advocate for a patient who is receiving prejudicial treatment and care. It is time for all prejudice to be eliminated from society in general and certainly from the work we do as nurses.

Elderly people in society also suffer a great deal of prejudicial treatment and discrimination, which is referred to as *ageism*. There are more people celebrating their 85th birthday than infants being born each day in the United States. This figure represents the large number of older people who are receiving such good health care that they are living rather than dying. Society has never had to deal with so many elderly persons before. It was a new phenomenon to have millions of elderly people asking for health-care services, and the system was not ready for it. As mentioned in Chapter 1, this phenomenon will continue.

Elderly people, especially the old-old (>80 years old), require a great deal of time and patience when receiving nursing care. They often do not hear or see well, they often have arthritis and need assistance when walking, and they generally move slowly. They have more than one chronic disease that complicates giving care focused on an acute illness. The elderly need an advocate. They need someone who speaks to them so they can hear and understand what is being said and who will take the time they need when giving care.

We all have been exposed to ageism. Look through the birthday cards at a local store; most cards that seem so funny really are making fun of old people. This is an example of ageism. If you entered a room with a beautifully dressed, cute baby in one corner and a well-dressed, older woman in a wheelchair in another corner, which corner would you migrate to? Most people would go to the baby. This symbolizes our ageist society.

If you are ageist, you will have a difficult time advocating for elderly persons in your care. I suggest you spend time with your grandparents or other older relatives and learn to enjoy them. Talk to older people in the community and see what their lives are like. Learn how they have survived life to their current point, and I think you will learn to admire and respect them.

It takes courage to live rather than die, and it is difficult to be old in our society. With just those two thoughts, you can take on the role of advocate for elderly persons.

The role of patient advocate calls for the highest level of nursing care that can be given, which requires an understanding of Maslow's and Watson's theories on human behavior. Every nurse is responsible for protecting patients from others infringing on their rights as human beings.

Before you finish this chapter, turn back to the statement by Einstein at the beginning of the chapter. Significant problems must be faced as the role of the LPN manager evolves and is defined. It is my hope that after reading this chapter you will recognize that your thinking has been altered forever by the information you absorbed. Einstein suggests that problems can be solved only if people change their thinking; that also is my challenge to you.

REAL-WORLD CASE STUDY

■ You are the LPN assigned to a newly admitted cardiac patient with rule out myocardial infarction. Mr. Ahmed is 48 years old and overweight, and he looks very ill. He is perspiring, moaning with pain, and pale despite his dark complexion; as you assist him to a position of comfort, you recognize that he is weak. He is receiving oxygen and cardiac monitoring and has an IV running. His wife and two small children are in the room. The day-shift nurse said the family had been with Mr. Ahmed since his admission. His wife looks tired and frustrated with the crying children. The day nurse also said Mr. Ahmed refused pain medication. The overall scene is not conducive to a cardiac patient or a critical care unit.

You sit down to talk to Mr. Ahmed before you do your assessment. It seems impossible. The children are crying and the wife is near tears. Mr. Ahmed climbs out of bed, pulling off his oxygen and most of the leads. He then kneels on the floor, faces east, and starts to pray.

You are shocked and very concerned. Your first reaction is to take charge of the situation by ordering the family out and getting assistance to put Mr. Ahmed back to bed. Then you remember some of the principles you learned in your introductory class more than a year ago. The most important thing you remember is that "there is a reason for every behavior." Then you remember the patient advocate principles you learned. None of them would be served if you raised your voice and started ordering people around. What can you do?

There are some immediate and essential things you should do, and then you will have time to consider the more long-term solutions to the problems you encountered. Define the problems you encountered in this situation and then resolve them while advocating for the patient. Use the categories of immediate and essential and long-term solutions.

Key Points

- There have been several major paradigm shifts that have impacted modern nursing care. Among them are germ theory and the knowledge that germs carry disease, the use of therapeutic touch as a healing modality, and the focus on diversity and cultural differences in the delivery of nursing care.
- Critical thinking is an important skill for a nurse to possess. There are four aspects of critical thinking: (1) Critical thinking is a productive and positive activity; (2) critical thinking is a process, not an outcome; (3) evidence of critical thinking depends on the context in which it occurs; and (4) critical thinking can be triggered by both positive and negative events.

- Maslow's theory states that a person's lower-level needs must be met before he or she can work toward meeting higher level needs. This applies to managers who must evaluate employees' needs to be safe and to feel acceptance before they are able to be effective in the work setting.
- Watson's theory addresses the art of nursing and places emphasis on caring for patients and for other nurses when someone is in a management position.
- There are many aspects of identity. Four aspects of identity that the LPN should advocate for are spirituality, sexuality, ethnicity, and age.

ANSWERS TO REAL-WORLD CASE STUDY

■ *Immediate and Essential Problems*

1. Get Mr. Ahmed back to bed, on oxygen, and hooked up to his cardiac leads.
2. Use an appropriate method to relieve Mr. Ahmed of his pain.
3. Identify and meet the needs of his wife and children.

■ *Long-Term Problems*

1. The family needs help. Assess to see if what the wife needs is information, childcare, permission to stay home, or something else that is important to her.
2. Develop a plan for managing Mr. Ahmed's pain.

Continued

3. Mr. Ahmed appears to be a religious man. How can you accommodate his religious needs without jeopardizing his health?

4. Spend time with the patient and family so that you can recognize or learn about the culturally specific care Mr. Ahmed needs.

■ *Essential and Immediate Problem Solutions*

1. It would be so easy to call for help and physically place Mr. Ahmed back in bed attached to the proper equipment. As a patient advocate, however, you have a responsibility to look at this man holistically and respect his religious needs. It is unacceptable to ignore his physiological needs while he is praying. Call for help to get an extension to the oxygen mask and quietly, respectfully put it on him while he prays. If Mr. Ahmed tolerates being out of bed, allow him to finish his prayer, then have people who are standing by quickly assist you in getting him back to bed with his leads in place. If he could not tolerate being out of bed, it would be your moral obligation to interrupt him quietly and assist him back to bed.

2. Quietly talk to Mr. Ahmed about having pain medication. Explain why it is important, especially for cardiac patients. Mr. Ahmed has the right to refuse the pain medication, but keep in mind that cardiac patients should not be having pain. Use your best skills, be quietly confident in what you are doing, and do not give up if there is any chance he will take the medication.

3. In the Arab culture, which is the Ahmed family's background, the family is highly valued. It is reasonable to assume Mrs. Ahmed has stayed because she is committed to keeping her family together. You need to talk to her to determine what her needs are and how you can help her. Ask her to accompany you to the conference room so that Mr. Ahmed can sleep (especially if he took the pain medication). You need to determine whether she has

money to feed herself and the children (she may have left the house in a panic without her purse). Then encourage her to go eat something. If there is a volunteer available, she might assist the tired Mrs. Ahmed with the children during the meal. If there is no money, call social services for a meal voucher for Mrs. Ahmed.

■ *Long-Term Problem Solutions*

1. Mrs. Ahmed may need a social worker to help her make decisions about childcare, travel to and from the hospital, or how much time she should spend with her husband. If you need assistance in helping Mrs. Ahmed solve her problems, call someone right away. It is important that the family be taken care of so that they are not a worry to the patient. One solution may be that Mrs. Ahmed would spend the afternoon with her husband. This would allow for physician visits and basic nursing care to be given in the morning without interruption.

2. Many Arab men are very stoic. It is a culture with thousands of years of history, and the strength and power of the Arab man has always been a part of that history. Perhaps Mr. Ahmed thinks it is weak of him to take pain medication. He might be afraid of IV medication because of fear of drug addiction or not knowing what the drug is; he may not want narcotics at all. You won't know until you talk to him about it when he is not in pain. Your best opportunity for this discussion is after the pain medication you have given him is effective and he is comfortable. When he is comfortable, ask him about his thoughts and feelings regarding pain and its management. He may want a patient-controlled analgesia pump so that he can have control over the amount of medication given. (A patient-controlled analgesia pump allows the patient to administer safe doses of the pain-relieving drug.) He may need to be taught what is happening to his heart when he is in pain. He may want to see the name and dosage of

the drug on the syringe or on the bottle as you draw it up where he can see it. Neither of us knows what would encourage him to take pain medication, but if you talk to him in a caring fashion with a focus on resolving the problem, you will soon know. *Note:* Many hospitals have pain management nurses who are experts. Do not hesitate to obtain a physician's order for a pain management nurse and call one in if one is available where you work.

3. Spirituality is important to many people. Apparently it is to Mr. Ahmed. If he is a devout Muslim and wants to be out of bed, facing east, and praying several times a day, you have a challenging nursing care problem to resolve. Talk to him. Ask him to explain to you what it is he is doing. You need to explain to him that he needs to do it with modification. Perhaps he would stay

in bed to pray if the bed faced east. Would he agree to get out of bed just once a day at a time identified beforehand so that you or another nurse could assist him and monitor him? For the few days he will be in the intensive care unit, would he consider just praying in bed? As you talk to Mr. Ahmed, he may come up with solutions himself. These discussions are a great opportunity to teach him about his heart and resolve problems. Use the time wisely.

4. When Mrs. Ahmed is with her husband, you should spend some time talking to them about their culture. What do they need to feel comfortable in the hospital? Are there things you need to know to give him the best care possible? It is a wonderful opportunity to talk to a person with a cultural background different from yours, so take advantage of it.

REVIEW QUESTIONS

1. What are the four components of identity for which nurses should advocate?
   1. Spirituality, sexuality, ethnicity, and age
   2. Mind, body, soul, and spirit
   3. Head, heart, ethnicity, and age
   4. Ethnicity, soul, age, and culture
2. What statement explains Dr. Maslow's theory?
   1. People should be well rounded and able to adjust to change.
   2. All aspects of development are equally important and required for progression.
   3. Basic needs of safety and acceptance must be met before a person can progress.
   4. Self-actualization is the first and most important step in human progression.
3. What is the definition of the word *paradigm?*
   1. A pyramid with aspects of human development arranged by order of importance
   2. The combination of mind, body, soul, and spirit
   3. The application of knowledge and skill that is the result of experience
   4. A pattern, model, or example of something

4. Which statement about critical thinking is correct?
   1. Critical thinking is a process, not an outcome.
   2. Critical thinkers are self-actualized.
   3. Critical thinking involves being critical of others.
   4. Critical thinking is only part of positive events.
5. According to the chapter readings, what are three changes that have resulted in paradigm shifts in modern nursing?
   1. Physician attitudes, germ theory, antibiotics
   2. Germ theory, therapeutic touch, focus on diversity
   3. Germ theory, critical thinking, health insurance
   4. Physician attitudes, critical thinking, focus on diversity

References

Bussard, M. E. (2015). Clinical judgment in reflective journals of prelicensure nursing students. *Journal of Nursing Education, 54*(1), 36–40. doi:10.3928/01484834-20141224-05

Gazarian, P. K., Fernberg, L. M., & Sheehan, K. D. (2016). Effectiveness of narrative pedagogy in developing student nurses' advocacy role. *Nursing Ethics,* 23(2), 132–141. doi:10.1177/0969733014557718

Kuhn, T. (1962). *The structure of scientific revolutions*. Chicago: University of Chicago Press.

Maslow, A. (1963). *Toward a psychology of being*. New York: Van Nostrand Reinhold.

Watson, J. (2012). *Human caring science: A theory of nursing* (2nd ed.). Sudbury, MA: Jones & Bartlett.

Wilkinson, J. M., & Treas, L. (2015). *Fundamentals of nursing* (3rd ed.). Philadelphia: F. A. Davis.

Web Resource

Patient Care Partnership www.aha.org/advocacy-issues/communicatingpts/pt-care-partnership.shtml

4

Health-Care Environment

KEY TERMS

Advocate
Clinician
Counselor
Educator
Manager
Primary health care
Secondary health care
Tertiary health care

CHAPTER CONCEPTS

Health-Care System
Collaboration

HOLLI SOWERBY

LEARNING OUTCOMES

1. Describe components of health-care systems that allow for access, treatment, and payment of services in the United States.
2. Identify the roles and tasks of the LPN in health-care agencies.
3. Identify agencies where the LPN provides health-care services.

The very essence of all good organization is that everybody should do her [or his] own work in such a way as to help and not hinder everyone else's work.

—Florence Nightingale

Health-care delivery in the United States is a combination of public and private organizations that attempt to provide citizens with access to cost-effective, quality health care. However, not all Americans are healthy, which means many need the services provided to enhance personal and community health. Even with the recent changes requiring all Americans to obtain health insurance, not all Americans have insurance, and because the health-care system is based on the ability to pay, this is a serious problem in the national health picture. Not all people in the United States are citizens; some are illegal aliens. Because they are not citizens, these people do not pay taxes that assist in paying the health-care needs for low-income persons. This situation places a payment burden (through the payment of taxes) on legal citizens. The health-care system in the United States has several major problems, yet it is one of the most effective health-care systems in the world.

I have a friend in Canada who has been waiting for nearly 1 year for "her turn" to have a total knee replacement. She has a great deal of difficulty walking because of the pain her arthritic knee gives her. This has a serious impact on her quality of life and ability to work to provide for herself. I have had two total knee replacements, and I can verify that people do not wait for their "turn" for such procedures in the United States. In a previous chapter I mentioned that in many developing countries families are responsible for providing the food and medications needed by their loved ones while hospitalized. This is not true in the United States (however, I remember having a friend smuggle me in a candy bar once when I was hospitalized!).

Although basic elements are provided for patients in U.S. health-care systems, these systems remain a challenge to navigate: "How do I find the best surgeon?" "How do I preauthorize for an admission?" "What happens when I have an emergency and I am not near a provider hospital?" "Do I need family members to stay with me?" These are common questions asked by individuals trying to access our health-care system. The U.S.

health-care system is fraught with challenges and stressful decisions. It is into such a conundrum that the licensed practical nurse (LPN) bravely goes to give the best of nursing care in myriad situations.

 HEALTH-CARE SYSTEMS

People enter a health-care system when they are seeking services to evaluate their current health status or to treat a health condition. The word *systems* is plural and implies that there is more than one health-care system available to service health-care needs.

Health care commonly is categorized into three levels of care: primary, secondary, and tertiary. *Primary* health-care services emphasize health promotion and the prevention of illness and disability; an example is a visit to the doctor's office. *Secondary* services involve detection and early treatment to prevent illness and disability; an example is a stay in a hospital. *Tertiary* services provide restorative and rehabilitative services for people with chronic or irreversible conditions; an example is a nursing home (D'Amico & Barbarito, 2016).

Financing of Health Care

The United States is the only industrialized country in the world that does not provide access to health care for all of its citizens by paying for most of the services. Health-care services in the United States are paid for in various ways. Employers pay for some health-care services through employee insurance benefits. The federal government pays for some health care for persons older than age 65 years through Medicare plans. State governments pay (with help from the federal government) for health care for low-income individuals through Medicaid plans. Individuals, churches, and charities may pay some health-care expenses. Health-care providers often forgive some expenses that are uncollectible. Commonly, patients, payers, and health-care providers work out payment for services in advance. Services during emergencies are seldom denied, but payment for care is sought later after the emergency is managed.

As the number of Americans without health insurance increased, political pressure to remedy that situation also increased. In March 2010, Congress passed and President Obama signed the Patient Protection and Affordable Care Act (PPACA). Some portions of the law went into effect in 2011; others went into effect in 2014. The main purpose of the act was to reduce the number of Americans who do not have health insurance. It did this by expanding Medicaid to cover more people, allowing parents to keep children on their plan until age 26, requiring most employers of more than 50 people to offer health insurance, forbidding insurance plans to exclude people with preexisting conditions, and requiring everyone to get health insurance. According to the Kaiser Family Foundation (2016), significant success has been achieved toward the goal of reducing the number of uninsured people. By the end of 2015, 12.7 million had enrolled through the insurance exchanges. Medicaid enrollment increased by 16.1 million after the ACA expansions went into effect.

It may seem difficult, or impossible, for every individual to get health insurance, but the law tried to make this practical in several ways. In addition to requiring larger employers to offer a group plan, it gives tax credits to smaller employers who do the same. States are required to establish exchanges that make it easier for individuals and small businesses to find coverage. The law also caps the percentage of income that a person would have to pay for insurance premiums and provides subsidies to persons whose income is not high enough to afford coverage.

The law has been controversial. Many people are in favor of the expanded coverage and support the law. Others are concerned about the cost and how it will impact the federal deficit, employers, and individuals. Several states even challenged the law in court by saying that the federal government does not have the authority to require employers, insurance companies, or individuals to do some of the things that are required. In the summer of 2012, the U.S. Supreme Court ruled that although the federal government does not have the authority to force people to buy health insurance, it does have the authority to tax people who do not have it. So, the law stands, including the parts that require employers or individuals to pay fines if they do not comply. The Supreme Court did change part of the law, however. States will not be required to expand their Medicaid programs. By 2015, 30 states had chosen to expand Medicaid coverage under the provisions of the ACA (Centers for Medicare and Medicaid Services, 2015).

Physicians and health-care administrators select what services will be available in their health-care settings and then negotiate with insurance companies to determine the prices that will be paid for each service. Employers and sometimes employees negotiate with insurance companies on what services they want to have provided and what the expectations will be for reimbursement for these services. Medicare (federal payment for citizens older than 65 years old) and Medicaid (state payments for citizens with low income) regulations determine health-care services and reimbursements for many persons.

Many health professionals who provide health-care services have their fees for reimbursement negotiated through health-care administrators. Box 4.1 provides a partial list of health-care professionals whose fees for services either are administered by a health-care agency or must be negotiated with an insurance payer.

As an LPN, you need to be aware that health-care agencies' policies determine what services you can provide that will be reimbursed by payers. Reimbursement often influences the services the agency where you work can offer to the public. Regardless of the reasons for health-care disparities in the United States, the LPN has a vital role in treating all patients holistically and with excellence.

Risks of Health Care

Medical and nursing procedures often involve certain risks; labor and delivery is a good example. Most Americans do not accept medical or nursing

---

Box 4.1 Health-Care Providers' Fees Administered by Agency or Negotiated With Insurance Company

• Physical therapists
• Nutritionists
• Pharmacists
• Nurses (nurse practitioners, registered nurses [RNs], and LPNs)
• Respiratory therapists
• Occupational therapists
• Social workers

FOCUSED LEARNING CHART
Agencies That Employ LPNs and Their Role in the Agency

AGENCY	ROLE OF THE LPN
Hospital	Providing direct bedside care, teaching, mentoring other LPNs and nursing assistants, administering medication, and performing complex procedures
Home Health Care	Providing direct patient care, teaching, and performing physician-ordered procedures without the direct supervision of an RN; requires strong assessment and problem-solving skills
Hospice	Keeping the patient clean and comfortable during the dying process and providing pain management; comforting patient and family members and encouraging them to express their feelings about death and dying
Extended Care Facility	Patients are less acutely ill than hospitalized patients, but the care rendered by the LPN is similar to the care provided to hospitalized patients
Assisted Living Center	Assisting patients in taking medications or assisting residents in performing activities of daily living
Public Health Department	Providing immunizations and education, investigating disease outbreaks, and screening for diseases
Physician's Office	Taking vital signs and interviewing the patient; often, LPNs in a physician's offices learn to draw blood and take x-rays
Emergent Care Center	Providing similar duties as those provided in a physician's office
Industrial Clinic	Providing similar duties as those provided in a physician's office, including the treatment of lacerations, orthopedic injuries, and chemical spills
School Health Clinic	Mainly providing the treatment of students' injuries and sudden illnesses
Inner-City Clinic	Taking vital signs and interviewing the patient; often, LPNs in inner-city clinics learn to draw blood and take x-rays

In all settings, the LPN is under supervision of a physician or RN and should report all assessment finds to the supervising licensed personnel.

mistakes or bad outcomes from procedures as part of their health care. Blaming and suing physicians, nurses, and health-care agencies can be costly to the system, and it is happening with increasing frequency Liability management is being addressed on national and local levels by physicians, health-care administrators, and attorneys. Safe practices by the LPN are crucial to ensure that nursing mistakes with bad outcomes are prevented.

Health-Care Technology

The United States is recognized worldwide for its advances in medical technologies. New technology has introduced effective ways for treating illness. Who will pay for expensive new medical procedures is problematic. Many people who would benefit from new processes do not have available health-care reimbursement funds; consequently, they often cannot access the benefits of new technology. It is important for you, as an LPN,

to stay current in new technology to continue to bring the best possible care to patients in the health-care systems where you work.

ROLES AND TASKS OF THE LICENSED PRACTICAL NURSE IN THE HEALTH-CARE SYSTEM

The scope of practice for LPNs is one that has grown over time. Originally educated to work at the bedside in hospitals, LPNs now can assume positions in a wide variety of settings. In addition to the diversity of places an LPN can work, there also are new and unique roles to be filled (Box 4.2). It is important to understand and recognize how to perform the tasks in each of the roles. Defining these tasks and roles is the purpose of this chapter. The tasks in each of the roles are assigned and supervised by an RN. An experienced LPN may

Box 4.2 Roles for the LPN in Health-Care Systems

1. Clinician
2. Manager
3. Advocate
4. Educator
5. Counselor
6. Consultant
7. Researcher as support staff
8. Collaborator

be in an agency where the supervisor is not always on site, but there always will be an RN supervisor on call for help or consultation. Protocols of the employer on how to report assignments and problems to the RN are crucial for you to understand as a practicing nurse.

Eight Roles of the Licensed Practical Nurse

Clinician

Being a clinician refers to what most people consider as nursing care. The basic tasks of the LPN are the skills learned in nursing fundamentals class and fundamental clinicals. As an LPN, you will provide services such as personal care, administering medications, dressing changes, ambulation, gathering vital signs, and reporting patient changes to the RN. The LPN often is the eyes and ears of the RN when doing ongoing patient assessments. The LPN needs to be attentive to the patient's condition to ensure that good-quality holistic care is being received.

Part of being a modern-day nurse is that you can be employed by a variety of agencies where the tasks may differ according to agency policies and needs. Despite working under the direction of an RN or physician, LPNs must be aware of licensing standards and the scope of practice for the state where they are practicing to prevent doing a task that may not be covered under LPN licensure. As a clinician, you need to continue to improve your nursing skills and stay current with updates on practice standards. Memberships in professional associations, such as the National Federation of Licensed Practical Nurses (NFLPN) and

National Association for Practical Nurse Education and Service (NAPNES), are important to remain current on new practice standards and regulations. In Chapter 6, you will learn about being a lifelong learner, an important aspect of being an excellent clinician.

Manager

The tasks of the LPN as a manager of care are the skills you use in following patient care plans and assessing, teaching, and educating the patient and the patient's family. This is management of patient care. Management of others involves being a team leader, unit manager, or charge nurse. This type of management includes the management skills you are learning in this book.

When managing patient care, the care plan outlines what tasks you will need to accomplish in meeting the needs of the patient in the home, nursing home, or hospital. You are responsible for organizing and prioritizing the tasks on the care plan and using your clinical skills and knowledge to provide holistic, personalized care. You can evaluate the care and teaching you give from the patient's care plan and report to the RN the patient's progress and responses to your work. If you are working for a home health agency, you will be the patient's care manager while you are in the home, and you will give your report to the RN case manager.

Advocate

The tasks of an advocate are to be an ally, supporter, and source of information for the patient and the patient's significant others. The LPN is an advocate for the patient by caring about how the patient feels and by having a willingness to help improve the health-care situation. How the LPN advocates for patients in diverse care settings depends on the setting itself. The hospital has its own personality and rules and regulations, as does each unit in the hospital. Working in the community in an assisted living facility requires a different approach to advocacy than working in home health or a skilled nursing facility. The LPN role as advocate in a physician's office is different from any of the others. In some agencies, you may have a closer contact with the patient than the RN and may need to suggest care options to promote quality care. You will always report the results of your assignments and nursing activities to an RN or a physician. As an advocate, you may be able to suggest changes in the care plans when you identify a more effective way to provide care. Additional information about advocacy can be found in Chapter 3.

Educator

The tasks of educator are outlined in the nursing care plans. In these plans, you will find what you need to teach the patient as identified by the RN and the unit or facility protocols. In the home, you may be teaching the patient or family about medications, wound care, or patient safety. In many community positions, your teaching would focus on health promotion and health maintenance. In the hospital, you generally would be teaching about disease management and appropriate care following discharge. Most teaching is given to the patient and the family members. In some situations, the LPN has additional educational responsibilities. In home care, you would not have an RN with you as you are providing care; instead, your instructions to patients would be guided by agency protocols and instructions of an RN. Your knowledge and skills as a nurse will direct you in your role as a patient educator. Any questions about your responsibilities as an educator should be discussed with your supervisor.

Counselor

In the role of a counselor, you as the LPN can help explore feelings and attitudes about wellness and illness with patients and their families. The LPN frequently uses the role of counselor in hospice, the home, or an extended care facility. Patients may need your support in accepting the options that have been selected for medical care. You may find that the care options are not satisfactory to the patient, and you need to confer with other health team members to determine whether treatment

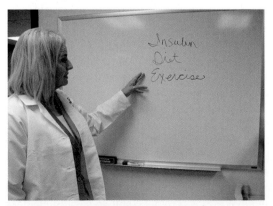
This LPN is educating a patient and his family.

plans need to be changed. In this situation, the role of counselor overlaps with the role of advocate. It is important that you report your observations concerning the patient's unease with the treatment plan to your supervisor. Your suggestions on revising the care plan would be helpful. If care plans cannot be changed, you can help the patient understand reasons for the current treatment plan and be supportive.

Consultant

The LPN consults with supervising RNs regarding patient care assignments. You use your knowledge to understand what health issues need close monitoring and follow-up. The tasks of a consultant are to be a communicator of patient assessments to the RN. If you are working in a physician's office, you may be consulting directly with the physician. In the home, nursing home, or hospital, your accurate assessment of the patient's responses to care is vital to determine the effectiveness of the care plan. If the care plan needs to be altered, your skills at doing a holistic assessment of the patient contribute to the revision of the care plan.

Researcher

LPNs participate in the research process when they identify a problem with a care plan or a patient who needs to be examined or evaluated. Research is focused on identifying new information or defining and supporting current practice. When something does not work or is a problem, it can be an indicator for the research team to study the situation. The research team accesses information in nursing and health-care journals and reviews standards of practice to find the best method to meet a patient's needs. This is known as evidence-based practice. In a home setting, your assessment of a problem provides information to the RN so that changes can be altered to serve the patient better. Your assessment tasks confirm when the care plan and your treatment have or have not been effective. When doing your assessments, you must be open-minded and able to communicate your findings to the RN.

There are some situations in which you will be asked to gather data for a research project. This data gathering could be in the form of an interview or taking biological information, such as vital signs. When you are asked to participate with the research team, be very detailed in what you do so that the resulting data are accurate and useful.

Collaborator

Many professionals make up the team involved in the care of each person; besides the LPN, there are RNs, certified nursing assistants (CNAs), and the physician. There also can be physical therapists, occupational therapists, a medical social worker, home health aides, recreational therapists, volunteers, and nutritionists. An LPN works, or collaborates, with other team members when providing care to a patient. In home care, you collaborate frequently with the RN as the case manager. In assisted living situations, you work with the resident and members of the community. Long-term care facilities and hospitals have the entire team as listed. Quality care is given when you and the team members work together in planning for the patient's care management. As you gain expertise in your practice skills and assessment abilities, your skill at collaboration increases. You become a successful collaborator when you have the respect of your supervising RN. You earn this respect by being knowledgeable, a good planner when providing patient care, and a good communicator of each patient's assessment. To be an effective collaborator, you need to work well with patients, families, and other team members.

REFLECTIVE THINKING

Describe your own strengths, limitations, and values in functioning as a member of a team. Do you feel it is important to work as a team to provide quality patient-focused care? What skills do you think you will need to function on a team? Write your thoughts in your class notebook.

Summary of Roles

The eight roles of the LPN can help you in becoming an effective manager of care for the patients to whom you give care. The roles described are used by LPNs in all health-care settings and agencies. As you review LPN practice standards in your state, see if you can identify the eight roles that you have learned about in this chapter.

HEALTH-CARE AGENCIES

Hospitals provide most of the health-care services in the United States. Other health-care agencies include home health, hospice care, extended care facilities, assisted living centers, public health departments, physician's offices, emergent centers, industrial clinics, school clinics, and inner-city clinics. The LPN always works under the direction of an RN or, in some clinic settings, a physician. It is possible that the RN or physician may request you to perform an assignment outside the licensing standards for LPN practice. It is crucial that you know the LPN practice standards so that your license would not be put in jeopardy with the state board of nursing. If you find yourself in this situation, you should refuse to do the task assigned and bring it to the attention to the facility administrator. An RN or physician may need to be reminded of the practice scope and standards of the LPN and alter the assignment.

Hospitals

Patients needing the most serious and intense care are admitted to hospitals, where health-care professionals and medical supplies are available for treatment. The LPN is an important member of this health-care team. The health-care team may include the physician, RNs, and CNAs. There also can be physical therapists, occupational therapists, a medical social worker, volunteers, and nutritionists. Your position involves providing direct bedside care, teaching, mentoring other LPNs and nursing assistants, administering medication, and performing complex procedures and other duties as assigned and that fit within your scope of practice. LPNs generally work on all units in a hospital. They may be assigned management duties or patient care. It is a compliment to LPN education that graduates can assume such diverse positions.

These LPN students are working together to investigate a variety of jobs available to them at graduation.

REFLECTIVE THINKING

Select a nursing practice setting (e.g., surgical floor, labor/delivery, physician's office, nursing home), and describe the eight LPN roles as they are fulfilled in the setting you selected. Record your information in your class notebook and come to class prepared to share it with others.

Home Health Care

Patients who do not require the intense health-care services of a hospital but continue to need nursing services could be discharged to home health care. The patient continues to receive state-of-the-art health care, but the family has some of the responsibility for patient care. RNs and LPNs provide the health-care services ordered by the physician. Although the LPN works under the supervision of an RN, LPNs often are in the home without the direct supervision of an RN. This role requires strong assessment and problem-solving skills. It also is necessary to know when to conference with the RN by phone if a question arises concerning the patient's status or care. The LPN has a history of being an important team player in home health care and is one of the reasons home health care has been successful in the health-care system.

Hospice

A patient who has a terminal health condition may desire to die at home. The patient and family can choose a hospice program through which care and comfort are given for a dying person in the home, inpatient setting, or extended care facility. The LPN works under the direction of the RN in providing care that keeps the patient clean and comfortable

Home health nurses plan their own schedule as they travel to the homes of their patients.

during the dying process. Pain management is a priority in hospice care. In addition to regular care, the patient and family members are comforted and encouraged to express feelings about death and dying. Working in a hospice organization gives the LPN an opportunity to provide care during one of the most intimate experiences human beings have—death. The LPN communication in this setting is focused on being supportive and understanding of the person dying and of the family and friends of the dying individual. This is an opportunity to give excellent emotional and physical nursing care in a holistic manner.

Extended Care Facility

An extended care facility provides specialized health-care services focused on long-term care, rehabilitation, or both. Patients are referred to as residents because they live in the "home" and are to be treated as if they were in their own home; for example, you should knock on the door before entering a resident's room. People are transferred to extended care facilities when they no longer need intense hospital services but continue to require care from a multidisciplinary team of health-care professionals. Residents may require extended care such as physical therapy after orthopedic surgery or a stroke. Respiratory therapy may be required for people on ventilators. Some people are frail and have multiple chronic diseases and can no longer live at home. According to the 2010 U.S. census data, only slightly over 5% of people older than age 65 are in nursing homes at any one time, but nearly 50% of those over 95 reside in nursing homes (U.S. Census Bureau, 2011). The rest are out living their lives with or without disabilities.

Residents in extended care facilities are less acutely ill than hospitalized patients, but the care rendered by the LPN is similar. The RN is in charge of making assignments, and the LPN must follow up immediately with the RN if there is a change in the resident's condition. Often, LPNs are shift charge nurses in nursing homes.

Assisted Living Centers

Some people are healthy enough not to require close medical or nursing involvement in managing their health-care requirements, but they need assistance in taking medications or performing activities of daily living. A home setting is not always an option for patients needing limited health care. Care is provided in a facility that usually allows for private or semiprivate rooms. The LPN is an important employee in assisted living centers. An RN may not always be present in the center; however, the LPN still works under the direction of an RN, and any questions or problems must be referred immediately to the RN on call.

Public Health Department

The purpose of a Public Health Department is to prevent diseases. Immunizations, education, investigating disease outbreaks, and screening for diseases are the major functions of health departments. Public Health Departments are located in most larger communities and are managed by individual states. Health care is provided to the public, but follow-up care for illnesses is referred to a health professional in the community. Each health department has protocols for the LPN's work assignments in the agency.

Physician's Office

A physician's office provides health care to patients seeking treatment, advice, or follow-up on illnesses. The LPN works under the direction of physicians or nurse practitioners and must refer assessment findings and questions to them. The LPN takes vital signs, interviews the patient, and performs other duties as assigned. Often, LPNs in physician's offices learn to draw blood and take x-rays; this depends on the physician.

Emergent Care Centers

Emergent care centers treat patients who have an immediate health concern and do not want to wait for an appointment in a physician's office or go to the emergency department. Health-care professionals in emergent care include physicians, RNs, and LPNs. The LPN works under the direction of the RN and reports all patients' assessments to the RN.

Industrial Clinics

Industrial clinics are located in industrial settings where accidents and medical incidents may occur. Industrial clinics may have facilities to treat injuries, such as orthopedic injuries, lacerations, chemical spills, and medical illnesses. The industrial clinic is equipped to treat immediate emergencies and illnesses and then refers the patient to another health-care setting. Each industrial clinic has protocols for the treatment of injuries and illnesses in its facilities. Not all industrial clinics have LPNs, but if LPNs are employed, they must work under the

direction of a physician or RN. The LPN always reports assessments and treatments to the supervising physician or RN.

School Health Clinics

School health clinics are located on school campuses. School clinics mainly treat students' injuries and sudden illnesses. When necessary, the nurse refers the student to the parent for care in the home or for care in another health-care setting. School districts have protocols in place for the treatment of emergencies and other responsibilities of nurses. An RN is usually the school nurse, but in some areas of the United States where there are limited numbers of RNs, an LPN may be the school nurse. The LPN must be aware of the health-care provider under whose direction responsibilities are given. The LPN reports all assessments and treatments to this person. The state licensing board must approve protocols for an LPN's practice standards in a school. In some inner cities where there is limited access to health care, schools are used as health-care clinics. The main health-care providers in these school health clinics are nurses. In the school health clinic, an LPN works with an RN to provide health-care services to the populations within the school

Nursing care in all settings allows the LPN to do holistic assessments.

boundary. The LPN works under the direction of the RN and reports all assessments and treatments.

Inner-City Clinics

Health clinics in inner cities are operated with funds from government agencies or charities. Physicians, RNs, and LPNs are the main providers of health care in these clinics. Each inner-city clinic has protocols for services that are offered in its clinic. The LPN works under the direction of a physician or an RN. All assessments and treatments are reported to the RN or physician.

This rich description of the LPN role in multiple settings is an exciting one! You have a great future ahead of you, and I strongly suggest you move forward with energy and define yourself in whatever becomes your niche. Take some time to explore different roles and environments; find the perfect place and enjoy what you are doing to fulfill your goal of being a licensed practical nurse!

REAL-WORLD CASE STUDY

Part A

■ Today is Brian Nelson's last clinical day before completing his LPN program. His assignment for the day is to work with Tom Brown, LPN, in the Star Home Health-Care Agency. Tom went over the day's visits with Brian. They reviewed the care plans for the patients together. Brian made notes on what he wanted to remember for the clinical journal he will give to Dr. George, his nursing instructor, at the end of the day.

The first home visit was to a patient who had been released from the hospital 3 days previously. The patient had an infected wound that needed to be irrigated. He also needed a dressing applied twice a day, once by his wife and once by the nurse. The care plan included assessing the wound, wound irrigation and dressing change, vital signs, monitoring medication compliance, diet intake, and evaluating pain. Tom asked Brian to take the patient's vital signs while he questioned the patient and his wife about the dressing changes, the patient's pain, medications, and diet. The patient's vital signs were the same as the day before except the temperature was elevated. Brian assisted Tom in changing the dressing. They both noted redness

around the wound and serosanguineous drainage on the dressing. The patient stated that the wound was more painful, and he did not want to walk around the house because of the pain. Tom said the wound was redder today than on the visit yesterday. Tom reviewed the wife's method for changing the dressing and discovered she was not washing her hands before changing the dressing, and she did not always use gloves.

What should you do to correct this situation? Outline in your class notebook the critical steps you need to take to educate the patient and his wife regarding the dressing change.

Part B

■ Tom and Brian asked about the patient's appetite and diet. The patient had not felt like eating yesterday and today. He had drunk about 16 ounces of grape juice yesterday. The patient was using pain medication about every 6 hours and was taking his antibiotic two times a day, as had been prescribed at the hospital.

What would Tom and Brian's patient assessment include? What is the "chain of information" for their assessment? In other words, to whom did they report their assessment, and where did the information go so that there could be appropriate assistance given to the patient and his wife?

Part C

■ Brian had a good experience working with Tom as he made four other home visits that day. After each visit, Tom discussed his care of the patients with Brian. Brian observed Tom as he made his entrances on the medical records and completed the paperwork required by the agency. Tom reported all of the home visits to the RN at the end of the shift. The RN and Tom suggested that Brian be included in updating the care plan on the patient who had the wound infection. Brian was pleased that he could have input in revising a care plan.

Dr. George read Brian's journal and asked Brian to identify the roles and tasks he and Tom had performed while caring for the patient with a wound infection. Brian reflected on his day's activities and could see that the LPN in a home health agency had more roles than that of a clinician.

What are the roles that Brian identified after his day as a home health nurse? Use examples from the patient with the infected wound.

Key Points

- The health-care delivery system in the United States is complex and changing. Even though new laws require everyone to have health insurance, 33 million Americans are still uninsured. Both public and private agencies provide health care in the United States.
- The LPN may function in many roles in the health-care system. Being a *clinician* refers to what most people consider as nursing care. The LPN may be a *manager* of care or a manager of other health-care providers. The LPN will be an *advocate* for patients in diverse settings. The LPN is also an *educator,* a *counselor,* and a *consultant* concerning patient care and disease process and management. Doing

research is another area that the LPN may find interesting. The LPN is also part of the health-care team and is a *collaborator* in patient care.
- Each state has its own nurse practice act that governs the LPN scope of practice. Most LPNs work in hospitals, but there are other health-care agencies that employ LPNs. These agencies include home health, hospice care, extended care facilities, assisted living centers, public health departments, physician's offices, emergent care centers, industrial clinics, school clinics, and inner-city clinics. LPNs are always supervised by an RN or, in some cases, a physician.

ANSWERS TO REAL-WORLD CASE STUDY

■ *Part A*

Brian and Tom discussed the correct way to care for the wound with the patient and his wife. Brian asked the wife to repeat his demonstration of changing the dressing. The wife washed her hands correctly, correctly assembled the wound care supplies, appropriately irrigated the wound, and applied the dressing. The wife seemed to understand the correct techniques to use when doing wound care. She had not understood the importance of following the principles of appropriate wound care to prevent infection. She was upset that she may have caused the wound to become infected and said she felt like she had let her husband down. Tom and Brian reassured her she was a good wife.

■ *Part B*

1. Elevated temperature
2. Increase in redness and tenderness around the wound
3. Serosanguineous drainage on the dressing
4. Increased pain
5. Medications being taken as ordered
6. Decreased ambulation
7. Decreased fluid and nutrition intake
8. Wife's poor technique in caring for the wound

Tom called the RN supervisor at the agency's office and reported the assessment findings. Tom suggested that the physician write an order for a nurse to visit the home twice a day for 2 days to assess the wife's ability to care for the wound. The RN would then call and report the elevated temperature and wound assessment to the physician. It is the physician's responsibility to write new orders and the RN's responsibility to see that they are carried out.

■ *Part C*

1. Clinician—he gave nursing care to the patient.
2. Manager—he assessed the situation with the wound and "managed" it by following the chain of command to get updated orders; he also did the teaching with the wife.
3. Advocate—he taught the wife while advocating for her as well. He did not allow her to feel like a failure; he advocated for the patient by doing a thorough assessment and making changes as needed.
4. Consultant—the suggestion to the RN, and eventually the physician, for the dressing wound teaching for the wife was the consultant role.

Continued

ANSWERS TO REAL-WORLD CASE
STUDY *continued*

5. Counselor—the teaching role and counselor role are similar here. The LPN had to counsel the patient and his wife to teach them.
6. Educator—teaching was done on the wound care, and a plan was made to reinforce the teaching over the next 2 days.
7. Researcher—there was not a formal research role.

8. Collaborator—the student, LPN, RN, physician, patient, and wife made a positive change in the treatment for this patient.

The LPN becomes the eyes and ears of the RN when providing nursing care in the home. The LPN needs to have the knowledge and skills to recognize signs and symptoms of the patient's condition that need to be reported immediately to the RN.

REVIEW QUESTIONS

1. Identify the three levels of primary care.
   1. Primary, secondary, tertiary
   2. Public, private, government
   3. Prevention, detection, treatment
   4. Aide, nurse, doctor
2. What statement explains how the federal government enforces the Affordable Care Act?
   1. The government charges participants a fee to enroll based on their income level.
   2. The government requires registration on the insurance exchange to declare coverage status.
   3. The government imposes a tax penalty on those persons who do not acquire coverage.
   4. The government deducts fees from income based on insurance coverage norms.
3. Identify the statement below that shows the LPN understands the correct reaction to an assignment that is outside of the LPN scope of practice.
   1. The LPN completes the task and documents in her charting that it is outside her scope but was assigned by her supervisor.
   2. The LPN asks the supervisor for authorization to function in a higher role in the current situation.
   3. The LPN calls the ombudsperson to register a formal complaint regarding unsafe practice at the health-care agency.
   4. The LPN refuses the assigned task and makes an appointment to discuss it with the facility administrator.

4. Which statement about the role of the LPN is correct?
   1. The tasks performed by an LPN are assigned and supervised by an RN.
   2. The LPN may work autonomously in some settings and report to a shift supervisor.
   3. As long as the LPN has experience, supervision is not required.
   4. LPNs must work in the line of sight of the supervising RN.
5. According to the chapter readings regarding the stated problems with the U.S. health-care system, identify the correct statement.
   1. The government now provides a central agency to control health care.
   2. All U.S. citizens now have access to insurance.
   3. Standardized treatment guarantees that new technology and treatments will be used.
   4. Insurance must reimburse for treatment and care provided.

References

Centers for Medicare and Medicaid Services. (2015). Brief summaries of Medicare and Medicaid. Retrieved from https://www.cms.gov/Research-Statistics-Data-and-Systems/Statistics-Trends-and-Reports/MedicareProgramRatesStats/Downloads/MedicareMedicaidSummaries2015.pdf

D'Amico, D., & Barbarito, C. (2016). *Health and physical assessment in nursing*. Boston: Pearson.

Kaiser Family Foundation. (2016). Total monthly Medicaid and CHIP enrollment. Retrieved from http://kff.org/health-reform/state-indicator/total-monthly-medicaid-and-chip-enrollment/

U.S. Census Bureau. (2011). Census Bureau releases comprehensive analysis of fast-growing 90-and-older population. Retrieved from https://www.census.gov/newsroom/releases/archives/aging_population/cb11-194.html

Web Resources

National Association for Practical Nurse Education and Service (NAPNES) http://napnes.org

National Council of State Boards of Nursing https://www.ncsbn.org

5

Nursing and Informatics

DIANE LEGGETT
AND JULIE RHODES

KEY TERMS

Electronic health record (EHR)
Electronic medical record (EMR)
Health information exchange (HIE)
Health information system (HIS)
Meaningful use (MU)
Nursing informatics (NI)
Telehealth
Telemedicine
Telenursing

CHAPTER CONCEPTS

Collaboration
Communication
Evidence-Based Practice
Health-Care System
Informatics
Safety

LEARNING OUTCOMES

1. Define nursing informatics.
2. Examine advantages of using informatics in the care of patients.
3. Identify basic skills needed for patient care using computers.
4. State methods of protecting health information in a work environment.
5. Describe the use of electronic tools to manage business in the workplace.
6. Describe health-care trends that are driving greater use of informatics in health care.
7. Understand the impact of meaningful use for patient outcomes.
8. Consider the use of telemedicine in patient care.

In attempting to arrive at the truth, I have applied everywhere for information, but in scarcely an instance have I been able to obtain hospital records fit for any purposes of comparison. If they could be obtained, they would enable us to decide many other questions besides the ones alluded to.

—Florence Nightingale

Much of the knowledge and information we have today comes from the fact that someone documented what he or she saw, heard, or experienced. Practically from the time humankind discovered the ability to make embellishments on cave walls, information has been transmitted to others. Symbols on rock, tablets, animal skins, or other material described hunting expeditions, farming, times of famine, or family histories. Journeys were documented with directions and possible dangers to avoid. Just imagine all the things that would need to be rediscovered without the information available to us from previous generations!

This same knowledge and information transfer is a form of communication used in health care and nursing. Think of Florence Nightingale and the challenges she faced as she and her nurses worked with the soldiers in the Crimean War. Despite the difficulties faced, she was astute at keeping records. She documented activities of the nurses and the patients, changes that occurred in the conditions of the facilities and the patients, nutritional status and intake, lighting, heat, sanitary conditions, and many other items. Because of the records and documentation she kept, we are able to learn about the effects of cleanliness, light, and fresh air on a patient's condition. We are also able to see how important records are for expanding knowledge in the nursing profession.

Documentation has always been a part of the nursing profession. A visit to a historical display showed records kept by student nurses and their instructors in the late 1800s. These records told a brief story of classes and learning hardships (grades), daily activities in the hospital setting, and even communication. It was interesting to read of the nursing duties of that time and think of the advancements that have brought us to where we are now. As nurses, we have more knowledge, technology, and responsibilities, which include even better record keeping.

Documentation is only part of what we do as nurses. We also must be able to find and use information in the care of patients. A remarkable amount of information is available to assist nurses in providing the best outcome. Accessing, applying, and using current information that is found through the use of computers is referred to as evidence-based practice. *Evidence-based practice* is a term you will hear when collaborating with other nurses or health-care team members. It refers to the use of current research that demonstrates improved outcomes in patient care.

LOOKING AT THE PAST

Before computers, records were kept in a chart with multiple papers and sections for things such as medical orders and doctor's notes, progress reports, laboratory results, and nurses' notes. These charts could quickly become full of papers that were time-consuming and laborious to go through to find pertinent information. After patient discharge, the charts were taken apart, put in a folder, and filed. I remember being asked frequently to retrieve the old charts of a patient when there was a readmission. It was not a great deal of fun looking through multiple files! The care provider wanted to examine the past records to assist in the present

---

 Evidence-Based Practice

Kerfoot, M. K. (2015). Intelligently managed data: Achieving excellence in nursing care. Nursing Economic$, 33(6), 342–343.

This article addresses how to achieve excellence in nursing care using intelligently managed data. Much information and data are available but not yet used for clinical decision making and management support in nursing. Competency in nursing informatics will help nurses become advocates in the workplace to help transition from traditional thinking to data-driven decision support and to ultimately improve patient outcomes.

Questions:

1. What are some ways that you can influence informatics use in your workplace?
2. What devices are you already using that collect data?
3. How could these data be used to make decisions about patient care?

care. This task was time-consuming for everyone involved. If a patient had multiple admissions, this could mean the retrieval of many charts. I remember a patient who had been admitted to the facility six times over the previous 2 years. I was asked to retrieve the charts, which were swollen with papers that would have filled a large laundry basket. These were taken to the care provider, who then asked me and another nurse to find the medication administration sheets, progress notes, physician's orders, and laboratory reports. This activity took time to complete, which was frustrating to us and the care provider who were trying to care for patients in the facility as well as the new admission.

Another time-consuming activity was the documentation and review of daily cares in the patient's chart. Documentation was entered into the patient's chart by nurses, other care providers visiting with the patient, or health providers from other disciplines (e.g., physical therapy). When the care provider came to visit with the patient, the chart was taken to the room, and each section with the documentation was reviewed (just think of going to five rooms with a stack of 9 inch by 12 inch metal chart holders full of papers). The review allowed the care provider to examine recent reports and nurses' charting and ask the patient questions. The review was a great process to keep current on what was happening with each patient, but took time for both the nurse and the care provider.

In 2004, President George W. Bush and his administration mandated that the health-care industry migrate paper records to electronic health records (EHRs) over a 10-year period. Officially known as the American Recovery and Reinvestment Act, the intent and purpose for this migration was to pave the way toward having health-care records that could be shared throughout the care continuum, regardless of who or where the care was delivered (Kirby, 2015). Since this mandate was enacted, health care has been involved in a digital revolution that includes the use of financial incentives in the form of rewards and penalties. By 2013, 50% of health-care providers, and 80% of hospitals had implemented EHRs (Kirby, 2015).

LOOKING AT TODAY

The tools we have acquired today to assist us in nursing care are amazing! Technology has provided methods of accessing patient information

with great accuracy and minimal time and effort. We have equipment that automatically records information such as vital signs without us ever having to go back to the desk or a patient chart. If a question arises regarding a medication (e.g., spelling, pronunciation, color, side effects), we are able to locate this information quickly using the medical center or hospital database, which has increased safety in health-care facilities. Sometimes patients will come to the facility or office armed with information about their condition that was found on the Internet. This can assist health-care personnel in providing answers to questions patients may have. I remember my grandmother's visits to the doctor's office when she wasn't feeling well. She would sit patiently in the waiting room, go to the examination room when called, and then let the doctor examine her and ask questions. On the way home, we would question her about the visit and ask her whether she had told the doctor what was hurting (or didn't feel right), to which she would reply, "No, he never asked me that!" Consider how useful it would have been for her to have some information in her hand to ask about before the examination.

If a patient comes to us with information from the Internet, it is important for us to verify the accuracy of the information. There are multiple sites providing answers to questions patients may have regarding health issues. Patients trust nurses to give them the best care and reliable information. When you are with someone who has information found on the Internet, take time to look at the papers they may have brought with them. This is an opportunity for teaching while helping the patient and family identify reliable sources.

Make a note of the information source. If it comes from medical centers (e.g., the Mayo Clinic) or a government Web site (e.g., HealthyPeople. gov), the information will be more accurate and reliable. Look for references to research that verifies claims made on the paper. This is also a clue to reliable health information. As you are examining the papers, talk to the patient and family, explaining to them what you are hoping to find. Take this opportunity to teach them how to find reliable information and how to avoid other information that may be misleading.

In addition to being able to find health care–related information on the Internet, we now have equipment that automatically records data such as vital signs for health-care providers who offer telemedicine and for mobile health-care providers who make health-care information available in a variety of ways on a multitude of devices. Information mobility is on the rise, with health-care providers and patients accessing information on smart devices. Nurses have had to adapt and become information-literate in order to work with these ever-evolving innovations. Recent studies report a direct positive impact on the quality of care as a result (Anderson & Sensmeier, 2015).

REFLECTIVE THINKING

Technology has changed much of nurses' work and continues to affect practice. An example is a surgical patient with a vital sign monitor set at regular intervals. Consider the effect technology has had on nursing care, such as the time it takes to perform nursing tasks, documentation, or patient interaction. Record these thoughts in your class notebook and be prepared to discuss them with others.

NURSING INFORMATICS

You may have heard the terms *informatics* and *nursing informatics (NI)*. This is a continually developing area in our health-care system and one that offers multiple benefits to individuals who are willing to learn and use this technology. A specialty in nursing for informatics was recognized by the American Nurses Association (ANA) in 1992. In 1994, the ANA released two documents outlining the standards of practice and scope of practice for nurses specializing in informatics. There have been several updates and revisions since then, with a definitive description released in 2015. NI utilizes multiple sciences to create electronic systems for information collection, organization, data analysis, and knowledge retention. NI supports the practice of nursing in the delivery of patient care as well as providing general health-related information for consumers and patients (Harrington, 2015). A nurse who has specialized in informatics focuses on the use of information technology for many aspects of nursing, including patient care data; education for self, patients, and families; locating research to improve patient care; or scheduling for employees or meetings. Some of you may find yourself questioning why anything like informatics for a nurse

is necessary; after all, don't nurses just provide patient care? We do care for patients, but realize that part of our care involves best practices, safety, and gaining new knowledge as needed. These aspects of our care are made easier with the use of informatics. As a beginning nurse, you are expected to have basic information to perform skills relating to patient care, management, and the use of information systems. As you become more experienced, you will gain proficiency in information technology that will assist in the daily care you provide and the decisions surrounding patient care. Some of you may even decide to continue and become a specialist in informatics that focuses on information management to support all areas of nursing.

Electronic Health Records

Today we have an enormous amount of information that is readily available because of relational databases and statistical software. One of the skills that is performed and recorded on a regular basis is the physical assessment of vital signs. The information gathered is referred to as data, and the data are entered into a clinical record on a computer terminal. The nurse is able to compare previous data entered at any time, which assists in quicker decision making regarding care of the individual. Before the use of computers, these data were entered on sheets in the patient chart. Separate sections were located in each chart for the vital signs, assessment, nurses' notes, laboratory tests, doctor's orders, and other information. When the nurse desired to compare previous entries, it was time-consuming to locate the correct section, find the appropriate dates, and compare information.

The advent of computers for recording and storing data has increased efficiency for many health-care workers and has increased interest in electronic health records to manage health-care information. The electronic health record provides access to information by all individuals involved in the care of the patient at the time and place needed rather than having to go back to the desk, find the chart, and search the sections for the required information. The electronic health record also allows more than one discipline or provider to access the information at the same time. In the past, the charts were carried into the rooms for reference when the provider came to visit. If an individual from any other discipline (e.g., physical therapy) needed the chart, that person had to wait until it was returned to the desk. Now the information can be easily accessed from the individual departments without even needing to go to the patient care area! This system also provides faster results from tests that have been ordered. If the care provider orders a laboratory test or an x-ray, the results can be entered from the department completing the test and be available in a short period of time. This has decreased wait time while increasing efficiency and safety.

The ability to use technology in patient care has many advantages for patients and individuals involved in patient care, including improved charting integrity and legibility, and the potential for reducing the numbers of errors. Have you ever received a handwritten note from a friend and been unable to decipher some of the words? This is what happened frequently with the handwritten notes in patient charts. We were not always able to read the words clearly and would frequently need another set of eyes to help us understand what had taken place during the previous shift. Electronic health records provide clear and legible information that is easy to follow. Accuracy is improved with well-defined sections, and a more complete record of events is provided. This also allows for better reporting when patient care is transferred to another area or to another nurse.

Some systems in health-care facilities have decreased the numbers of errors through the use of electronic health records and computer charting. An example of this is medication administration. Prompts may appear on the patient's record to remind the nurse of any medications or treatments and the time they are to be administered. Before a medication is given, the computer asks for verification of the patient, room number, medication, and dosage. If any of those do not match with the order, the computer will ask the nurse to check the order and verify before proceeding. I can remember when this system was first introduced. We all complained about the extra time it was going to take us to get the medications out to the patients, but a reduction in the number of adverse medicine incidents has been far greater than any extra time we may have spent.

Integration of Sciences

With all the data that are gathered on every patient using health information systems (HIS), the opportunity is at hand to integrate sciences (Kerfoot, 2015). Direct care nurses are being required to integrate their knowledge of nursing science (critical thinking and reasoning) with computer science (information technology) and information science (information management) in order to use these data to drive decisions. In addition, many medical devices, such as insulin pumps, glucose monitors, and medication scanners, currently have embedded technology that requires the integration of these sciences to successfully operate the devices, retrieve the data, and then analyze them for patient-centered care. The integration of data from all these sources into one seamless source, such as the EHR, can provide relevant data to the nurse in an immediate manner, improving clinical decision making and reducing medical errors (Gideon & DiPersio, 2015).

Clinical decision support (CDS) systems are currently aimed at providing intelligent support to physicians; however, many nurses are advocating and working toward smart solutions to support nursing and nursing care as well. Across the country, more than 3 million nurses make up the bulk of the EHR users (Kirby, 2015). Usability of these systems must be adoptable by all users with a certain degree of ease, with an overall sense of efficiency and satisfaction following their use (Shultz, 2015).

Data, Knowledge, and Wisdom

In 2009, the Health Information Technology for Economic and Clinical Health (HITECH) Act was legislated, outlining the need to use data in a meaningful manner and thus leading to the term *meaningful use (MU)* (Gideon & DiPersio, 2015). The use of electronic health records increases the amount of data that can be documented. Using data in a meaningful manner can improve patient care by synthesizing data to provide knowledge and wisdom about the patient's history and current condition. The meaningful use of data can be accomplished if the focus is on the value of the data versus the volume of data (Thede, 2015).

An electronic health record (EHR) is used to store data. Typically, these data can be retrieved from within the health-care company who stored the data. However, the United States is on a path toward meaningful health information exchange (HIE) and access to data is needed from all health-care providers across the health-care continuum. This is done by having the health-care company who gathered the data submit meaningful data to an HIE in a commonly defined format. The outside health-care company can now retrieve the meaningful data for use in the continuing care of the patient. For example, Clinic A stored data on a patient and then submitted the meaningful data to an HIE. The patient is now at Hospital B (a non-affiliate of Clinic A), and data are needed to continue care. Hospital B is able to retrieve data from the HIE.

The overall goal of the meaningful use of an EHR is the ability to access and retrieve data in a manner that is timely, safe, efficient, and patient-centered. The use of data can increase knowledge and wisdom in health-care practices as a whole, including evidence-based research, disease prevention, health promotion, and overall wellness, thus improving patient outcomes in a variety of circumstances (Greenberger, 2015).

Telehealth

Advances in telecommunication have allowed for telehealth services to enhance patient care. Telehealth can be as simple as storing information and then sending it to a provider, such as having a diagnostic test done in a remote location and then having a radiologist in another location read the data and provide results. It can also include real-time interaction through telephone conversations, texting, FaceTime®, or even videoconferencing. Telehealth can use specialized equipment and robotics that allow a physician to see images, such as the throat or an ear of a patient, in a location different from the patient's. Specialized portable devices are used to gather information, as are new devices worn by patients that use applications to monitor and transmit data. This technology is also used in intensive care settings to connect patients with off-site intensivists (physicians with additional training in critical care) and trauma specialists.

Telenursing is also a nursing specialty and is slowly making its way into community nursing courses. The newest trends in telehealth focus on the patient in order to provide patient care in patients' homes instead of the provider's setting. A simple example of a licensed practical nurse (LPN) using telenursing occurs when an order is requested and received via text or e-mail. Another example of telenursing is an LPN in a physician's office who coaches a patient with a chronic condition over the phone. A more in-depth example of telenursing is an LPN who is physically in a remote location with a patient and is able to attach monitoring equipment to the patient for a

physician in another location to monitor that patient's disease or condition. These types of telenursing allow for more frequent contact, frequent monitoring of compliance, and identifying potential problems before they occur. It also tends to eliminate unnecessary visits, emergency room visits, and some hospitalizations. It is cost effective and is starting to be recognized for reimbursement by insurance companies and Medicare. The biggest stumbling blocks to this technology currently are reimbursement, research, legal, and technical issues. Can you imagine the impact this kind of care is currently having in allowing for follow-up appointments for veterans and in providing health care in disaster areas? Imagine the impact it could have on overall health promotion and on our nation's current mental health care crisis. The use of telehealth has the potential to revolutionize many areas of health care by reaching more patients in a timely and effective manner.

HIPAA

Privacy is such an important aspect of caring for patients that a law was passed requiring the protection of private information (Box 5.1). The Health Insurance Portability and Accountability Act of 1996 (HIPAA) provides "standards protecting the confidentiality, integrity, and availability of data, and standards defining appropriate disclosures of identifiable health information and client rights protection" (Berman & Snyder, 2015, p. 103). Even the age of a patient can be considered

Box 5.1 Examples of Identifiable Health Information

- Name
- Age
- Gender
- Social security number
- Address
- Telephone number
- Employer
- Physical health condition
- Mental health status
- Provision of health care
- Health-care payments

identifiable health information! Patients place a great deal of trust in the nurses who care for them, and it is important that we follow the policies and procedures of each facility to maintain the patient's confidentiality and trust. When working with a computer, it is important to turn the computer monitor to a position so that only you can see the screen as you type in the information. You also need to remember to log off whenever you are not at the computer. Doing this prevents others from accessing private information.

With the increasing use of technology to care for patients, it is imperative that all health-care professionals maintain the confidentiality of patient information. Designers of electronic medical records are diligent about building in safety protocols to ensure the continued confidentiality of patient data as they are transmitted from one place to another. What are our responsibilities as nurses in protecting these data? Professionalism has always dictated that patient information not be shared verbally. How do we translate this to our current digital environment? A few simple answers are keeping login information private and secure, logging out of screens before leaving any documentation station, and positioning the computer screen away from eyes that might be watching but do not have a need to know. These questions also have implications on how and when we use our personal and employer-issued electronic devices and what we post to social media.

Computers and Systems

Some of you may feel apprehension, fear, or frustration at the thought of using a computer to assist in patient care. It is important to acknowledge your feelings and then work to overcome whatever is impeding your acceptance of something new. Facilities offer training for individuals involved in patient care, and employees familiar with the systems are usually available for assistance as needed. Positive experiences will help you to feel more competent in your skills. I can remember the introduction of computers for patient care at my regional hospital. My initial reaction was what has been described—I was a nurse and not a computer person! I did not want to interact with a computer; I wanted to be in the room with the patient. I soon learned how advantageous it was to use the computer to help me get the work done in less time and with greater accuracy.

As a beginning nurse, you will need to know basic competencies for the computer to integrate nursing science, information, knowledge, and to communicate with other providers that may be involved in the care of the patient. Some of the basic skills include knowing how to use a keyboard, how to navigate from one area of the system to another to access or enter data, how to retrieve data, and how to protect information that is confidential or private. Most facilities have a system in place for use in patient care, and although not all systems are the same, there are similarities.

FOCUSED LEARNING CHART
Nursing Informatics and Patient Care

DATABASE
Provides a central reference for patient information.

DOCUMENTATION
Allows for improved efficiency and legibility for better patient care.

MEDICATION ADMINISTRATION
Increases safety by checking orders and patient information at the bedside.

EDUCATION
Provides a method of obtaining and delivering education for self, families, and patients.

RESEARCH
Gives health-care workers the ability to access current research to improve outcomes.

You will need to spend time at the computer to enter the information you have gathered from your patient. Remember to use good body mechanics during those times so you will not have sore and tired joints or an aching back. Your body is very important for the work you do, so take good care of it in all your activities! If you will be spending extended lengths of time at the computer, take a brief break to walk, stretch, and refresh yourself. Such breaks will improve your concentration and assist in preventing poor posture. Infection control for the computer often goes unnoticed, but think of how many hands use the keyboard and mouse in an hour. Cleaning the keyboard and mouse on a regular basis and cleaning your hands after use help protect the patients and yourself from infections.

REFLECTIVE THINKING

When working, you will be caring for more than one patient. Most facilities have EHRs that contain the patient information. Some of this information will be needed by you in your daily care. How will you keep needed information for each patient without compromising confidentiality? Some nurses use report sheets or cards to take notes throughout the day. Record suggestions and come prepared to discuss with others.

Papers and Presentations

In addition to computer use for patient care, as an employee or manager, you may be asked to write a paper or give a presentation for other staff members or administration. Use of the computer allows you to prepare papers and presentations. Presentations can range from delivery of information to administrative personnel to general education for specific staff members or presentation of research to improve patient care. It is important to be aware of what you will be presenting, the time frame for the presentation, and the audience.

It is helpful to begin with an organized outline of the information. Begin with the basic information you want to communicate to the group. If you do not have a clear understanding of what you want the group to know, the group will be unsure of what knowledge is pertinent. Research reports generally follow a specific format with an abstract, introduction, methods, results, and discussion. This format is helpful as an outline for you to follow when presenting. An outline assists in organizing thoughts. Stating or defining objectives is a good method of clarifying the purpose of the presentation and what it is you want the audience to know at the conclusion. Objectives are also valuable as you plan the closing or ending of your presentation because you will be able to emphasize what the group should know.

With objectives, an outline, and an approximate time frame, you will be able to determine the amount of information to include. Timing is also a consideration for activities to enhance learning and maintain audience interest. Now you can begin planning what you want to say and how you will present the information. The introduction, or opening, of the presentation should be planned to grab the attention of the audience and let them know from the beginning what is to be learned. Think of this as making a good first impression. The body or main points are covered in the next section of the presentation. Do not overwhelm the audience with full slides or posters; this can distract from learning. Keep the points simple, but be sure to have references and facts to verify the information. Examples are another good method of helping audiences remember the main points. Finally, practice what you have prepared. Do this in front of a mirror, with an audience, or both. A brief outline or reminder sheet for your reference during the presentation will keep things flowing smoothly. Following your practice presentation, you or your practice audience may have noticed changes you could make that would improve your presentation.

Presentation of research contributes to improved patient care. *Evidence-based practice (EBP)* is a term you will hear in the care of patients. EBP is a process used to make clinical decisions based on research and other evidence. Nurses also include patient preferences as an integral part of EBP (Williams & Hopper, 2015). This process requires you as a nurse or manager to be aware of current research information that is relevant to your place of employment and to share with colleagues and staff. Research and review articles applicable to your place of employment, verify information by comparing it with other research and reviews, and then prepare to share what you learned.

Health Literacy

When developing educational materials, it is important to assess the health literacy or level of comprehension of your patients. Health literacy refers to "the degree to which individuals have the capacity to obtain, process, and understand basic health information and services needed to make appropriate health decisions" (U.S. Department of Health and Human Services, 2016). Your patients, their families, and others you may work with need to be able to understand any instructions you may give them—instructions from their care provider, consent forms they will be asked to sign, or instructions on medication bottles. Health literacy refers not only to being able to read information but also to being able to listen and process the information and use it to make decisions. If you provide written material, it must be written at a level the patient can read and comprehend. What about individuals with a language barrier? They may be unable to read, listen, or comprehend information if it is presented only in English. Learn the policy in your facility for working with patients who have limited English-speaking skills, and when you are in a situation with a patient speaking another language you will be prepared to offer the best health education opportunities.

Language may not be the only barrier encountered regarding health literacy issues. Remember my grandmother and her doctor's office visits? She was a functional, independent adult who was able to navigate decisions regarding transportation, money, meals, and daily care, but when it came to understanding what she needed to do to obtain the best health care possible, she was unable to function. She was not illiterate, but she became dependent during her time in the health-care system. You may also encounter individuals who function well in their own environment, but on entering the health-care system they become dependent

and may not display the ability to make choices regarding their health care. The health literacy of these individuals changes depending on the situation and context.

Spreadsheets

As a nurse manager, you will be managing volumes of information. This information may include staffing and budgetary data as well as information related to patient safety and satisfaction, all information having to do with numbers. Spreadsheets are the most common form of numerical data management in the workplace. Spreadsheets are basically a table with columns and rows that allow entry of numbers. The unique aspect of spreadsheets is the ability to enter formulas for analyzing the numbers that have been entered. Do any of you remember making a row of numbers, trying to keep them in a line, and then adding them one at a time? I would find myself going over the numbers many times and adding more than one time to make sure I had the correct answer! The spreadsheet will do all of this for you and is much better at keeping the numbers in a line. Think of the possibilities for using spreadsheets in your place of employment. As a manager, you want to know how many employees have been working the past week. By using a spreadsheet to enter the numbers, you will be able to view the total number of employees for the week easily. Now you want to know just how many nurses worked during the past week. Again, you put in the numbers from each shift, a formula, and you have the answer. Spreadsheets are useful for analyzing data such as infections treated, patient falls that may have occurred over a certain length of time, calculating length of stay in a facility, and many other items.

Spreadsheets also help in the preparation of a budget. The spreadsheet allows the user to view a wide range at one time, make comparisons, and adjust as necessary without having multiple pages spread out. The use of a spreadsheet reduces errors in calculations and provides a more efficient use of time. The information on a spreadsheet can also be used to produce a picture representation of the information such as a graph or pie chart. This format is a good way to present numbers visually to management or other employees. As a nurse manager, you will want to learn how to use spreadsheets to your advantage.

A nurse educating a patient.

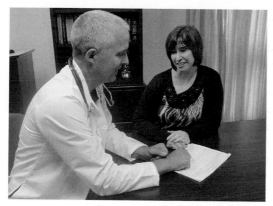

A nurse manager discussing his budget with the administrator.

Presentation Software

Another application that is useful in the workplace is the ability to prepare presentations that can be viewed as slides for managers, other employees, families, or patients. Presentation software is usually a part of the application package installed on a computer with the most common being Microsoft PowerPoint (Microsoft Office, n.d.). There are several online presentation tools available, such as Prezi, Google Slides, SlideRocket, Haiku Deck, and many others. The benefit of using these tools is being able to access them online anywhere you have access to the Internet. Some facilities use this type of presentation for patient education or staff meetings. There are multiple uses, and you may be asked to develop a presentation for your facility.

It is important to keep in mind the purpose of the presentation as well as the audience and amount of information to be delivered. Will this be used as support for a lecture, or will the slides replace the lecture? Audience involvement will decrease the amount of information placed on the slides; in fact, you may have only a question to stimulate discussion on a slide. If there will be limited involvement from the audience, more information will be included on each slide. After you have decided on the information for the slides, you will need to choose a color scheme for the slides. A background will appear on each slide for consistency and should be examined to ensure it does not detract from the information presented on the slides. Stark contrasts in colors may make it difficult for the viewer to follow the presentation. When you have prepared a few slides with the background color and lettering, display them as

you will be doing for your presentation to assess ease of viewing for the audience.

Slides offer areas to place the title or text. The font you use should be easy to read and large enough that the participants in the back row will not need a telescope to follow what you are presenting! Again, displaying the slides may assist you in determining the best font and size. Take care not to place too many items on one slide, which can be distracting. See Box 5.2 for suggestions on formatting slides. Pictures can be added to slides for viewing enhancement but should not detract from the points of the presentation. Pictures may be the central object for a slide. If a picture is the main topic on a slide, keep the font (if any is used for the picture) small enough not to detract but large enough for the audience to read easily.

Many fun things can be added to a presentation to increase interest. Some of the things that can be included on slides are sound, video clips, or animations. The slides can be prepared to transition in a variety of ways, such as fading in, appearing as blinds opening, or starting at the center and gradually filling the screen. These transitions can be spectacular but can also detract from the presentation. Be careful how much emphasis you put on the extras and use them sparingly (Sewell, 2015; Thede, 2015).

One thing that has been a great help to me in presentations is the speaker notes section at the bottom of the slides. I have been able to write notes about what needs to be included in the discussion, references for any research being discussed, and questions to ask the audience. These can be printed

---

Box 5.2 Tips for Developing Presentation Slides

1. Keep the number of slides to a minimum.
2. Select a font style and size that is easy to read, especially from a distance.
3. Use short sentences with no more than five to six words per line.
4. Include only five to six lines of text per slide.
5. Use contrasting color for slide background and text.
6. Use only graphics that help convey your message.

to have as a guide when presenting and have been a good reminder when I get nervous in front of a group! When it is time to give your presentation, the slides can be printed as a handout with room for the audience to take notes, as a full-page slide, or as a page with the slide and the notes together for use during the presentation.

Teleconferencing

Have there been times you wished you would be able to attend a special conference or presentation, but it was taking place in a distant city? Computers and the Internet have made it possible for us to participate in conferences, allowing us to view slides, listen to the presenter, or even participate through live conversation or by typing in questions or responses. This same technology provides opportunities to work with individuals in other geographic areas. Think of how wonderful it is to be able to get ideas and opinions from multiple sources. You could even participate on committees and not be required to live close to the actual venue!

Other Issues

There will be times the computers and electronic systems will not be available for use in patient care. As great as they are, there are occurrences that crash the system, and nurses need to be able to continue caring for the patients under such circumstances. An important point to remember to preserve information is to have a backup system in place and to use the backup features each time you enter information in the computer. Know what the facility policy is for times when the system goes down. You may need to put your information on paper to be transferred into the system when it is running again, so find out what forms you will need to use during the down time. Know the process for data entry when the system is functional again, or if the papers used during the down time will be kept in storage. Finally, ensure you understand your facility's document retention policy and abide by it. This policy would include any data entered on paper during times the computer was not functioning.

Managers need to stay in touch with other health-care professionals and employees. E-mail is an efficient method of communication but needs to be used appropriately. E-mail can arrive much more quickly than a letter, allows for a reply that may include the original message (for those who may forget why the message was sent), and can be sent to multiple recipients. This method of communication can save time in tracking down people and waiting for replies and can improve communication. When creating a message, examine the boxes at the top of the e-mail. There will be a box for the name or address of the recipient, one for the sender, and one for the subject of the e-mail. The subject line can be a few brief words or just one word, but be sure to enter something to alert the recipient to the purpose of the e-mail and to prevent the e-mail server from moving the message to a junk mail section.

When creating the message, write clearly, be brief, and keep the message to the point. Although e-mail is a wonderful tool for communication, lengthy messages may not be appreciated or even read in a busy work environment. An e-mail that is too short, however, may leave the reader feeling as if you were too abrupt or that some information may have been excluded. Abbreviations, signs or pictures, and sarcasm may be misunderstood by the recipient, so be judicious in your use of something that could be misinterpreted. The font's size and color are another aspect that can enhance or detract from the message. It is not wise to use all capital letters, which can convey that the sender is "shouting," or a light-colored font, which may not be legible. Before sending the message, read it, correct any errors, and verify the information to ensure it will be understood.

Professional networking and communicating with coworkers is a wonderful opportunity available through the use of computer systems. Computers provide a method of keeping up to date on current information needed to provide state-of-the-art care for patients. Computers also offer the possibility of illegal transfer of patient data when communicating with others outside the facility. This possibility puts private information at risk, so most facilities have restrictions for accessing anything outside of the facility. Be careful in your use of the technology in your facility by maintaining a professional attitude in all of your communication on whatever electronic device you are using. Enjoy the possibilities that come with this technology, but be a wise consumer to protect yourself, your patients, and your health-care facility!

LOOKING FORWARD

Technology use and innovative solutions to problems will continue and expand as clinicians learn how to transform data into knowledge. Technology will be the key that enables care delivery models of the future that are even more focused on providing the best individualized care that is supported by evidence-based research (Anderson & Sensmeier, 2015).

REAL-WORLD CASE STUDY

■ You recently graduated from an LPN program and were hired to work the afternoon-to-evening shift as a charge nurse for one area under the supervision of a registered nurse (RN) in a long-term care facility. The facility has recently introduced computer charting and medication passes to improve efficiency. Management spent time investigating systems and training employees before introducing the new system. You have found it helpful to get patient information and have even had the system catch a medication error before you gave the medication to the patient.

Despite the positive approach by management, on several shifts you have heard some of the other nurses complaining about the amount of time it is taking them to get the information into the computer and especially how much more time it has taken them to get the medications out to the patients. Although there has been complaining, you have observed other activities at the computers, such as online games, shopping, and personal e-mails. This afternoon, when you went to ask another nurse a question, you discovered the desk void of any personnel, but you could see a patient chart still on the computer screen. You returned to your medication pass assignment, and one of the patients asked you why you always had to put that machine on his armband when the other nurses didn't.

Do you see any problems with the management of the computer in the work environment? How should you handle the situation with the other nurses and with the patient?

Key Points

- The specialty of nursing informatics was first recognized by the American Nurses Association in 1992. Nurses who specialize in informatics focus on the use of information technology for many aspects of nursing, including patient care documentation and decision making, education of self and patients, and locating research to improve patient care.
- Through the integration of multiple sciences, EHRs have been developed to improve the integrity of the documentation process. This integrity combined with analysis allows for data-driven clinical decisions that impact patient outcomes.
- Records have always been an important part of nursing, but retrieval of that data has been extremely problematic. Digital data and the information and knowledge about patients that can be derived from that data hold great promise. The information allows nurses and other health-care providers to make better decisions regarding patient care, ultimately improving patient care.
- Information systems are ever changing for health-care workers. Data are being recorded in large volumes, and efficient tools to provide

real-time analysis are being developed. Masses of consumer information are readily available; however, the reliability of this information needs governance.
- Because privacy is such an important aspect of caring for patients, the HIPAA law was passed to require the protection of private information. Steps LPNs can use to protect health information in a work environment include keeping login information private and secure, logging out of screens before leaving any documentation station, and positioning the computer screen away from eyes that might be watching but do not have a need to know.
- Many types of telehealth programs are available, allowing patients to be served electronically in remote health-care facilities as well as their homes at an ever-increasing rate. Smart devices are now being used by patients and health-care providers to document and retrieve health information. The use of this technology reduces errors and makes information more easily accessible.
- Nurses today will need to know how to use computers in order to do their jobs. Skills will

include the ability to use a keyboard, word processing, and spreadsheet software; access reliable health information on the Internet; and know basic computer hardware and software troubleshooting strategies. Nurses will also be the resource to support patients with their use of health-care technology.

■ The Health Information Technology for Economic and Clinical Health (HITECH)

Act outlines the need to use data in a meaningful manner, thus leading to the term *meaningful use*. Using data in a meaningful manner can improve patient care by synthesizing data to provide knowledge and wisdom about the patient's history and current condition. The meaningful use of data can be accomplished if the focus is on the value of the data versus the volume of data.

ANSWERS TO REAL-WORLD CASE STUDY

Unfortunately, these situations do occur in health-care facilities. Some nurses are resistant to change and will find ways to override systems to get the work done in what they consider less time. Charting changes in patient status, treatments, medications, vital signs, and many other items in the computer provides a method of easy access for data retrieval and review. It standardizes readability for any items that need to be clarified and increases safety in patient care. Computer systems in facilities benefit both the nurse and the patient and should not be used for personal business. Overriding the system for what some may consider efficiency compromises patient safety, and using the computer for personal business compromises the security of patient personal information.

The best approach would be to talk to the other nurses regarding your concerns of patient information. There have been times when I talked to a nurse and discovered the nurse had been called to a room for what appeared to be an emergency. The urgent call had directed the attention from the computer to the emergency, and the computer had been left on without thinking of the possible consequences. It takes time to incorporate a new habit, such as turning off the computer or exiting the patient screen, so helping each other without undue criticism is appreciated.

Talking about the use of computers for personal business can be more difficult. You may want to talk about getting work done first, then locating a private area with a computer for personal business during a break, letting the nurse know how important it is to protect the integrity of the system for the patients. You could also suggest to management the need for further training to understand the importance of computer use in the facility. One facility had to remove access to anything but patient information because of the overuse of computers for nonwork activities!

REVIEW QUESTIONS

1. Which of the following statements is true?
   1. Nurses should only spend time caring for patients, not documenting.
   2. The original nurse documenter was Florence Nightingale.
   3. Documentation does not help patient outcomes.
   4. Electronic documentation does not improve patient safety.

2. Whose presidential administration is responsible for starting the meaningful use transitions?
   1. President Barack Obama
   2. President George W. Bush
   3. President Bill Clinton
   4. President Ronald Regan

3. Meaningful use is defined as:
   1. Data that are collected for each patient in any health-care setting.
   2. Information that is collected on paper and scanned into the medical record.
   3. The use of collected data to make clinical decisions.
   4. Improving patient outcomes in any way possible.
4. Telemedicine can be used for all of the following types of care, *except:*
   1. Remote consultation by an intensivist or trauma specialist.
   2. Robotic examination of a patient by a remotely located provider.
   3. Phone calls, FaceTime®, video-conferencing, and texting.
   4. Hands-on surgical intervention that is not assisted by robotics or other personnel.

5. Health care is going through a digital revolution, allowing for decisions to move from traditional care decisions to:
   1. Data-driven decisions.
   2. Decisions based completely on patient choices.
   3. Decisions made solely by physicians.
   4. Nontraditional decisions.

References

Abdrbo, A. A. (2015). Nursing informatics competencies among nursing students and their relationship to patient safety competencies. *CIN: Computers, Information, Nursing, 33*(11), 509–514.

Anderson, C., & Sensmeier, J. (2015). Survey shows how informatics supports quality nursing care. *Nursing, 45*(8), 25–26.

Berman, A., & Snyder, S. J. (2015). *Kozier & Erb's fundamentals of nursing: Concepts, process, and practice* (10th ed.). Upper Saddle River, NJ: Pearson Prentice Hall.

Bickford, C. J. (2015). The standards of nursing informatics: New scope and standards practice. *CIN: Computers, Information, Nursing, 33*(4), 129–131.

Centers for Disease Control and Prevention. (2015). Learn about health literacy. Retrieved from www.cdc.gov/healthliteracy/learn.

Gideon, A. C., & DiPersio, D. M. (2015). Medical order entry and clinical decision support: Current nursing informatics issues. *Nursing Clinics of North America, 50*(2), 315–325.

Greenberger, M. (2015). Understanding health information exchange. *Nursing Management, 46*(12), 14–15.

Harrington, L. (2015). American Nurses Association release new scope and standards of nursing informatics practice. *Technology Today, 26*(2), 93–95.

Kerfoot, M. K. (2015). Intelligently managed data: Achieving excellence in nursing care. *Nursing Economic$, 33*(6), 342–343.

Kirby, S. B. (2015). Informatics leadership: The role of the CNIO. *Nursing, 45*(4), 21–22.

Microsoft Office. (n.d.). http://office.microsoft.com

Nightingale, F. (1859). *Notes on hospitals.* London: John W. Parker & Son.

Sewell, J. P. (2015). *Informatics and nursing: Opportunities and challenges* (5th ed.). Philadelphia: Wolters Kluwer.

Shultz, S. (2015). Usability: A concept analysis. *The Journal of Theory Construction & Testing, 19*(2), 65–70.

Thede, L. Q. (2015). Central trends in nursing informatics: Students' reflections from International Congress on Nursing Informatics 2014. *CIN: Computers, Informatics, Nursing, 33*(3), 85–89.

U.S. Department of Health and Human Services. (2016). Health literacy. Retrieved from http://www.hrsa.gov/publichealth/healthliteracy/

Venes, D. (Ed.). (2013). *Taber's cyclopedic medical dictionary* (22nd ed.). Philadelphia: F. A. Davis.

Williams, L. S., & Hopper, P. D. (2015). *Understanding medical surgical nursing* (5th ed.). Philadelphia: F. A. Davis.

Web Resources

American Nursing Informatics Association www.ania-caring.org

Health Information Management Systems Society (HIMSS) www.himss.org

National League for Nursing www.nln.org

Nursing Informatics Learning Center nursing-informatics.com

U.S .Department of Health and Human Services Administration (HRSA) www.hrsa.gov/healthit/meaningfuluse/MU%20Stage1%20CQM/whatis.html

From Student to Nurse

6

Fulfill Your Role as a Student

AMY STEGEN

KEY TERMS

APA
Confidentiality
Honesty
Learning styles
Paraphrase
Percolate
Plagiarism
Self-talk
Sexism
Ways of knowing

CHAPTER CONCEPTS

Communication
Ethics
Patient-Centered Care
Professionalism

LEARNING OUTCOMES

1. Name nursing's four ways of knowing as identified by Dr. Barbara Carper (1978).
2. List four expectations of students in the classroom.
3. Discuss the academic code or code of honor at the school you are attending.
4. Apply the concept of percolated thinking and its importance in studying for a test.
5. List and describe three study strategies for test taking.
6. Describe the four basic types of test questions and the critical aspects of each type.
7. List three methods for decreasing test-taking stress.
8. Interpret the importance of effective writing to nursing practice.
9. Demonstrate the use of three common grammar rules.
10. List the steps to writing a successful paper.
11. Define plagiarism.
12. Describe how to avoid sexist language when writing.

Let us be anxious to do well, not for selfish praise, but to honour and advance the cause, the work we have taken up [as nurses].

—Florence Nightingale

This chapter is unique compared with the others in this book. The focus is on assisting you in being an excellent student. This chapter discusses how to do well in the classroom and in the clinical arena and provides information on how to take tests and write papers. These skills and socialization will assist you in being successful in your nursing program. You cannot be a nurse manager without becoming a licensed practical nurse (LPN) first.

The foundation of this chapter is the concept referred to as *nurses' ways of knowing,* which was developed by Dr. Barbara Carper (1978). Her work is based on the way nurses learn and know information. The "survival" or study information in this chapter is based on Carper's ways of knowing to assist you in learning her principles for your future as a nurse manager. This is your first-aid or survival chapter, so enjoy and use what you are about to learn.

KNOWING YOURSELF AND UNDERSTANDING NURSES' WAYS OF KNOWING

Knowing yourself is an important aspect of nursing. One of the most effective tools that you need in nursing is you. There are times in nursing when you are the only tool available, and you can use it wisely only if you understand yourself. Using yourself wisely as you give patient care is known as the *therapeutic use of self.*

Carper (1978) described nursing's four ways of knowing as aesthetic, empirical, ethical, and personal. To know yourself as a therapeutic person, you need to understand these concepts. Since 1978, practicing nurses, nursing educators, leaders, and researchers have been using the four ways of knowing to understand nurses and nursing better. Although the four ways of knowing interact and overlap with each other and need to be considered together, it is easier at first to learn and think of them separately.

Aesthetic knowing refers to the art of nursing and complements empirical knowing, which is about the science of nursing. Aesthetic ways of

knowing are similar to the caring theory on which this book is based. Dr. Jean Watson teaches about the art of nursing when she discusses transpersonal caring. The art of nursing is the kind, sensitive nursing care that is the hallmark of what the profession represents. Current modern practices, with the focus on the financial "bottom line," try to push out the time necessary to be an aesthetic nurse. I sincerely hope you work hard to resist that trend. Without aesthetics in nursing practice, we do not have a profession.

Empirical knowing is having skill in the "how to do" of nursing. Do you know "how to" irrigate a colostomy, do cardiopulmonary resuscitation effectively, and manage all of the tubes and lines that critically ill patients need? If so, congratulations! You are an excellent technical or empirical nurse.

Ethical knowing deals with the moral components of nursing and decision making based on doing the right thing. Ethical ways of knowing are the concepts that provide integrity and reliability to nursing. Everyone expects a nurse to be honest, to be able to make ethical decisions, and to see the world in a way that promotes what is right. These are all aspects of ethical ways of knowing.

Personal knowing involves ongoing learning about yourself and your continuing development as a genuine, fully aware, therapeutic person (Chinn & Kramer, 2015). Personal ways of knowing are exciting. Some additions to your personal ways of knowing (i.e., studying, writing, and communicating) are shared with you in this chapter. This concept of knowing relates to getting to know yourself better. Now, while you are in school, is a good time for you to start a conscious examination of what you do through the lens of Carper. You will learn many ways to consider and improve yourself as you learn more about nursing and leadership.

An effective nurse cannot be technically competent only or moral only but also must be able to provide transpersonal caring. Nurses need to work to develop all four ways of knowing to be truly effective.

LEARNING IN THE CLASSROOM

Some instructors provide more entertainment value than others do, but they all know something you need to know. As a contemporary student, you

---

FOCUSED LEARNING CHART
Nurses' Ways of Knowing

AESTHETIC

Art of nursing
_____

Transpersonal caring
_____

Holistic management of care
_____

EMPIRICAL

Science of nursing
_____

Technical skills
_____

Expert physical care
_____

ETHICAL

Science of ethics
_____

Ethical integrity
_____

Ethical decision making
_____

PERSONAL

Self-awareness
_____

Self-management
_____

Positive decisions for self
_____

---

are probably a sophisticated TV and movie viewer, accustomed to the fast pace and special effects developed by professional entertainment specialists. When you are in the classroom, you are not there to be entertained. Listening to instructors requires skill, concentration, and experience.

Another responsibility of students is to get the information they need to be successful. There is a rule about questions in the classroom: There are no dumb questions! Generally, when a student has a question, it is one that several others in the class wanted to ask but were afraid to do so. Remember, there are no "dumb" questions, simply questions that need to be answered.

If your question is about an assignment or test, be sure you review the syllabus first to see whether the information you need is already there. Do not go to the instructor with a question about information that he or she has carefully spelled out in the syllabus. If you have questions after reviewing the syllabus, however, go to the instructor. You should be confident and pleasant. You should be empowered enough not to preface your question with, "This is a dumb question, but . . ." You should be clear on what you want to ask and not leave the conversation without getting the information you

need. The indicator of successful communication is when all involved achieve their goal.

Learning Styles

Learning style refers to the ways an individual processes information. Each person is unique and generally uses a distinct learning style. Some individuals may use more than one style depending on the concept or information they need to learn. There are three main learning styles: visual, auditory, and kinesthetic (movement). Table 6-1 provides information about each learning style.

Do you know which learning style you most commonly use? I am definitely a visual learner. I learn best by seeing written material or graphics related to the content. I prefer it when a presenter uses slides to complement a lecture. Without the visuals, I find myself watching the other people in the room and tuning out the presenter. Although I know I am a visual learner, I may not always be in a situation where my learning style will be met. When developing classroom activities, most instructors try to incorporate learning activities that meet the various learning needs of students in the classroom. However, this may not always be the case. If you are an auditory learner, you may want

TABLE 6.1 LEARNING STYLES

Visual	Individuals learn through written language such as reading and writing. They also prefer visual materials such as pictures, charts, and graphs.
Auditory	Individuals learn best by just listening to information. They prefer listening to someone speak such as in a lecture or recording or discussing information with someone else.
Kinesthetic	Individuals learn best by doing or participating. They prefer to manipulate things as part of the learning process and need the opportunity to move around in a learning environment.

to ask the instructor whether you can record the lecture so you can play it back while you are studying for the test. If you are a visual learner and you have an instructor who does not include any visuals with his or her lecture, you may need to draw your own pictures and diagrams to help you remember the information. Mind mapping is a technique that may help you. If you are a kinesthetic learner, drawing pictures or highlighting information during lectures may help. You may also want to spend more time in the nursing practice laboratory. Although no learning style is either better or worse, given the same content, most students can learn the content at an acceptable level. How they master the content is determined by their individual learning style (Beischel, 2013). Identifying your personal learning style may help you with your education as well as your future career goals.

Organization and Note Taking

On the first day of class, you probably were given some form of an outline, syllabus, or list of objectives for the class. Nursing instructors generally are well organized and share their expectations with students about what they think the students should learn. Keep class handouts and place them in your notebook so that you will be able to refer to them when you are studying. Put your name and the date you received the handout somewhere on the first page.

Keep a calendar in your notebook and write in the dates you have to remember, such as examination dates, when papers are due, and any other dates important to being successful in the class. Some instructors may use an online course management system to support their course. The management system will include a course calendar that lists the important course due dates. Assignments accumulate quickly, so be organized and timely in the work you do.

Listen carefully to your instructor and try to understand what is being told to you. *Memorizing is not enough in nursing.* You need to understand and use the concepts you are being taught. Learning classroom content is a principal way of accumulating the essential aesthetic and technical knowledge that relates to nursing. Rather than taking notes on every word, listen attentively and jot down key words that will help you remember the lecture. Put a star or an arrow next to the topics the instructor talks about more than once because they may have more importance.

Study Habits

Studying is a personal thing. People have different ways of studying. If studying is something you have not been good at in the past, you need to think about the many possible ways of studying. If sitting alone with your book and your notes starts your mind wandering, you may need to try some new methods to get yourself started. Some people find that typing their notes or rewriting them gets them into a focused study mode. They are able to concentrate on the more difficult parts, reread confusing parts, and review topics in the textbook. If your instructor provides lecture videos, be sure to schedule time to view the videos as often as necessary.

Many students find that a study group works best only after all members have studied alone for a while. The group can offer a review or some clarification of topics. Sometimes group members write out test questions for each other. Writing and answering questions are good learning techniques.

Your Health and Lifestyle

Sleepiness or other physical or emotional discomfort may cause you to be inattentive in class. If the room is too hot or too cold, ask the instructor about it. It may be that the instructor is unaware of the problem. If you did not sleep well the night before class, it will be difficult to sit still and stay awake. Sit in a cool part of the room, near a bright window, and stay as attentive as possible. Try to get enough rest before class so that this will not be a problem again. If you are not feeling well, it may be better to ask to be excused from the class. You can arrange to borrow and copy notes from two people in the class. If you are getting ill, it is better to be home taking care of yourself for the first day or two rather than spreading your illness to the whole class. Nurses and nursing students need to be role models for a healthy lifestyle.

Thoughts About Attire and Time

As a student in the classroom, your clothing needs to be comfortable but conservative in style. When working in a health-care setting, your attire needs to be appropriate for the setting. In most cases, a clean and pressed set of scrubs is appropriate. Excess jewelry should not be worn. Hair should be clean and pulled back away from the face and shoulders. People tend to be more anxious than usual when they are sick. Although you will not usually interact with patients in the classroom, the conservative dress expectation applies to the nursing classroom. Dressing appropriately is an aspect of developing your professional personality.

Punctuality is an expectation of nursing students. People do have emergencies or oversleep and are late for class now and then. If this happens to you, go to class late rather than miss the class. When there is a break or at the end of class, go to your instructor and apologize. You do not have to give long explanations, just say you are sorry. If you know ahead of time that you might be late for class, tell the instructor in advance. It is courteous to be on time, but if you have to be late, it is best to be direct about it.

YOU AS A STUDENT IN THE CLINICAL AREA

When you are working in the clinical area as a student nurse, you are working under the licensure of a registered nurse (RN) who is acting as your clinical preceptor. You are given this privilege so that you can take the time to learn how to do nursing and be socialized into nursing as a profession. If you were working as a nursing assistant, you would be rushed and your day would be filled with responsibility. As a student, you are given the time to work through the things you are learning. You should take advantage of your clinical opportunities to learn all you can and practice the skills you have been taught.

The clinical area can be the most stressful place where you will need to function as a nurse. You may become tense or anxious in the clinical setting because you are dealing with real people who are quite ill. Everything about the care you give a sick person is crucial and places the necessity of knowledge from all four ways of knowing at the forefront of what you do. Your care must be ethical, aesthetic, and technically correct. While you are in the clinical area, you also are enhancing your personal way of knowing.

Preparing for Clinical Assignments

Your clinical instructor is there to help you, teach you, guide you, and supervise you. You need to be attentive to the instructor and keep him or her well informed about your patient. The instructor is responsible for all students and their patients and for clear and effective communication with the agency staff about patient care.

Dress

The type of clothing you need to wear will be explained to you in your student handbook or by your instructor. Remember to keep your attire neat and clean. If your style of dress is sloppy, your patients will expect that you will be sloppy about your patient care, too. Even if they are wrong, the thought will make them anxious, which is not therapeutic.

You should not use perfumed soap, shaving lotion, or cologne. People who are ill are sensitive to odors and may become nauseous or even short of breath because of cologne you are wearing. If you smoke or if you just sat next to someone who smokes, your clothing will pick up the smoke smell and that odor can make your patients feel ill. Most clinical facilities now require noticeable tattoos and piercings to be covered. Be especially careful about odors and your appearance on clinical days.

Being Well Prepared

You need to prepare well for your clinical day. Use your textbooks to review the procedures you expect to be doing. Even if you believe that you know the procedures, you need to study and review them. The clinical area is where all four ways of knowing come together to help you become a nurse. It is a rich learning experience. The textbook information becomes much more clear when you are thinking of it in terms of specific patients.

COMMUNICATION IN THE CLINICAL SETTING

As a future licensed nurse, you have a major responsibility to communicate effectively with all people necessary to provide the highest level of care to the patients in your charge.

Communication Principles for the Clinical Setting

While you are in a patient care area, ask only appropriate questions. You are encouraged to ask all possible questions you have about the patient for whom you are giving care, but do not ask questions about other patients. Sometimes a famous or

infamous person (e.g., an athletic star or a criminal) is admitted to the unit. If you are not giving care to that person, it is inappropriate and unprofessional for you to ask questions about him or her. It also is wrong for you to review the person's chart or look up information on the computer. This behavior is unethical (not an ethical way of knowing) and violates Health Insurance Portability and Accountability Act policies and in most facilities is a reason for dismissal.

Be respectful in your communication with others. Treat physicians and nursing assistants with equal respect (aesthetic knowing). Treating patients and their families with respect is essential and should quickly become automatic.

Do not hesitate to find out what you don't know (technical way of knowing). This may be information about a drug you are asked to give or what laboratory results might mean. Don't pretend you know things and through this behavior possibly harm a patient. One of the principles of being a professional is being a lifelong learner. You should find out what you don't know or obtain correct information about which you are unsure; this could be summarized as "get to the truth!" The importance of what you do in the clinical area cannot be overemphasized.

Confidentiality

The things you learn about your patients are personal and confidential. You can discuss them with your faculty member and your classmates as a learning experience, but you need to be careful about where and how loudly you are talking. It is a breach of professional ethics to ask a patient personal questions that do not pertain to the person's health care. If you write notes about your patient anywhere other than the clinical record, do not use the patient's name. You could use initials on your notes to distinguish between your assigned patients. Tear up or shred your notes before discarding them.

In small communities, even with no use of names, other people can easily identify the person about whom you are talking. If you describe an 18-year-old football player who was in an automobile accident and was crying because he fears his girlfriend is pregnant, you can be sure that everyone within hearing distance will identify the people involved even if no names are used. Do not be careless. There are legal, ethical, caring, and professional issues involved here, and you need to be

LPN in appropriate attire.

mindful of them all. It is your professional obligation to maintain confidentiality. If you have questions, take them to your instructor for clarification.

REFLECTIVE THINKING

During your last clinical day, did you observe any breeches of patient confidentiality? Did the nurse talk about patients at the nurse's desk or in the elevator? Did nurses share information about patients who were not in their care? Write your observations in your class notebook.

Honesty

Honesty is an expectation of nursing students and nursing professionals that goes beyond the normal expectation of other people. In many social situations, if you do not know the exact answer, people may think it is all right for you to guess. If someone asks whether the local pizza place is open late Saturday night, many people will take a stand and say yes or no, even if they are not sure. A nurse needs to be sure of any answer. If you guess about the hours of the pizza place, people will expect that you also will guess about the hours of the hospital pharmacy or the side effects of a medication. Do not bluff or guess about anything. If you are guessing, say it is just a guess. You need to be known as a meticulously honest person.

Your choice of profession may have brought you into an entirely new setting. That choice may be demanding new behaviors and even different kinds of thinking from you. How can you adapt? What beliefs do you need to hang on to? What behaviors can you change without losing your own identity? All of these questions, along with all that you are trying to learn while meeting your personal responsibilities, involve all four of Carper's (1978) ways of knowing. Try to learn to think of what you are doing within the framework of those four components. I assure you it will be helpful.

SUCCESSFUL STUDY STRATEGIES

I recognize that students lead busy lives. As one of the few fortunate enough to be in a nursing program, you need to make school your priority; to do so takes time. I have advised many students who are deeply concerned about their inability to

do well in a class. The most frequently stated reason for not doing well is that they do not have time. Most of the students who come to me work full-time, attend school full-time, and have families. I understand how important those responsibilities are. But this is your chance to become an LPN. It is an opportunity that does not come to everyone and may not come to you a second time.

Ask your extended family whether they can help you in any way. Could they take some responsibility for the children or assist you by buying books? Talk to your spouse or partner about arrangements that can be made so that you need to work only part-time for the year you are in school. If you are a single parent, you may need to look into school loans. If you don't have a car, develop a plan for getting to school and have a backup plan so that you can get there every day. Being a successful student takes time, and you need to work with those who love you and respect what you are doing to give you the time you need. Sacrifices made now can reap tremendous rewards later in your life.

Time Management

Discussing the time required by your school and studies with your family and friends may help them to realize that they need to excuse you for a while from at least some of your usual routines. You may be able to take some of your courses during the summer, giving you more free time in the fall and spring. Talk with your employer about schedule changes. You may need to change jobs to meet your student responsibilities.

Setting Priorities

Setting priorities takes a great deal of thought and focus on problem-solving. You may need to develop a list of temporary priorities. Getting high grades may take precedence over some other things that you like to do. You may have to give up movies or some favorite TV shows in favor of study time. You may have to give up some things that are even more important to you, but if it is just for 1 or 2 years, you need to consider it. Education often requires sacrifice.

It is not a good idea to reduce your sleeping time. Do not stay up late to study or do written assignments. Make a plan to have regular study time when you are alert and able to concentrate. Schedule frequent study times during the week to remain current in your assignments. Sleep is important for your physical and emotional health as well as your learning abilities.

Developing Test-Taking Skills

Your presence in a nursing program proves that you have successfully demonstrated test-taking skills. It is not an easy task to be admitted to a nursing program, and it is even more challenging to remain there. The stakes are higher in nursing school; the tests may be more complex, and the content is challenging. Perhaps you have more responsibilities than you had in high school, such as having a spouse, children, or a full-time job. All of these things affect your ability to take tests successfully. Subsequent sections in this chapter give you information to assist you in preparing for and passing tests.

Academic or Honor Codes

All schools have an academic code or code of honor that addresses the issues of academic freedom, honesty, and integrity. One way to be prepared for test taking at your college or vocational school is to identify the principles expressed in the school's academic code or code of honor. Ask your instructor where to find the code, and take the time to locate and read it. Perhaps discussing the academic code could be a class activity. If that is not possible, talk to classmates about it to ensure you understand exactly what the code means. You now are part of the higher education system, and you need to be both aware and supportive of the standards that exist for you.

Attend Class and Do the Reading

Attending class and doing the reading may seem too obvious to mention, but they are not. You need to be in class to get to know the instructor and how he or she thinks. Understanding the general thinking process of the instructor helps you pinpoint areas of priority and ways to think about those priorities that will be on a test. There are other advantages of going to class. It is a characteristic of a good student, someone who is motivated and interested. The information given by the instructor reinforces and clarifies what you are studying. It generally is fun to get to know your classmates, and, most important, it is an optimal way to learn.

Reading the assignments is a time-consuming aspect of studying. Unless you read, however, you will not learn the material or know what will be on a test. I suggest that you plan time to read each week. If you read early in the week, your mind will have time to "percolate" the information you have read. *Percolate* means that the ideas have time to penetrate or seep into your brain. Do you remember the old percolator coffee pots? They often are used on camping trips where I live. The water goes up the stem of the percolator to the coffee beans, where it is diffused over the coffee. The new ideas you learn in class and through the reading need time to percolate. This concept makes a strong case for not cramming in your reading the night before class. When you do that, there is no time for percolating, which encourages critical thinking. By cramming just before class or a test, you are missing out on a great opportunity to learn.

Create Study Tools

Few people can attend class, read the text, and do well on the examinations without having specialized study tools. The truth is that it generally takes more than attending class and reading to be successful. When you take the time to create study tools that are effective for you, the entire study and test process becomes much easier.

Flash Cards

Flash cards are a commonly used study tool. You should always have blank cards with you to write down new and creative ideas. You can use this method in class to write down new information or anything that "sounds" like a test question. Sometimes the instructor will say, "This will be on the test." Be sure to write the information that follows on a card. Or the instructor may make a comment

Some learning takes "percolating" time to master.

that you recognize as something that is a priority for her or him. (How do you know the instructor's priorities? You go to class and listen.) Write those ideas down.

REFLECTIVE THINKING

In your class notebook, write the points of your school's academic or honor code that interest you the most. What aspect of the code do you support? Is there something you either do not understand or disagree with as it is written? Be prepared to discuss the academic or honor code for your school in class.

Flash cards are crucial to use while you do your reading. You should think of flash cards as portable test questions. Use flash cards to record anything new, things you don't understand and need to ask about after class or look up in the library, formulas for drug administration, definitions, theories, key words, and sample problems. You can use notecards to make regular flash cards; there are programs online that allow you to make electronic flash cards to use on your phone or other electronic devices. Take the cards with you wherever you go and pull them out to study. You may find time while riding the bus, waiting in line, or between classes. If your flash cards are well thought out and you master the information on them, you will not need to worry about a test.

Study Checklists

Some students find study checklists useful in preparing for an examination. A study checklist is not a review sheet for a test but rather a "to-do" list. Checklists contain the briefest possible description of each item to be studied. The list should include the required reading, listing chapters and page numbers; the concepts you need to memorize; and the definitions, nursing theories, and formulas you need to know. Check the list items off when you have learned them. When everything is checked off, you are ready for a test.

Mind Maps

A mind map is a study method that allows you to test yourself by creating an outline, or map, for the information you need to master. It allows you to

recognize what you do and do not know before a test because you create it from memory. A sample mind map is provided. It shows one way to list the major topics or content you have been studying. This is done without reference to any of your study aids. When you are through, check the material to see what you missed. If you need to review a specific content area, it will show on the mind map.

How to Review for a Test

Being a successful student takes time. In addition to attending class, doing all the reading, preparing and studying flash cards, using checklists, and drawing mind maps, you still must review for an examination. Although flash cards and mind maps are forms of review, there are additional strategies you should know about.

Daily review is done with your reading, class notes, and flash cards. You should be adding to your flash cards while you read, then spend time reviewing them on your own a few minutes every day. You should allot 1 hour per class for weekly reviews—structured time in which you focus on nothing but the week's material for that class. When a subject is complex, as nursing classes tend to be, the brain requires more time to establish thinking patterns regarding the new material. The weekly reviews should include assigned reading and lecture notes or videos, flash cards, and mind maps.

Major reviews generally are conducted the week before a major examination or finals week. Many students conduct this review with other students. You may want to try this type of study group to decide whether it is helpful for you. A comprehensive study session may last 3 to 5 hours. The study session is a time to strengthen and deepen understanding of the concepts you have been studying. Determine which study strategies are most beneficial to you. Talk out loud to yourself or others, reread something you are unsure of, go over your flash cards one more time, and do complete mind maps. If you're working with a group, you may want to ask each other practice questions. All of these strategies help. The night before an examination, take a break. Go to a movie or out to dinner. Go to bed early and sleep well because you are prepared. Do not cram all night or get up early to review. If you are prepared, you do not need to do any more than go into the examination room and take the test.

Mind Map on Critical Thinking

Mind map of a critical thinking chapter. *(Source: Anderson, M. A. [2000]. To be a nurse [p. 145]. Philadelphia: F. A. Davis.)*

 ## UNDERSTANDING TEST QUESTIONS

When I went to high school, I simply took whatever test was given to me and hoped I did well; I had no test-taking strategy. That changed when I went to college; it had to if I wanted to be successful. This section gives you the best information possible regarding how to take specific types of examinations.

Multiple-Choice Tests

Nursing school faculty generally give multiple-choice tests to give you as much experience as possible with this format because multiple-choice questions are used on the National Council Licensure Examination for Practical Nurses (NCLEX®-PN). There are some important things to know about a multiple-choice examination that will help you improve your overall score. Noting the strategies presented here and practicing them will eventually help you become more knowledgeable and confident when you take the NCLEX-PN. There are specific strategies for taking the NCLEX-PN examination, but you shouldn't worry about them now. Instead, focus on being good at the tests you are taking this semester as a way to improve your overall test-taking ability.

Most multiple-choice test questions are written to a specific formula. The following is a sample multiple-choice question:

1. You are assigned to obtain informed consent from a patient who is 78 years old and who has had a severe stroke. The patient cannot respond, but you sense that he can hear you. What strategy will you use to obtain informed consent?
   a. Because the patient cannot discuss the issue, prepare the form as a DNR, have the patient sign an X, and witness it for him.
   b. Talk privately with the daughter who comes in on your shift. Record her decision on the form. Have her sign the form for her father.
   c. Ask the social worker to call a family meeting. Hold the meeting in the father's room with the social worker conducting the meeting.
   d. Notify the RN to take care of the problem.

This is a classic multiple-choice question. Do you know the answer? The question is designed to require you to think critically. Let me explain the anatomy of a multiple-choice question.

The *stem* of a multiple-choice question is the information that follows the number of the test question. In this question, the stem is "You are assigned to obtain informed consent from a patient who is 78 years old and who has had a severe stroke. The patient cannot respond, but you sense he can hear you. What strategy will you use to obtain informed consent?"

Read the stem carefully. It is important that you understand what is asked in the stem and what information the stem contains. At first reading, our sample question seems to be asking about informed consent. But as you read on, you learn that the question is specifically about doing the ethical thing in terms of obtaining informed consent for this man. This is true even though the word *ethics* is not used in the question. To be a critical thinker, you have to integrate information from two different areas of the ethics chapter. Read the stem carefully so that you don't go to the responses with the wrong idea. You also need to recognize there is only one right answer. Some tests want you to make more than one response. It also is important to note that the word *except* or *only* is not in the stem. If you focus on learning to read question stems clearly now, you will be doing them automatically and quickly by the end of the year.

Most multiple-choice questions have four responses. Some instructors may use three or five responses. Even if you are sure of the answer, read all of the responses carefully because a critical thinker always does. It is important for you to examine or assess the question carefully before you make a response. Most multiple-choice questions have an answer that is obviously the wrong answer. Which one is it in the sample question?

Response *A* is incorrect. By simply applying ethical thinking to this response, you can see that it is the wrong thing to do because it is absolutely against the basic principle of informed consent.

There should be two responses that are "almost right." They have a component of what could be a right answer, but they are not entirely correct. By finding and eliminating the obviously wrong and the "almost" right responses, you can choose the correct answer. What are the two "almost right" answers in our sample question?

The almost right answers are *B* and *D*. The action in item *B* is also unethical because it does not involve the patient in a meaningful way, which is the purpose of informed consent. The action in item *D* is not wrong, but it is incomplete because it doesn't resolve the issue. The correct answer to our question is *C*.

Some instructors use "all of the above" or "none of the above" as the final response in the possible response choices. Always look at such responses carefully; they generally are incorrect responses. Do not assume this to always be true, however. Use your critical thinking skills and read each response carefully, cross out the obvious wrong answer, find the two most likely to be correct, and then trust in your excellent study skills to assist you in determining which answer is correct.

Some multiple-choice questions do not require critical thinking. Instead, they simply ask you to recall information rather than apply knowledge. An example of such a knowledge question is, "What is a bed bath?" An example of a critical thinking question on the same topic is, "In situation 'X,' what type of bath would you give? State your rationale." Be prepared for either knowledge or critical thinking questions on any test.

True-or-False Questions

True-or-false questions are easy for instructors to write, and most students like them because there is a 50% chance of getting the right answer. Usually these questions are clearly written, and you have to rely on your knowledge to determine whether the information is correct or incorrect. To pass a true-or-false examination, you need to know the content. The following is a sample true-or-false question:

1. Florence Nightingale was a British nurse born in Florence, Italy.

Unless you have taken a nursing history class, I do not expect you to know the answer to this question. It is true. Florence was conceived and born during her wealthy parents' 2-year honeymoon; they were in Florence, Italy, when she was born.

When taking a true-or-false examination, the key to success, in addition to thorough studying, is to read the question carefully. What if the question had been written as:

1. Florence Nightingale was a German nurse who was born in Florence, Italy.

You now know this is the wrong answer. But if you had read it first, would you have been tempted to mark it as true? Suppose you knew where Florence was born and in your mind you remembered something about Germany (that is where she went to school). Careful, unhurried reading will help you get true-or-false questions correct.

As you are carefully reading the question, look for key words such as *some, all,* and *always.* They change the meaning of the question and should be considered. Ask your instructor whether there is a penalty for guessing. If there is not, answer every question even if you don't know the answer. You do have a 50% chance of getting it correct. Don't let a statement that seems to be true confuse you with what you know. Study well and answer the questions with confidence.

Completion and Matching Questions

Completion questions are those that require you to fill in the blank, as follows:

1. Florence Nightingale was born in: _____

_____

Usually one or two words are all that is required to fill in the blank. The question is not a short essay, so keep your response brief and specific. Look for hints about the type of answer wanted by carefully reading the statement. For example, should the response be singular or plural? Generally you either know the answer to a completion question or you don't. It is difficult to make a guess.

Matching test questions are questions that have two columns and require you to match concepts or definitions. Read both columns through completely before making any matches. Then reread the left column and find the match in the right column. To make your next selection more efficient, cross out the answers you have used so that you don't have to consider them again.

Essay Questions

Essay examinations are the most challenging for instructors to grade. The grade is subjective, so do all you can to assist the instructor grading your paper. The following strategies will assist you in being successful.

- **Write** so that it is **easy to read** your answer. Think of the number of papers the instructor is grading and how tired he or she may become.
- Use **ink.** In some cases, you may be using a computerized testing system, so you will be typing your responses.
- Write on **one side of the paper** only. If using a computerized testing system, be sure to double-space your information.
- **Read the directions for the test questions carefully!** The directions explain the number of points assigned for each question and provide other information that is important to the person grading the test. *Follow the directions.*
- **Compare** the number of questions with the time allowed for the test. Then determine how much time you have for each question, assuming that the points for each question are the same.
- **Start** with the questions you know best; this will give you confidence for the rest of the test.
- Before you write, **make a quick outline.** An outline helps you stay focused on what is important and assists you in avoiding overwriting.
- Now you are ready to write, **so get to the point!** Don't write an introduction or use flowery statements. One way to get to the point is to use part of the question in your answer.
- **Be brief and use pertinent information.** Write as if the person grading your paper were tired and bored. Perhaps your paper is the last one being graded. Just get to the important part of the answer and state your position and ideas clearly.

Box 6.1 contains words you should understand as they relate to examinations. These words often are part of the instructions given in an essay question. If you don't know the meaning of the

---

Box 6.1 Words to Understand When Taking Examinations

- **Analyze:** Break into separate parts and discuss, then examine or interpret each part.
- **Compare:** Look at two or more ideas or concepts by identifying their similarities and differences.
- **Contrast:** Explain what makes the difference between two or more ideas.
- **Define:** Give the exact meaning; make your definition brief.
- **Describe:** Create a picture with words by giving a detailed account.
- **Discuss:** Debate or argue the pros and cons of an issue.
- **Summarize:** Give a brief, condensed account; make a strong conclusion; avoid unnecessary detail.

words, it is hard to write a correct answer. Take some time to learn them.

MANAGING TEST ANXIETY

If you are experiencing feelings of stress before or during a test, you will not be doing your best on the test. There are ways to combat test anxiety, one of which is to be well prepared; this already has been discussed. Review the following approaches for managing test anxiety.

Psychological First-Aid Kit for Test Preparation

Negative self-talk can be a test-taking stress. A common scenario for negative self-talk is for you to be trying to study yet the negative self-talk continually intrudes on your thoughts, and you are unable to study at all. The way to stop this from happening is to say to yourself, "Stop!" This is an example of using self-discipline to stop the unproductive thinking. It takes more than one time to get the negative self-talk to stop. Every time the negative thoughts come to your mind, you need to say, "Stop!" and go back to your studying. Changing one's behavior is challenging but worthwhile.

Another idea for your first-aid kit is the 10-minute to 2-hour vacation. I have gone to school most of my life, either part-time or full-time, and I learned early on that the luxurious, 2-week vacation was not going to happen while I was in school. So I learned to enjoy "mini-vacations."

The 10-minute vacation allows one to daydream. I have an active imagination and have no trouble thinking about what it would be like to be a cliff jumper in Borneo or Amelia Earhart. What was she thinking all alone in the sky? It is fun for me to do that for a brief period. When my 10 minutes are up, I can return to my studying and make great progress. A 10-minute vacation is helpful because when I fill my mind with pleasant or questioning thoughts, I leave no room for anxiety or worry. It is a restful event for my mind, and when the rest is over, I am able to work again.

The 2-hour vacation often is a movie. I am a movie buff and really enjoy going to the theater. I find it is an effective stress reliever. You will do better on a test if you can relax while you study and prepare for it.

If you don't do well on a test, consider the following:

1. Einstein's parents thought he was mentally challenged. He spoke haltingly until age 9, and as he grew older, he answered questions only after giving them a great deal of thought. He was advised to drop out of high school because the teacher thought he would never amount to anything. My favorite story about Einstein is when someone asked him for his telephone number, he went to a telephone book and looked it up. Then he commented that he never cluttered his mind with information that was recorded elsewhere.
2. Jonas Salk developed the polio vaccine. To do so, he spent 98% of his time documenting the things that didn't work (his failures) until he found the process that did work and essentially eradicated a devastating disease from the planet.

Physiological First-Aid Kit for Test Taking

Before taking the test, you need to ensure that you get a good night's sleep (no cramming and no worrying because you are so well prepared). Eat a nourishing, high-protein breakfast, and do something different, such as driving to school a different way. If you live close enough to the school, perhaps you could walk. Don't get to the test early because being around all the other students generally causes anxiety. You don't need their anxiety. Arrive at the test in time to walk into the room, no earlier. Then take the test just as you have prepared to do.

It is wonderful to fill one's mind with new and exciting information. It is even more wonderful to be rewarded for what you learn by getting good grades and, more important, by being able to give quality patient care based on a sound knowledge base. To move forward in your career, you need to study hard and learn to enjoy it. You also need to learn to write effectively to be successful.

WRITING SUCCESSFUL PAPERS

Being able to use the English language meaningfully is crucial to "getting things done" for patients and their families. Also, a measure of an educated person is the ability to read and write. Writing is one of the things I love to do, so I am better at it than other things. Because I love to write, I have done it a great deal and have learned to do it well. As a nurse, you will spend 85% to 90% of your time communicating verbally and through the written word. If writing and speaking have not been "favorites" of yours, you may want to consider working them into the things you like to do so that you can continue to develop your skills.

Basics of Writing

I have read and graded at least "a million" student papers during my lifetime and it can be challenging work. Students who know how to write properly always get better grades than students who do not know basic grammar and writing skills. A student who has learned how to write can express ideas clearly and make a more convincing argument. These are two things you need to be able to do well as a nurse.

Types of Papers

You will be asked to write two basic types of papers in nursing school: formal and informal papers. Most of the papers you write will be informal. You are likely to write many informal papers before you graduate. An informal paper is one that does not require extensive use of the *Publication Manual of the American Psychological Association* (APA manual). The APA manual is a book of guidelines for professionals. There are several types of writing style manuals. The APA manual is referenced here because it is the one most commonly used in nursing. An informal paper could be a chapter summary or a book report. It could be a written description of your first day in the clinical area as a student nurse; it could be on any topic the instructor thinks is important for you to express your thoughts about.

Do you remember what I said at the beginning of this section? It was that I love to write, so I do it often. I also mentioned that the more I write, the better I become at it. The same is true for you. Your instructor may assign a weekly informal paper that is a reflection of your thoughts on the nursing care you gave that week. In it you could practice using correct grammar and putting your thoughts on paper in a clear and understandable way. You can also use the Reflective Thinking exercises throughout the book to practice your writing skills. Doing a writing assignment with this as your focus is as important to your nursing career as learning to give intramuscular injections.

Using original reference sources is the only way to write a formal paper properly.

Writing, like giving injections, is something you will do almost every day you work. Use school to perfect your writing skills.

Principles of Writing

The principles of writing a paper are effective habits to develop and are worth your time and attention. Remember your goal: maximum learning and maximum grade. The following principles will help you achieve this goal.

Write Your Papers Early and Review Them

The first principle of good paper writing is to write all papers early so that you and others can review them. If you are writing a paper the night or even the weekend before it is due, you are cheating yourself of the learning you deserve and possibly a good grade. Start papers early in the semester so that you have time to maximize your learning.

The way to improve your writing skills and your knowledge is to have someone else review your work and then review it yourself after taking a break from it for a short time. It may also be helpful to use the writing center on your campus if one is available. Remember when I told you about ideas being able to percolate like the coffee in old coffee pots? This is an example of that concept. While a classmate is reviewing your paper, your mind has time to percolate over the information you wrote, and when you get the paper back, there will be things you want to improve by rewriting.

I recognize that some of you may be amused by what I have to say. You might be thinking that you're lucky to get your papers in on time, let alone organize and plan when you will write and review them. This often is how students feel when they are caught between school assignments and work or family commitments. It takes a great deal of organization to work out such problems.

Make an Outline

Many people write without an outline and consequently have a disorganized and unclear paper (not a good way to get a good grade). An outline may seem restrictive to many novice writers, but it is the very thing that keeps you headed in the right direction and gets you there in a meaningful way. My strong recommendation is to write an outline. Outlines organize your thinking and can be a time saver.

Formula for Writing a Paper

Writing a paper is not as simple as it sounds. There is a formula to follow that I discuss later in the chapter, but it is important for you to recognize that if you have gathered information and done your research, started early so that there is time to percolate your thinking and review your paper, and have written a clear outline, you have done the hardest work. Now it is time to write, delete, revise, proof, polish, and submit. I use the acronym *W-DRPPS* and remember it by thinking of it as "writing-drops." The idea is not to "drop" any part of the writing process. If your life is so busy that you can't do one or more steps in the writing process, you have "dropped" one. It is best to use all the steps of the formula:

- **W**rite
- **D**elete
- **R**evise
- **P**roof
- **P**olish
- **S**ubmit

Potential Problems in All Writing

There are three serious potential problems that can occur in writing of any type—the use of sexist language, plagiarism, and paraphrasing without correctly citing the original reference. You need to understand these problems and avoid them in your writing.

Sexism is an outcome of the lack of empowerment of women. Because of this lack of empowerment, much of the common language used in speaking and writing in the United States is biased toward men. Spend some time reading magazines and books, and you will encounter the vocabulary I mean. Avoiding the use of sexist language is challenging because it requires changing long-held habits of thinking, speaking, and writing. Some common sexist terms are *mankind, chairman,* and *policeman* and colloquialisms such as referring to both men and women as "guys." The following concepts may help you write in a nonsexist style:

1. Learn to use gender-neutral terms. Why does a driver need to be identified as either male or female? Why is a doctor identified as a lady doctor? Why can't she just be a doctor? Don't use the terms *little lady* or *girls* when referring to women; these terms are demeaning. Use *police officer* instead of policeman, *humankind* instead of mankind, and *chairperson* instead of chairman.

2. Use examples that include both genders. When you are writing, you may use stories to make a point or illustrate a concept. When you do, use both genders in the story. List the accomplishments of men and women. Make the physician a woman and the nurse a man to assist people in changing their paradigm of thinking.

3. Use plural forms of nouns and verbs. This concept saved me hours of struggling to get the gender issue right. In the past, male pronouns were used (i.e., *he, him,* and *his*) to represent all of humankind. An example is, "The physician has many instruments on his surgical table." To correct this, you can write: "Physicians have many instruments on their surgical tables." It is much easier to make everything plural.

4. Do not use sexually stereotypical words or concepts. Examples are "sissy," "momma's boy," "man-eater," "old lady," "powder puff," or "tomboy." Such words and phrases simply encourage sexist thinking.

5. Use parallel names. For example, instead of "President Barack Obama and his wife," use "President Barack Obama and First Lady Michelle Obama" so as not to devalue the woman as a nonentity.

Nonsexist writing is simply one more thing to learn while you are in school. As you write papers, you need to be aware of this concept and read for sexist errors as you do for punctuation errors.

Another problem in writing is plagiarism. This problem can get you expelled from school or sued or both. *Plagiarism* is using another person's words, thoughts, ideas, and expressions without giving appropriate and complete credit. Suppose you found a great chapter on diabetes mellitus in the library and copied from it for a one-page paper you needed to complete? It was a different book from what everyone else was using, so you thought the instructor would not notice. What is wrong with this picture?

Plagiarizing is stealing, which is why it is something for which you can be expelled from school. Instructors also can be terminated for plagiarizing. Plagiarism is a form of academic dishonesty and can damage not only your reputation but the reputation of the school (Reisig & Bain, 2016). To avoid plagiarism, give appropriate credit to the person whose work you use, adapt, or modify. If you have any questions regarding what constitutes plagiarism, consult your instructor.

Paraphrasing is restating another's ideas or thoughts using a different form. If you paraphrase someone, you also must cite the complete reference used. You should build your own thinking on the thinking of others. This is a normal way to learn and progress intellectually. I am simply recommending that you do it with integrity by accurately citing and referencing all works you use.

Properly citing references is an important part of the writing process. When citing information, it is best to use the original research source rather than citing from a textbook that addresses the same information. This ensures the information you are including in your paper is accurate and you are using the correct citation. Most nursing programs will use the APA manual to guide citations and referencing. Your instructors will instruct you on which format to use to properly cite and reference your papers.

CONCLUSION

Now you are ready to proceed into the world of tests and writing projects. If you have paid attention to the information in this chapter, you are capable of proceeding with confidence. If you have problems, go to your faculty person for suggestions and seek out the student learning center. It may have a different name on your campus, but there should be some type of support system for you. My best wishes for your success!

REAL-WORLD CASE STUDY

■ Melinda Sandavol and Sally Fredrickson have been friends since high school. They shared everything, including dating the same boy at the same time during their junior year! While they were in high school, they were busy being socialites and going to dances instead of studying. They both had part-time jobs, and they were determined not to allow that to interfere with their play time. There was little time left for homework. They found their classes easy and got good grades with minimal need to study.

Both friends applied for admittance into the LPN program at the local community college and were thrilled when they were accepted. They played hard the summer before school started (they each live at home with their parents and have part-time jobs), and they went to school ready to discover what college was like. They were bitterly disappointed, however, to find that they were failing their nursing classes by midterm of the first semester. They had skipped some classes and worked instead of studying. They were unprepared for their tests and were shocked when they found they did poorly. That was not what had happened to them in high school!

Their nursing instructor referred them to the study resource center on campus. You have been assigned to work with both young women to salvage their first semester and get them on the right study track. What are you going to do to help them? Write the solution to the case study in your class notebook, and be prepared to discuss it in class.

Key Points

- Know yourself and understand the nursing way of knowing (aesthetically, empirically, ethically, and personally). These different components of knowing are what make a nurse truly effective and able to provide transpersonal caring.

- Identify your preferred learning style —visual, auditory, or kinesthetic—to best utilize it. Being organized and developing good study techniques around your learning style will help you master the content. In addition to developing and practicing good study habits, it is important to take care of yourself by eating right and getting enough sleep so that you can do your best in class and clinicals. Practicing good self-care will keep you healthy and mentally sharp, which will help you study and test better.

- Practice good professional behaviors by being punctual and prepared for class and clinicals. Make sure to dress professionally for clinicals and avoid perfumes or colognes, which patients may be sensitive to. Maintaining confidentiality and being honest at all times is essential for the nursing professional, both ethically and legally.

- Create study tools and develop a test-taking strategy based on the different types of questions. Make sure to review for tests often and regularly, and avoid cramming. This will help information "percolate" and become clear in your mind. It is also important to learn how to manage your stress before and during testing in order to perform well.

- Develop strong writing skills, including good grammar and spelling. Start writing papers early and use an outline for organization. It will make writing easier if you become familiar and competent with the APA style of writing. In addition, it is important to avoid sexist language, plagiarism, and paraphrasing without proper citation when writing.

ANSWERS TO REAL-WORLD CASE STUDY

Everything you need to know to help these young women be successful in their test taking is in this chapter. You simply need to pick the solutions that you think would be the most helpful to them and support them in fulfilling them.

Because these young women are right out of high school and seem inexperienced in college classes, I would strongly emphasize they attend class and read the material as their first step to poor test score recovery. It will take more than a mere suggestion for these students to change their test scores. Remember the chapter on motivation? They need to come to an understanding of how important it is for them to complete school if they really want careers as LPNs. Perhaps you could have an experienced LPN meet with them for 30 minutes or so in your office. That may encourage them to renew their motivation to become nurses. Spend additional time talking to them about strategies to increase their study time. Because both women are single and living at home, perhaps they could quit work for the rest of the semester. Would their parents support them in their financial needs until the next term? They need motivation, time, and study skills to be successful.

If you are able to assist the young women with motivation and time, proceed to the study skills in the chapter. Because they are doing so poorly and do not have a great deal of time to make a significant change, I would call their nursing instructor to see what the areas of emphasis are for the next test. What types of test questions will be used, what is the content, how much time will be allowed for the test, and is there a penalty for guessing? When you know these answers, work with the women closely to prepare them for the next test and each future test until the end of the semester. It will be a challenging, but I hope successful adventure.

REVIEW QUESTIONS

1. As a student, you find that pictures and drawing mind maps help you understand and remember the information from class. What type of learning style are you most likely exhibiting?
   1. Auditory
   2. Visual
   3. Kinesthetic
   4. Written

2. Carper (1978) described what four types of knowing as essential for nurses?
   1. Aesthetic, empathetic, ethical, personal
   2. Empirical, ethical, personal, transcendental
   3. Aesthetic, empirical, ethical, perpetual
   4. Aesthetic, empirical, ethical, personal

3. The student reads the chapter, mind maps the information, and participates in a study group during the week prior to the test. This represents which idea?
   1. Empirical knowing
   2. Kinesthetic learning
   3. Percolated thinking
   4. Personal knowing

4. Your neighbor shares some personal health information with you because she knows you are in nursing school. What should you do with that information?
   1. Call her physician
   2. Speak with her husband
   3. Keep it confidential
   4. Provide for privacy

5. Which of the following is not an example of sexist language?
   1. Chairperson
   2. Sissy
   3. Mankind
   4. Policeman

References

American Psychological Association. (2010). *Publication manual of the American Psychological Association* (6th ed.). Washington, DC: Author.

Beischel, K. P. (2013). Variables affecting learning in a simulation experience: A mixed methods study. *Western Journal of Nursing Research, 35*(2), 226–247. doi:10.1177/0193945911408444

Carper, B. (1978). Fundamental patterns of knowing in nursing. *Advances in Nursing Science, 1*(1), 13–23.

Chinn, P. L., & Kramer, M. K. (2015). *Integrated theory and knowledge development in nursing* (8th ed.). St. Louis: Elsevier.

Reisig, M. D., & Bain, S. N. (2016). University legitimacy and student compliance with academic dishonesty codes: A partial test of the process-based model of self-regulation. *Criminal Justice and Behavior, 43*(1), 83–101. doi:10.1177/0093854815611165

Web Resources

APA Style www.apastyle.org

Purdue Online Writing Lab http://owl.english.purdue.edu/owl/resource/560/01/

7

The Importance of Critical Thinking

KEY TERMS

Brainstorming
Serendipity
Thorough thinking

CHAPTER CONCEPT

Patient-Centered Care

LEARNING OUTCOMES

1. Define critical thinking.
2. Discuss the importance of developing critical thinking skills.
3. Demonstrate the skills of a creative thinker.

Creativity comes from "Action out of the center of one's own experience" coupled with the responsibility to receive both consequence and happiness.

—Knodal

The term *critical thinking* may be new to you. Perhaps you are wondering how critical thinking differs from just plain thinking. Being a critical thinker is the hallmark of being an educated person. People who do not think critically generally are obedient to what is asked of them; they consider neither the consequences of their actions nor alternatives. Living in a modern society, we are presented with unlimited choices about who to be, what to buy, and what to do. We have to make decisions, and so we must learn the skills of critical thinking (Pitt, Powis, Levett-Jones, & Hunter, 2015)

In school, you are given many opportunities to develop and use critical thinking skills. When you register for your classes, write a paper, make an oral presentation, or simply think through a problem, you are participating in school-related critical thinking activities. You may pick the most boring class on campus, give an unsatisfactory oral presentation, or say something awkward in a nursing class, but you will learn from each experience and use this knowledge to make better decisions in the future. Learning critical thinking skills so that you can apply them to clinical nursing should be a powerful motivation for you to learn them well. As a nurse, you will use the process of critical thinking to facilitate clinical reasoning, clinical judgment, and decision making (Zuriguel Perez et al., 2015). You need critical thinking ability to be able to think through a patient emergency or other patient-related problems. If you don't have critical thinking abilities, there is a high probability that you will harm a patient.

WHAT IS CRITICAL THINKING?

You are taking care of an older patient ready to be discharged from your hospital who will require daily dressing changes as well as the coordination of multiple medications. When his spouse comes to take him home, you notice that she has severe arthritis in her hands. When giving her the discharge papers to sign, she states, "Show me where to sign. I can't see very well." The charge nurse told you this patient is ready to go home, but you are concerned that your patient will not have the support at home he will need to manage his dressing changes and medications. You recognize that your patient is going to need additional resources to meet his health needs, so you speak with the patient to see whether he has other family in the area who can assist with his care. You also consult with the social worker and charge nurse to see whether your patient would qualify for follow-up care through a home care agency. Finally, you do some research to find other community resources available to assist your patient.

By asking questions and looking for alternatives, you find out that the patient has an adult son who is willing to assist his father. You help the family make arrangements for home care to do the daily dressing changes and monitor his medication schedule. There is also a community organization that will send a volunteer to assist your patient with his personal care. You now feel comfortable discharging your patient. This is an example of critical thinking.

People demonstrate *critical thinking* when they show the ability (1) to think beyond what has been said or shown to them, (2) to consider options related to the information they have received, and (3) to evaluate and make decisions based on multiple sources of information. Do you make mental connections? Forge links in your mind? Go beyond the given? See patterns, relationships, and context? Such mental abilities can be learned, making critical thinking a normal part of your thought process.

In nursing school, you learn about medications and you learn about the individuality of people. If you are unable to think of alternatives for a patient who is having a serious drug reaction based on his or her individual metabolism, the patient will suffer from your inability to integrate information, which is one aspect of critical thinking (Box 7.1). Critical thinking is much more than knowing the facts to pass a test. It is knowing the facts and being able to apply them accurately, with an awareness of personhood for each individual. Being able to think critically is one attribute of a competent nurse.

REFLECTIVE THINKING

Think of a time when you were a critical thinker. The experience could have been when you were a child, new parent, or a nursing assistant. It was a time when you thought "outside of the box." What happened to you when you thought the problem or concern through and arrived at a place different from any place you had gone to before in your mind? Describe the experience and how you felt about it. Be prepared to share it in classroom discussion.

Critical thinking allows you to move beyond the here and now and build new realities. Do you remember studying Christopher Columbus? Among other things, he had the courage to sail to the edge of a flat world. We now know the world is round, but Columbus didn't. He had a vision, however; he had listened to other sailors and studied maps, and he critically examined all of the information he received. Then he sailed on a world that was round instead of flat. Other erroneous thoughts that have occurred throughout history include the following:

1. "Bleeding" people will make them better.
2. Illnesses result from an imbalance in the four vital fluids: blood, phlegm, water, and bile.
3. Blood originated in the liver where it was mixed with air.
4. Fingernails continue to grow after you die.
5. Going outside in the cold will make you sick.

As a student nurse, you are not spending hours each week learning to "bleed" patients because someone looked critically at the procedure and found it did not work. Critical thinking is a path to freedom from half-truths and deception. It is the path to defining and redesigning concepts of truth.

 THOROUGH THINKING

Many people respond negatively to the term *critical thinking*. Perhaps you could consider replacing it with the term *thorough thinking*. I am not sure the term should be replaced, but thorough thinking is a concept well worth exploring. Both terms are valuable. When you consider a moral dilemma, you need to do thorough thinking. You are asked to examine values for yourself and the patient, look at all possible options, consider the alternatives, and make a decision that could be evaluated after it had been implemented. This is an example of thorough thinking. It is neither "gut" reaction response nor unquestioningly following the rules. It is complex, takes time, and considers the needs of all persons in the situation.

The modern world is fast-paced. It asks us to make decisions almost immediately, which generally is at odds with thorough thinking. In all probability, you need to talk to people, check your facts, and spend time pondering whether you are going to make the right decision on a complex issue. Thorough thinking does not allow for immediate "yes" or "no" responses. In answer to requests for an immediate decision, you need to develop the courage to say, "I don't know." Then find out what the answer is by applying thorough thinking. Just as skilled students are thorough thinkers, so are skilled nurses.

THOROUGH OR CRITICAL THINKING AS APPLIED TO SCIENCE

Consider the following: Most famous scientists and mathematicians probably made lucky guesses at one time or another about the truths they're credited with discovering. The reason for their fame is that they were able to prove their discoveries to others. You may experience an important insight, but unless you can prove to others that it's new as well as valid, not many people are going to accept it. Insights, no matter how profound they may be to those who experience them, must be backed up by evidence.

Basic college geometry is modeled on principles developed 23 centuries ago by the Greek mathematician Euclid, often referred to as the "Father of Geometry." He defined his terms carefully and proposed statements that were readily acceptable to the scientific community of his day. Every carpenter and mechanic today recognizes that the sum of the angles of a triangle must equal two right angles and must total 180 degrees. The applied science of surveying is based in great measure on the truths of Euclid.

Box 7.1 Aspects of Critical Thinking

1. Thinking beyond the known information
2. Considering options
3. Looking at information from multiple sources
4. Identifying patterns and relationships
5. Integrating information from various sources

FOCUSED LEARNING CHART

Thorough Thinking Is an Essential Aspect of Critical Thinking

DO	DON'T
Look at all possible options.	Use your gut reaction as a solution.
Consider at least three alternatives or possible solutions.	Unquestioningly follow the rules.
Have the courage to say, "I don't know."	Respond to the pressures of our fast-paced society for quick decisions.
Take the time to determine the most effective solution to a problem by checking with others, doing a literature review, and spending time thinking about it.	

The astronomer Edmund Halley, for whom a comet was named, observed his comet in 1682 and recorded data concerning its motion through the solar system. Based on these data, Halley concluded, in a work published in 1705, that the comet would return at approximately 75-year intervals. Using both his own observations and the work on gravitation published by the physicist-philosopher Isaac Newton, Halley was able to infer that the comet would return at some point in December 1758. Halley died in 1743, but 15 years later, on Christmas Day 1758, the comet appeared. What a success, and what a triumph of reason! Halley's observations, coupled with Newton's work, taken as axioms and postulates, allowed him to calculate a prediction accurate to 1 month in 75 years. The motion of comets, which previously had been considered erratic and even mysterious, was resolved to a system of laws that could predict their behavior.

Halley's Comet makes its appearance every 75 years. (Source: *Courtesy of Mt. Wilson Observatory.*)

I saw Halley's Comet in 1986, which was the last time it appeared. It was beautiful, and my appreciation for it increased when I realized a man who didn't have a computer or modern telescopes defined the comet's motions in the 1600s. What Halley did with the resources available to him is amazing. His finest resource was his mind.

THOROUGH OR CRITICAL THINKING AS APPLIED TO NURSING

Thorough thinking has strong roots in the growth and refinement of nursing as a profession. Florence Nightingale was a statistician, innovator, and teacher. She took women who were poor and abused and envisaged what an education could do for them. Then she gave them the education they needed to be nurses. Nightingale's vision developed into schools of nursing throughout Great Britain and the United States. When Nightingale went to Kaiserworth Deaconess Institution in Germany, she spent her first few weeks learning how to scrub floors. Such were the duties and limitations of nurses during that era. Nightingale foresaw a different era and educated women to come in contact with patients and administer care. She developed an entirely new type of nursing.

When Jean Watson critically reviewed nursing in the medical model and believed it was lacking the principles inherent to every nurse, she was referring to holistic care. Watson's work developed the concept of nursing as a profession that could define its own practice rather than a profession that modeled itself after medicine. (See Chapter 2.)

The point of this chapter is not simply to teach you how to gain and use knowledge but rather to use original thinking to create new knowledge. Critical thinking is thorough thinking, which cannot be done well without the skill of creative thinking.

Have you ever had the "aha" experience in your education? The "aha" is that moment when, as a nurse, you pick up symptoms that no one else did. It could also be a teacher finding the perfect topic to engage a student in research, or a parent finally understanding a child's behavior. The "aha" experience comes from thinking creatively and critically so that a new idea—one you have never had before—emerges.

 ## CREATIVE THINKING

Creative thinking is the hallmark of being a critical thinker. I am amazed at my 2-year-old granddaughter and her ability to play creatively. She can be a dog on all fours using her tongue to lick milk from a dish or convert the pantry into a home for her toy zebras (I have to knock to gain admittance!). I have hope that she will continue to be creative as she learns and grows! There are a variety of ways to be creative; some are listed in Box 7.2 for you.

REFLECTIVE THINKING

I am sure you have had "aha" moments in your life. Take some time to identify one and record it in your class notebook. Explain the problem that caused you to discover the new information that was the "aha." What impact did it have on your life? How did you feel about coming up with a new idea? Was the idea effective for your problem?

Box 7.2 Ways to Be Creative

1. Conduct brainstorming sessions.
2. Focus and let go.
3. Cultivate creative serendipity.
4. Keep idea files.

Conduct a Brainstorming Session

There are rules associated with brainstorming:

- **Rule 1** is that every idea is a good idea, so write it down.
- **Rule 2** is to set a time limit for the session.

Some purposes of brainstorming are to find solutions, create plans, and discover new ideas. Brainstorming can be done alone or with a small group; you may want to try both approaches. You could brainstorm with yourself to choose a topic for your next term paper. You may brainstorm with the interdisciplinary team for solutions to a home care patient who is noncompliant with medications.

Another purpose of brainstorming is to generate as many ideas as possible. Some of your ideas may be outlandish, but the process can be fruitful. I often assign a term paper to students in the Leadership and Management class I teach in which the students are to determine what they want to learn and then are to document their learning. I have received some wonderful papers describing the learning experiences of students who did something they really wanted to do. For example, two women chose to go to Washington, DC, to learn all they could about the proposed changes in the Medicare laws. They made appointments to interview their state's senators and representatives and arranged for a tour of the National Archives where they learned how to research Medicare laws and obtain copies of the documents. They also got special passes for a tour of the White House from one of the senators and scheduled time to tour the historic sites. How did they think of such a creative and meaningful approach to their topic? They brainstormed!

Before you begin your brainstorming session, sit quietly for a minute or two to relax your mind so that new ideas can come to the forefront. Then set your timer for the allotted time and begin writing as fast as you can. If you are brainstorming in a group, assign a scribe to record all of the ideas so that the group process is not hindered. The purpose of brainstorming is to come up with as many ideas as possible, so every idea is valued and recorded. Many of us would have rejected the idea of traveling to Washington, DC, to gather data for a paper as "crazy." We would have missed a great idea; every idea is to be recorded no matter how implausible it sounds!

After the brainstorming session, review all of the ideas and determine which are not workable.

These students are brainstorming.

These can be tossed. Edit the remaining ideas until they are usable. By looking at a large variety of possible solutions, you are enhancing your ability to be a creative thinker.

Focus and Let Go

Being creative requires energy. When you are in the creative mode, you are focused. Your mind is working on nothing but the creative idea that has come to you. You may recognize it as a great idea but need to spend time struggling with how to implement it. Perhaps the idea needs to be developed into a larger project or made clearer and more focused. These and other aspects of creative activities take time and energy.

When you are intensely focused, you are using your conscious mind. If your idea is to travel to Washington, DC, for your paper, you need to work consciously on identifying the funding, planning the itinerary, and reserving a hotel room. When you "let go," or leave the creative idea, you are allowing your subconscious mind to work. You can't determine what your subconscious mind will be doing while you are out buying groceries, attending your child's PTA meeting, or sleeping. If you have been consciously working on something important to you, however, your subconscious mind generally continues the work while you are letting go, and later a good idea comes to your conscious mind.

When you work so there is free time to focus as well as to let go, your work will be much more creative than if you worked at it endlessly. This is one reason why students generally do not do better when they pull "all-nighters" for a test. They have been in focus mode for so long with no letting-go time that their mind is tired. When I work on time-consuming projects, such as this textbook, I may

be sitting at my computer for 8 to 10 hours a day. That would not be an effective strategy if I were not good at focusing and letting go. When I write for hours, I do get mentally tired. One of the ways I maintain my focus is to type with my eyes closed. I write while I listen to the soft tapping of the keys. When I feel really tired, I stop. I may put in a load of laundry (it just feels good to do something else), prepare a meal, or go for a short ride. When I return, I have rested my mind with a letting-go activity, and I can write again.

What works for you when your mind is tired? What letting-go activities are effective for you? For some, it is pacing while listening to music. Others exercise; some take a short nap. You need to determine what your letting-go activities are and consciously use them to rest your mind. Letting go enhances your creativity, lessens your mental fatigue, and moves you along the road to being a critical thinker.

Cultivate Creative Serendipity

Serendipity is the ability to see something of value when you weren't looking for it. History is full of serendipitous events. Here are two to consider.

- Edward Jenner discovered the smallpox vaccine, but he was not looking for it! Jenner noticed that milkmaids seldom got the dreaded disease, and by investigating such a serendipitous idea, he determined that cows with mild cases of cowpox immunized the women. Today, smallpox is all but eradicated.
- Alexander Fleming discovered penicillin because of a serendipitous event. Fleming was testing bacteria in Petri dishes in a room with an open window (the era before air conditioning). A spore of *Penicillium notatum,* a type of mold, blew in the window and landed in Fleming's Petri dish, killing the bacteria. Fleming did not lament the destruction of his original experiment. Instead, he creatively looked at what happened by isolating the mold. Because of his serendipity, penicillin was discovered. Over time, penicillin has saved millions of lives, and the drug is currently in its fourth and fifth generation of development from Fleming's original mold.

What if Jenner and Fleming had not been creative thinkers? The thought of not having penicillin to combat infection or of not having the smallpox vaccine changes the entire scope of health care as we know it.

You too can experience serendipity. To learn this skill, be attentive to the world in which you live. Read more than your textbooks (think of it as subconscious brain work or letting go). Reach out to diverse people. Talk to people you meet on the street and waiting with you in lines. Read a magazine that's new to you. Then give yourself time to think consciously and subconsciously about these many new ideas. Let searching for new ideas become a habit. It is a fun way to look at the world, and I find it takes some of the pressure off the high performance demands made on most of us. Go through life expecting to make discoveries, and you will.

Keep Idea Files

I realize the notion of keeping an idea file may seem like just too much for a busy nursing student. Remember, the goal is to be an outstanding nurse and critical thinker. This goal can be achieved when you have developed creative thinking skills. It is important for you to expose yourself to new ideas (i.e., people, reading, classes), and it is just as important to find a way to preserve the new ideas so that you can use them now and in the future. This is the purpose of an idea file.

Carry a small notebook with you in your book bag or purse or use an app on your smart phone so that you have a convenient place to record all of the great new ideas you encounter. It is such a waste to have the courage to talk to a perfect stranger in the grocery line, have the stranger tell you the greatest joke, and forget the joke by the time you get home because you didn't take the time to record the thought or idea. Or you may be sitting next to a pond, listening to the delightful sounds of nature, enjoying this perfect scene when the solution to a major problem comes to you. Because you have nothing to write it on, you lose it almost immediately. Some great ideas are just that fragile, so make note of them.

In addition to documenting information in a notebook or on your phone, you might also collect newspaper or journal articles (photocopy them) or comments made by a teacher during your clinical work. Once you have a system for recording your ideas, review them occasionally. By reviewing your file, you may find the joke you need for a presentation in your speech class or the perfect reference for a paper you are writing. The message is to value and take care of creative ideas, both yours and those of others.

Refine Ideas and Follow Through

Taking an idea to a productive place—refining ideas and following through—requires real genius. Examples include raising the money to go to Washington, DC, or writing the short story that you dreamed about last night. Don't lose your ideas. Take the time and energy to implement them.

Being creative within a safe framework is important for being a nurse. You may be the person who figures out how to position Mr. Carrigan, a challenging orthopedic patient, or you may be the creative person who designs a staffing schedule that changes the existing paradigm and makes staff members much happier. (Remember *paradigm* is a way of thinking or looking at things from a broad perspective.)

Don't go to the trouble to learn creative thinking and then never use your wonderful ideas. Keep adding to your file and use the information you have gathered in every possible situation. The purpose of learning creative thinking skills is to enhance your critical thinking ability.

CRITICAL THINKING

You are not a critical thinker if you accept the information given to you without questioning it or evaluating it for clarity and accuracy. Critical thinking is the way to make thinking an adventure.

You should question everything you read in this book. Don't just accept what I write as the truth. Critically examine the content and think it through. Critical thinking is paradigm-shifting work. You may never think the same way after reading this

This LPN is working with a team to develop a care plan for her patient.

chapter. That would be good because critical thinking is about analyzing and evaluating information, which may entail changing your views. As a student, you have instructors to assist and support you in learning to think critically. In Box 7.3, you will find some critical thinking concepts you may want to consider.

Be Willing to Say, "I Don't Know"

As mentioned previously, it is important to be able to say, "I don't know." I am not encouraging you to use this response when a teacher asks you about content you should have studied for class. It is not an excuse for not studying or not doing your homework. "I don't know" also is an inappropriate response when you are asked whether your patient has been administered his or her medications. When asked a question to which you honestly do not know the answer, however, you need to say, "I don't know." Then you need to find the answer. Brainstorm, or ask someone with more experience to help you, or perform a library search to obtain the information you need. If you have the courage to admit you don't know, perhaps others will be honest enough to do so as well.

Mr. Carrigan Revisited

Earlier in this chapter, I mentioned Mr. Carrigan and the need to position him. Mr. Carrigan is an 80-year-old man with a fractured hip and femur from a fall. He has a Foley catheter, intravenous (IV) fluids, and a low pain tolerance. It is his first postoperative day, and he is on bedrest until the surgeon thinks he can bear weight on his fragile leg. Mr. Carrigan doesn't

---

Box 7.3 **Critical Thinking Concepts**

1. Be willing to say, "I don't know."
2. Define your terms to allow for clear communication.
3. Practice tolerance.
4. Understand before criticizing.
5. Consider the source of your information.
6. Ask questions.
7. Look for all possible solutions.
8. Be willing to change your mind given new information.

---

want to move because it hurts. If you don't position him well and reposition him frequently, he is a likely candidate for pneumonia or a blood clot. A fellow student is assigned to Mr. Carrigan and calls you in to help decide how to position him. Rather than cause unnecessary pain for Mr. Carrigan by trying to move him without more information, you say, "I don't know."

Your fellow student likely will not like your answer. In our fast-paced world, everyone wants an immediate answer to questions, without requiring thought or planning. You are a critical thinker, however, so you are honest in your response. Your answer is based on the patient's need not to suffer unnecessary pain. You believe that you need someone with more experience to teach you how to care for Mr. Carrigan.

Mr. Carrigan needs to be turned. What clinical reasoning process will you use to gather enough information to solve the problem? Based on your clinical reasoning, what is your plan for Mr. Carrigan? My thought process is detailed in the following list, but this list reflects my thinking only. In your creative mind, you may have other ways to resolve the problem. If your list meets the overall objective of safety and care, you should use your list. Being creative and being critical in your thinking mean that there is more than one way to solve a problem. Here is my list of things I would do as a student to get Mr. Carrigan turned and positioned:

1. Talk to Mr. Carrigan. Is he alert? Does he have ideas about how to position him? How much pain is he in at the moment?
2. I have determined that Mr. Carrigan is alert and in pain. Ask the medication nurse to give him something for the pain. By doing this first, the medication will have time to be effective (approximately 20 minutes) when you return with a solution for turning and positioning Mr. Carrigan.
3. Find your clinical preceptor. This is the person who is responsible for you and the patients to whom you are assigned. He or she also is a registered nurse (RN) with education and experience. Don't neglect to use such a valuable resource.
4. The faculty person teaches you about turning sheets, back supports, and the power of a well-positioned pillow. You also are cautioned about the fragility of Mr. Carrigan's leg and how important it is to have enough people to

turn him so that someone holds and supports his leg at all times.

5. You now need to gather your supplies: four people (because this is the first time Mr. Carrigan is being turned, you want enough people to keep him safe and to prevent additional pain), four to six pillows for support, a back support obtained from central supply, and a turning sheet and other clean linens because this is the opportune time to change the bedding.

Saying "I don't know" means you don't have the knowledge, information, or experience needed to respond to the question or request, but it also means you will find the answer.

Define Your Terms

Any interaction has the potential for miscommunication. When you are interacting with someone and things seem to become uncomfortable or tense, one practical thing to do is to make sure you are talking about the same thing or that you are defining your terms in the same way. As an educated person, you do not want tense conversations to turn into arguments. You want to examine critically what is going on and do something productive with the interaction. Defining your terms is helpful in this type of situation.

When things are tense, take a deep breath to allow yourself to get enough oxygen in your system so you can relax, and sit down, if standing, and invite the person with whom you are speaking to do the same. Then ask an appropriate question, such as, "What do you consider effective pain control?" assuming that is your topic of discussion. Many nurses disagree about this issue. As a nurse who practices caring theory, your definition of pain management may be different from that of a nurse who does not practice caring. Is this the time to determine which approach is correct? No. Both of you simply define the terms and move on from there with renewed understanding.

Practice Tolerance

You have opinions about many things. Some of your opinions are strong, and others could easily be modified. Would you cheat on a test to pass a class, work in an AIDS clinic, or participate in euthanasia? Other highly charged opinions tend to be formed around notions of freedom and democracy, parenthood, and religious beliefs. Although you may have strong opinions about these and other issues, a critical thinker practices tolerance of other people's opinions.

Throughout U.S. history, society has been intolerant of various ethnic and racial groups—African Americans, Chinese, Irish, Germans, Italians, Jews, Hispanics, and so on. Yet it is obvious that slavery and all racism and prejudice are appalling aspects of human behavior. The world is a place of exciting diversity, and as a critical thinker, you would do well to learn to embrace diversity and practice tolerance. How else are you going to learn about other cultures? Remember our discussion about the courage of Christopher Columbus to sail on a world that everyone else thought was flat? His crew had tolerance for a new idea and look what happened! It is a challenge to value diverse people and ideas, and it is a crucial aspect of critical thinking.

Understand Before Criticizing

The phrase "there is a reason for every behavior" fits well under this topic. Someone may be holding you at gunpoint. Even during such a terrifying event, you must understand there is a reason for what the person is doing. As a critical thinker you need to understand that the behavior of the person holding you hostage makes sense for that person.

REFLECTIVE THINKING

Take some time and determine whether you have feelings of intolerance for an individual or group. If you do, consider how to change your thinking. Do you need to gather more information about the person or group so that you can understand them better? Do you need to talk to the individual or a member of the group? Do you need to evaluate thoughtfully why you have feelings of intolerance? You cannot have feelings of intolerance and be a successful nurse. The two simply are incompatible. I suggest you take some time now and work through any feelings you may have. Your faculty person may be a good resource as well. Best wishes!

How do people come to develop the "reason" for the behavior they exhibit? It is what makes each of us an individual. We are products of our parents' gene pool, culture, environment, experiences, and thinking. A person who thinks critically needs to understand some of that individuality before being able to act as an informed person. For example, a nurse assesses and talks to a patient before giving a treatment or even ambulating. By talking to the patient and listening with an open mind, the nurse can learn about the uniqueness of the patient, and quality care can be given. A teacher takes time to get to know his or her students. Based on initial information and additional experiences and time with the class, the teacher decides on the best teaching approach for that unique group of people. Physicians diagnose before they prescribe. Lawyers brief themselves on an opponent's case before going to trial. Open-minded listening is how you understand before criticizing.

If you are defensive or angry, you are not being open-minded. Open-minded listening calls for your energy to be focused on the other person, not you. You should not be having feelings that are in any way critical.

What Pushes Your Buttons?

Every person I know has issues that "push their buttons" or can cause a powerful negative reaction. As a critical thinker, you need to be aware of your own issues. Take some time to identify them and think of strategies for not reacting to people or situations that are evocative. If someone has identified your buttons and keeps pushing them (children are famous for this) to get a reaction, you need to practice tolerance and understanding of the person and avoid being critical.

If you learn to recognize your issues and strengthen yourself so that you do not respond to them, you can improve your life immensely. Think of the reactive arguments you would not participate in, the patient families you would learn to value and support, and the angry and the defensive interactions you would never engage in again because you have learned to control your "buttons."

Consider the Source

I feel uncomfortable when my sister brings me the latest fad for losing weight and says, "The research says this is true." She never looks at the source of the research, however. Her assumption is that if it's printed, it must be true. Never just accept what you are told or what you read, whether in print or on the Internet. Consider the source carefully, especially if you are thinking about changing your opinion or activity (such as eating) based on the information. Who wrote or said what you are interested in exploring? Is the individual a respected person in the field? Is the research legitimate? Do

you need to explore further and determine who else has something to say about the topic? Critical thinkers *think* about things rather than simply accepting them as truth.

Ask Questions

The essence of critical thinking is to ask questions. Don't accept the information that is given to you without exploring it. Get more information. First, discipline yourself to think in terms of questions. As you sit in class, consider what questions you would like answered. The second step is to have the courage to ask the questions. I delight in the critical thinkers I have in class. They are full of questions and often ask things that I would never have thought about myself. It is exciting to see what comes from their minds. "Don't waste a question" is my motto. If you practice thinking about and asking questions, you will get better at asking meaningful questions that pertain to a specific situation. When that happens, you will know you are a critical thinker.

To become a critical thinker, you need to consider what has been said: Is it true, and if so, what does it mean to you? The challenge is to be open-minded enough to change your opinion or thinking based on what you have heard or read, once you've established its validity. Critical thinkers always reserve the right to reject what they hear as well.

Look for at Least Three Solutions

Now that you have thoroughly explored a question and have a solution with which you are comfortable, you may think you are done. Whoops! Sorry! You need to consider at least two additional solutions. By looking at more than one solution to the question, you are able to fuel your own creativity and stimulate your mental energy. Never give up on the quest for the truth to any question. In other words, don't settle early, and don't close your mind to other possibilities.

Be Willing to Change Your Mind

Being willing to change your mind is the highest level of critical thinking. Have you thought through a situation or problem to the point at which you can change your mind? Have you listened to the other person without being judgmental or defensive and, after personal consideration, determined the other person's idea was a great one? I am not talking about changing your mind because someone in power (e.g., teacher, police officer) told you to change it. I am talking about the entire process discussed in this chapter that allows you freedom of thought and the truest form of empowerment. It all ties together. If you can think critically and act on those thoughts, you are empowered. You are able to contribute significantly to a study group, your family, and the nursing team.

I suggest you take a break now (subconscious time) and go to a movie, play basketball, or take a nap. Then come back to this chapter and read it again. You have just read a formula for critical thinking that calls for a new way of thinking. It is important to your life's success. So rest or play, reread the chapter, and then go try it out. It takes practice and time to change your paradigm of thinking, but people do it every day. Your goal is to be an effective critical thinker when you graduate.

Critical thinking is the way educated, professional people think. It is a challenging way to consider life and generally needs to be learned. It is not intuitive. To be a critical thinker, a person must be a creative thinker as well. This is a challenging prestep to critical thinking and is not a stage in the development that can be skipped.

In light of today's downsizing and lower LPN-to-patient ratios in many health-care organizations, the need to be a critical thinker is much more significant than ever before for nursing. As an LPN, you need to develop this skill over the academic year. Being a critical thinker is where you want to be when you graduate because of the power and ability it will give you as a practicing nurse.

REAL-WORLD CASE STUDY

■ You enter a patient's room to answer a call light and are surprised to walk in on a physician who put on the call light because he needed help. The physician is doing a procedure unknown to you that involves IV solutions and medications. You are a new LPN graduate and have not yet been certified in IV therapy. There is an LPN student in the room looking frustrated and possibly frightened. The patient appears to be in pain and looks at you as though she hopes to be rescued. The physician seems frustrated and is tense and raising his voice. He appears to be unable to complete the procedure he has undertaken because both of his hands are full, and he needs one more thing done. You wonder whether he asked the student to assist with the IV medications and became frustrated when she said she couldn't. All of these observations and considerations race through your mind in seconds. In addition, your blood pressure and heart rate increase because of the adrenaline release caused by the situation. Then the physician says to you, "Finally, a nurse! Grab that medication [a syringe filled with 'something' sitting on the over bed table] and give it in the second IV port."

What do you do, and, more important, how do you think it through? Write the solution to the case study in your class notebook and be prepared to share it in class.

Key Points

■ Nurses must be able to think critically to provide safe care to their patients. Critical thinking requires a nurse to think beyond what is known about the patient and consider options or alternatives that will help in meeting patient outcomes. The nurse must also be able to identify patterns and relationships in the patient's symptoms and behaviors and integrate information from multiple sources to best identify appropriate care for patients.

■ An "aha'" moment comes from thinking creatively and critically. Creative thinking is the hallmark of being a critical thinker and time should be allowed for that creative process. If you allow time to focus on your work and then take a break, the end result will be more creative. It is helpful to keep a file of ideas that you collect from newspapers, journals, or other sources to use for future projects.

■ To avoid miscommunication, be sure to "define your terms" so those with whom you are communicating will understand the true meaning of what you are trying to say. Be willing to say, "I don't know" if you honestly do not know the answer to a question. Then you need to take the time to find the answers by looking up the answer in an appropriate resource or asking a more experienced person

■ Critical thinkers think about and consider information they are provided rather than simply accepting the information as being true. Critical thinkers also practice tolerance of other people's opinions by listening to what they have to say and trying to understand the reason behind their thoughts.

ANSWERS TO REAL-WORLD CASE STUDY

What a potentially traumatic situation! This situation happened to one of my students, so don't discount it as something that would never happen. What would you do? A possible course of action follows. You may have other ideas that are just as valid. List them in your class notebook and come to class prepared to share your thinking.

Do *not* give the medication just because the physician told you to give it. You have visually evaluated the situation, and except for the patient's apparent mental stress, you determine the patient is not in any danger; there is a brief amount of time to get more information.

Before asking any questions, ask the student to go find an RN. Whatever the outcome, an RN is needed because of the IV medication. The RN should make the necessary decisions and administer the medication if it is deemed appropriate.

Ask questions! What is the procedure? What is the medication? What is the overall purpose for what is being done? While you are asking the questions, move in close to the frightened patient and touch her, give her some comfort and a feeling of security rather than the negative feelings coming from the physician's anxiety. This is *caring*.

It is possible that the physician is going to raise his voice at you in stress and frustration. He is in a less than ideal situation. Because you are a critical thinker, you can listen to his anxiety without becoming defensive. At this point, your concern is the patient. Is she safe? Is she anxious? Is she in need of medical attention other than what she is receiving?

When the RN arrives, he or she can determine a solution to the problem with the physician. You have gathered information and should share it with the nurse. With the RN on the scene, you should focus all of your attention on the patient, who is probably concerned. There is a temptation for people to gather around what is exciting. In this case, it could be the interaction between the nurse and the physician or the procedure that is being done. Where you are needed is with the patient, not the procedure, unless you are doing it.

REVIEW QUESTIONS

1. Which statement by the nurse indicates he is a critical thinker?
   1. The charge nurse told me to do it this way.
   2. I checked with several nurses and the patient's family for suggestions to help the patient sleep better.
   3. I have been a nurse for a long time and this is the way I have always done it.
   4. I collaborated with the physician to determine the best plan of care.

2. When using the process of thorough thinking, the nurse will:
   1. Go with her "gut" reaction to the situation.
   2. Follow the rules without questioning them.
   3. Consider all possible options.
   4. Consider only her thoughts about the situation.

3. Critical thinking includes the following concepts:
   1. Willingness to say, "I don't know"
   2. Practicing tolerance for others opinions
   3. Asking questions
   4. All of the above

4. A group of students want to use the process of brainstorming to come up with an idea for the class project. They will:
   1. Write down all possible ideas no matter how silly they may sound.
   2. Look though their class notebooks and textbooks for ideas.
   3. Scan the Internet for possible topics.
   4. Ask the instructor what other students have done in the past.

5. Having the ability to critically think can assist the LPN with decision making.
   1. True
   2. False

References

Pitt, V., Powis, D., Levett-Jones, T., & Hunter, S. (2015). The influence of critical thinking skills on performance and progression in a pre-registration nursing program. *Nurse Education Today, 35*(1), 125–131. Retrieved from http://dx.doi.org. hal.weber.edu:2200/10.1016/j.nedt.2014.08.006

Zuriguel Pérez, E., Lluch Canut, M. T., Falcó Pegueroles, A., Puig Llobet, M., Moreno Arroyo, C., & Roldán Merino, J. (2015). Critical thinking in nursing: Scoping review of the literature. *International Journal of Nursing Practice, 21*(6), 820–830. doi:10.1111/ijn.12347

Web Resource

Foundation for Critical Thinking *www.criticalthinking. org/pages/our-concept-of-critical-thinking/411*

8

Entry Into Practice

LEARNING OUTCOMES

1. Explain the difference between "knowing that" and "knowing how" knowledge.
2. Define the purpose and importance of the nurse practice act acknowledging laws that are specific to the state where you are to practice as an LPN.
3. Draw a correlation between Maslow's hierarchy of needs and role transition from student to practicing nurse.
4. List the three major questions that should be answered when searching for the perfect job.
5. Define self-evaluation and self-monitoring from the perspective of an LPN.
6. Describe successful mentoring (of both self and others) and identify at least four characteristics of toxic mentoring that can occur.
7. List three advantages of being a member of a professional organization for LPNs.
8. Describe the process and advantages of professional networking.

Expertise develops when the clinician (nurse) tests and refines . . . [nursing] expectations in actual clinical practice. Experience is therefore a requisite for expertise.

—Dr. Patricia Benner

Developing "knowing that" knowledge is crucial to being a successful LPN. This is generally done in the classroom and at preconference and postconference sessions.

When a new graduate from any educational experience enters the workforce, a major paradigm shift occurs. For the licensed practical nurse (LPN), the change can be challenging. This chapter explains some of the paradigms that you will encounter and assists you in working with them effectively. Dr. Patricia Benner has spent a great deal of her nursing career studying the process of moving from being a novice to being an expert in clinical practice.

According to Benner (2000), there is a difference between theoretical learning (classroom) and clinical practice. What you learn in school is the theory of nursing. You study scientific concepts, read case studies of real and imaginary people, and take tests on hundreds of pages of information that pertain to your future role as a nurse. Benner refers to the information you learn in school as the "knowing that" information. It is the foundation of your knowledge base for practicing nursing. For example, you "know that" low blood sugar causes hypoglycemia and that a glass of orange juice generally causes the blood sugar to elevate to a safe level for the patient. Your time spent in clinical experiences as a student involves developing "knowing that" knowledge. When doing a student clinical assignment, you have only one or two patients to whom you give care, or you pass medications to a small group of people instead of the entire team as an LPN does.

Benner explains that the second type of knowledge that is necessary to move from being a novice to being an expert nurse is "knowing how," or the information that nurses learn while practicing their art in the real world of nursing. You develop "knowing how" knowledge when you care for a patient or a category of patients over time and learn, for example, that a small piece of candy is better for a particular individual's hypoglycemic reaction than orange juice. This information evolves while you are performing the day-to-day responsibilities of your profession. Often it cannot be explained, similar to how a person learns how to ride a bicycle or swim cannot be explained. The swimmer or bike rider can receive a great deal of "knowing that" knowledge but still can't swim or ride a bike until he or she gets in the water or on the bike and does it.

The practice of nursing requires extensive "knowing that" knowledge. That is why you are in school. After your graduation, you will proceed to the "knowing how" part of your education. Expect challenges because not everyone follows the textbook procedures you so carefully learned in school, and not everyone you work with is an expert nurse. Your challenge is to develop the ability to work with a wide variety of professionals and paraprofessionals to promote the health and wellness of all people in your care while developing your own nursing expertise.

NURSE PRACTICE ACT

An important "knowing that" concept is understanding the laws that govern your practice as a nurse. After you graduate and pass the National Council Licensure Examination for Practical Nurses (NCLEX-PN), you are permitted to practice nursing within the framework of the LPN nurse practice act in your state. The nurse practice act is the most significant law governing your practice. A nurse practice act is the law of each state that defines nursing and what the various levels of nurses legally may do in their practice. The state board of nursing consists of nurses and others who generally are appointed by the governor to serve as the enforcement arm of the nurse practice act.

Every procedure LPNs perform must be done within the statutes of the law as it is outlined in the state nurse practice act. Although I have just defined the new graduate as a person who is still learning, that clinical learning must be done within the guidelines of the law. There is no room for error or misunderstanding after you graduate and are practicing as an LPN.

The nurse practice laws differ from state to state; some laws are specific, and some laws are general. It is essential that you assume the responsibility to understand thoroughly the role of the LPN in the state where you work. Most often the wording of a nurse practice act is purposefully general to allow for changes and growth in the organization without enacting new legislation for each change. In general, the scope of practice for an LPN focuses on the health needs of patients in hospitals, residents in nursing homes, and members of the community. In most situations, it is required that LPNs work under the supervision of a registered nurse (RN) or physician.

In addition to defining what nursing is for a state, a nurse practice act directs the state board of nursing in establishing the criteria for licensure and defining violations that can be disciplined by the board. It is common for a nurse practice act to require additional education regarding a specified standard for an LPN to work with intravenous (IV) solutions. If this is part of the nurse practice act in your state, it is unacceptable for the hospital where you work to write in their policies that an LPN can start an IV without the additional education. The policies and procedures of all employers should follow the nurse practice act. If they don't, it is your responsibility to know the law and follow it despite the hospital's policies. If you do not follow the law as outlined, you may be in violation, which would put your license in jeopardy. You can access the nurse practice act for your state by going to the National Council of State Boards of Nursing Web site at https://www.ncsbn.org/npa.htm.

Another example of accountability to a nurse practice act is the requirement that an LPN is answerable to the orders given by a physician or an RN. The ethics of nursing also state that you have a responsibility to give only safe and reasonable care to the people for whom you are responsible. A classic controversy can occur when a medication is ordered that you, as a charge nurse in a nursing home, believe would be unsafe for the frail 92-year-old resident in your care. You look at the chart and realize that the physician has not been in to see this woman for 36 days, and her condition has changed markedly. She has lost weight and is much more confused. You think that the dosage of medication is too high for a woman in her condition. What do you do? The law says that you are obligated to follow the physician's orders.

Nursing ethics say that you are obligated to practice safe and reasonable care.

The key in this situation is to obey the law without jeopardizing the resident. You should be sure you have expressed your concerns clearly to the physician. If the physician still insists that you give the medication, you are obligated to contact the RN, director of nursing, or administrator to share your concerns. This type of contact is important to make even if it is on a Sunday afternoon or at midnight. You have the right and responsibility to protect all persons under your care from what you consider unsafe practice. You also have the obligation to communicate that information to your supervisor so the problem can be resolved. Carefully document your decision and your basis for it—that you informed the physician of your concerns and which supervisor you called. Do not assume that the problem is then resolved. Keep in touch with your supervisor to ensure that the situation is being negotiated with the physician. You have the right to refuse to give any medication or treatment that you believe may be detrimental to a patient. You need to exercise that right, however, within the framework of the law.

It is an ongoing responsibility to maintain nursing practice within the framework of the laws governing that practice. The previous section on nurse practice acts may seem a bit serious, and perhaps it makes you uncomfortable. It is common for a new graduate to feel that way. It has to do with two concepts discussed in this book. First, your knowledge base while you are in school is focused on "knowing that" information. When you are in actual practice, you develop more confidence in working within the laws of your profession because you are developing your "knowing how" knowledge. It is important to give yourself time for "knowing how." Your clinical expertise gives you more information on "knowing how" to talk to a physician; how to assess medications for a frail, elderly person; and how to communicate with your supervisor.

REFLECTIVE THINKING

What would you like to know about your state's nurse practice act? Can LPNs in your state start IV lines when they graduate? List in your class notebook three items of information you would like to know regarding your license and legal practice when you graduate. Where can you find the answers to your questions?

Maslow Revisited

The second concept that has an impact on your successful entry into the practice of nursing is applying your understanding of Maslow's hierarchy of needs. Do you remember that the first need on his pyramid is survival or basic physiological needs? Generally, going to work as an LPN does not have a negative impact on your ability to breathe, eat, and move. The second level of needs—safety—may be threatened, however, as you make your transition from student to practicing nurse.

A basic concept of living in the 21st century is that you have the right to manage your life so that you are safe. People live in homes to protect themselves from the inclement weather, streets are dotted with fast-food restaurants to provide for immediate gratification of hunger, and there are managerial strategies to keep one feeling safe while at work. The most vulnerable time for unsafe feelings at work is the transition from student to LPN. You are approaching that time in your career. The information given in the next section on finding the perfect job is to assist you, as a new nurse, in finding a level of safety while at work.

For you to feel safe in your environment you should have an understanding of your own ego and how important it is to protect your ego from unnecessary damage. Every person goes through personal maneuvers to avoid embarrassing moments or incidents in which they feel inadequate. A situation in which you feel inadequate in your job as an LPN could result in a serious mistake that would hurt a patient and possibly jeopardize your nursing license. Such situations could occur on a new job.

As a new graduate, you could embarrass yourself by arriving late to work on the first day because you did not know how heavy the traffic would be that time of the morning or evening. That is damage to your ego. You could be assigned a patient with total parenteral nutrition who is on a home ventilator. If you are not skilled at either one of these modalities, because of your lack of "knowing how" knowledge you are going to be inadequate, and your care may endanger the patient. If you are handed an unlabeled syringe and asked to give it IV push during a code, this would be a serious mistake and would be breaking the law in

most states. These are just some possible scenarios. There also are many safety situations that can be essentially eliminated by the new graduate who knows how to make successful professional transitions.

FINDING THE PERFECT JOB

Be Objective

When I was a young nurse, I would daydream about being a wartime nurse. I watched movies that portrayed war nurses as having a glamorous job and opportunities to travel the world. What I didn't pay much attention to was the reality of the job: working in undesirable situations with limited resources. Wounded soldiers would be coming in for care at all hours of the day and night, including some with little hope of surviving. Think for a moment of my perception of the wartime nurse. I focused only on the exciting scenes in the movies, and I ignored the actual working and living conditions. It was a skewed view of what being a nurse during wartime might entail. I am sharing this story with you because the first step to identifying the perfect job is to be objective. This involves answering three major questions:

1. What is the job really like on a day-to-day basis?
2. What skills and experience do you need to learn as you gain "knowing how" clinical experience?
3. What are the support systems available at the job for a new graduate (i.e., orientation, preceptorship, and additional classes)?

Worst-Case Scenario Example

A worst-case scenario example follows. You are an excited new graduate who really wants a career as a nurse manager in a prestigious nursing home in your community. You know you have to work as a staff nurse for a time before being promoted to a charge nurse position, but you are eager to develop your "knowing how" knowledge during that time. You already have determined that working with elderly people and the high level of nursing practice at this particular nursing home constitute the type of job you want. The facility is so popular, however, that no additional openings are available for a new graduate. (Their orientation program allows them only a certain number of new graduates at a time because the orientation is so thorough.)

In the meantime, you have a husband finishing his degree and a 2-year-old child. It is your turn to get a job and support the family so that your husband can work part-time and earn his degree more quickly. The bottom line is that you need a job, and the local hospital has an opening in the newborn nursery. The nurse manager states that LPNs in the obstetric area are never placed in management positions; however, they do get to take care of "the cutest babies born in this city." Because of the recent loss of three LPNs, you are needed desperately; you are told you can start right away on the night shift and are to be "trained on the job."

The day-to-day work at the newborn nursery job may be with cute newborns, but if your focus is on elderly people, the cute babies will not keep your interest at work. Also, because of your own 2-year-old, it is possible, but disadvantageous, to work the night shift. The day-to-day reality of the job with the hospital looks inconvenient for your family situation and has the potential of being boring. The knowledge you would gain admitting and monitoring newborns would be valuable information for any nurse. This type of "knowing how" information does not help you in getting the type of job you really want, however. The work is important, and the knowledge is meaningful but not for your career track.

Not enough substantial support systems are available for you to be successful at this job. On-the-job training is not the same as an orientation or a preceptorship program. I also would be concerned about that training if you are on the night shift, when there are generally fewer people to assist you in learning the skills of the job. When you ask about a class to become IV certified, the nurse manager states that you wouldn't need IV skills in the nursery, so the class wouldn't be available to you. This is a job you should not take because it does not meet your criteria for knowledge growth, and it does not fit with your future career plans.

It may be easy to understand the previous example, but the reality is that you still need a job. What can you do? Unless you feel safe on a job (ego safety, safe from abuse from others, safe from dangerous practice, safe knowledge development), you cannot do a good job. This is the basic principle of Maslow's theory. If your safety needs are not met, you are not going to advance to the next level of the pyramid—social needs. This level involves the ability to interact with others at work and in social environments. If you do not feel safe, your ability to work on a health-care team and with families and other staff members does not evolve because this need is a step above the safety need. With this insight, you should not take the job in the newborn nursery. It does not meet your interest needs and does not fit into your career plans.

Where do you find a job? Generally, jobs are available for an LPN in many fields of nursing. If you really want the management job at the prestigious nursing home in your future, you need to take a job in a quality nursing home now. This gives you experience with the type of clients you desire to work with and knowledge of the nursing home system. Be sure it is a facility that gives an excellent orientation with the additional educational opportunities that you want and an opportunity to do some management in the future. While working hard at mastering the "knowing how" knowledge that the job offers, you should remain in contact with the personnel department at the nursing home where you want to work in the future. Keep updating your file, get to know the personnel director through your visits, and let that person know about the great opportunities you are taking advantage of at your current job.

While you are paving the way for the job you want, be careful to value the job you are currently doing. It is markedly unprofessional to devalue or be disloyal to a current job while seeking a different job. Don't get caught in that situation; nursing standards require commitment to your job. This commitment involves loyalty to the organization, genuine commitment to the patients, support of other staff members and administration, and an active approach to problem-solving instead of whining, backbiting, or making disloyal comments.

Think for a moment how you would feel if you had the newborn nursery job. I've mentioned the possibility of the work being boring because it isn't what you want to do. Most people complain when they are bored. You wouldn't be getting the continuing education you wanted, which could be another cause for complaints. The list could go on, including a shift you don't want and the lack of orientation. If you take the newborn nursery job, not only would you be unable to meet your safety needs but most people in that situation also would end up being disloyal to their employers. The bottom line: Don't take a job without knowing the answers to the questions listed earlier under "Be Objective."

To take a job that doesn't meet these criteria would not be a good transition for you as you move from student to nurse. In all positions that you take, you should keep your career goals clearly in mind. If you have the job you really want, you will continue moving up Maslow's pyramid of needs. As you meet your social needs with coworkers, you will develop a stronger self-esteem and potentially achieve self-actualization. It all starts with the right job application.

Other Concepts to Consider

Other concepts to consider in identifying the perfect job include self-evaluation and self-monitoring of progress.

Self-Evaluation

You are your best evaluator because no one knows more about you and your abilities than you do. Part of your self-evaluation should be focused on a career plan. To develop such a plan, you need to answer the following questions:

1. What do you want to be doing next year?
2. What do you want to be doing 3 years from now?
3. What is your 5-year plan?

The answers to these questions may involve time out of your career track because you are having a baby. It could mean part-time work because you have decided to earn your RN licensure. It could mean a rigorous schedule of continuing education courses so you can work on an RN and LPN dyad. A career plan needs advance planning and effort to achieve.

You may want to seek out someone to assist you in understanding the options available to you as an LPN and to learn the most effective way to achieve your goals. Every nurse on every licensure level started out as a new graduate. Perhaps working for a time was necessary to determine the career plan for some people, and others knew from their first day as an LPN where they wanted to go with their careers. Whatever your decisions are, you are the person who knows them best, and you understand the motivation behind them. You are your own best career monitor.

Self-Monitoring

I strongly encourage new graduates to make a 5-year plan. It needs to be written with flexibility because people get married and move to new settings with different opportunities, they have children and choose to stay home with them for a while, or they redefine their career goals after achieving additional "knowing how" information as they work. Nevertheless, a 5-year career plan is advisable. Do you want to be an RN in 5 years? How long should it take you to develop the skills and knowledge to work in a nursing specialty area? How much time do you need to work as a staff nurse before the nursing home places you in a charge nurse position? How long should it take for you to be recognized as an outstanding caregiver to the patients assigned to you? Time and planning are required for you to achieve these and other professional goals.

When the plan is established (with flexibility built into the plan), you are the monitor. At the end of year one, have you achieved the level of what you planned? If you have, congratulations! If you haven't, you need to examine why not. There may be an excellent reason for not being on schedule, such as an unplanned opportunity that surfaced during the year. If you haven't achieved your goal, it is crucial that you determine why. Was it the wrong goal? Was it an unrealistic goal? Was the problem a lack of people to assist you in achieving your goal? You need to evaluate your professional self on an annual basis and, through self-monitoring, determine what the next year should bring for you. If you find that this is difficult for you or that the planning and implementation of your plans are unsuccessful, you may need to seek out a mentor.

REFLECTIVE THINKING

To be effective in the self-evaluation process with your career, it is necessary for you to have a career plan. Take some "serious" time and decide what you want to be doing next year, in 3 years, and in 5 years. What do you need to do to achieve your goals? This could mean clinical experiences, more education, or time out for personal matters (i.e., having a family). List in your class notebook the following items related to your career plans:
1. One year from now, I would like to be:
2. What I need to do to achieve that goal is:
3. Three years from now, I would like to be:
4. What I need to do to achieve that goal is:
5. Five years from now, I would like to be:
6. What I need to achieve that goal is:

MENTORING

It is common to hear nurses on all levels complain about the lack of support they receive as they try to master a new role. Novice nurses are merely that, novice nurses, and they can learn and practice the profession much better if they have someone to guide them through the process of their new job.

Nurses have the notorious reputation of "eating their young." It is a horrible phrase, and the concept behind it is even worse because it indicates a lack of support and even aggressive negative attention to other nurses, especially novice nurses. This negative behavior can be attributed to the lack of professionalism in nursing in the United States at its beginning more than 100 years ago. At that time, Florence Nightingale started the three original hospital schools of nursing on the East Coast. These students were "used" to fulfill staffing needs at the hospitals without pay and then were required to do their studies "on the side." This situation occurred because there wasn't an established profession of nursing in the United States. I sincerely believe that the nurses of long ago did the best they could in the existing environment. This environment did establish a precedent, however, for nurses to devalue one another. That has been one of the saddest realities in the nursing profession—not only by not providing support for each other but also being aggressively negative at times.

The most powerful antidote for this "inherited" problem is that of mentorship. A *mentor* is a nurse with more experience and knowledge who is willing to assist a novice to learn the skills of the profession. A good mentor can increase your knowledge, help you socialize into your new work environment, assist you with improving your work performance, and support the success of your nursing career (Bozionelos et al., 2016). Mentoring is done through several different modalities, such as counseling, role modeling, and teaching. It is a behavior that is soundly grounded in Watson's theory of caring. Nurses need to demonstrate caring behaviors for themselves, each other, and patients. Instead of being a profession known for "eating our young," we should be the caring profession that nurtures our young. You can be an active factor in making that change as you grow in the profession.

Most nurses are fortunate if they have one or two mentors throughout their careers. This does not commonly happen. I encourage all who read this text to decide to be a mentor several times during your working life. As you mature in the art and science of nursing, you will have more and more to give to other nurses. I encourage you to commit to sharing what you know.

Your challenge as a new graduate is to look for a mentor. I realize this may elicit a groan from you as the reader, "How can I find a mentor when there are so few and I am so inexperienced?" My reply is, "Look around and see whether you can identify one." The benefit for you to have a mentor, as you move from student to LPN, is of far more value than you can imagine. New nursing graduates are novices, but even experienced nurses can be considered novices. An experienced nurse who changes job roles, from labor and delivery to an emergency department, for example, and works in that new role with only basic nursing background is, in that context, a novice. Every new job has a great deal of new information and many skills to master, and a mentor is an important person to assist in that mastery (Box 8.1).

Identifying a mentor is the first challenge. Look around and locate someone who shows interest in your area and the behaviors that you want to achieve. Evaluate the person to determine whether he or she is receptive to your questions and takes time to explain and clarify information to you as you are learning and developing. You have found someone you can approach about being your mentor if this person meets the following criteria:

- Has an interest in the same clinical practice you are interested in learning
- Demonstrates a high level of skill in your area of interest

Identifying and working with a mentor are important parts of successfully entering into nursing practice.

Box 8.1 Qualities of a Good Mentor

- Experienced
- Confident
- Competent
- Approachable
- Empathetic
- Accessible
- Honest
- Patient
- Respected by peers

- Is receptive to questions from you and others
- Integrates teaching into the questions being answered or explanations being made

It is an honor to be asked to mentor someone in the nuances of nursing. Some people may react with surprise, and others may express concern over their ability to meet your needs. Others may discredit themselves and state that they do not have the ability to do what you are asking. Your responsibility is to be clear in what you are asking and to ask in a pleasant and undemanding manner.

Some examples of approaches that could be used follow. Always remember to talk to your potential mentor in private, perhaps at a meal break or after work when both of you are not rushed or feeling stressed over meeting patient needs. An invitation or appointment to talk would be appropriate. This could be simply saying, "There is something I would like to talk to you about, Nadine. It would take 30 minutes or less. Is there some time this week we could go to lunch or get together?" It takes courage to ask people for their time, but I encourage you to do it. When the person you talk to understands what you are asking for, he or she may or may not accept the invitation to be your mentor, but that individual may always remember the tremendous compliment you have given by asking.

When you have the appointment with a potential mentor, you should be specific about what you would like from the person. You may make a direct request to learn how to do physical assessments as thoroughly as that person does, or you may be less specific and ask for suggestions and insights into how to do the overall job as effectively as your mentor does. Perhaps your need is to have someone help you clarify your 5-year goals and the best way to achieve them. These requests represent actions that range from specific to less well defined. Nevertheless, all are appropriate requests to make when you have identified the right person to work with you.

Most professionals are aware of the need to mentor the less experienced people on a healthcare team. It is just good business. Because of nursing's history, however, nurses may not know how to go about mentoring because they have not seen many role models. Another possibility involves people who are *toxic mentors*. This term seems extreme, but it is used frequently to describe four types of mentors who are destructive or "toxic." Toxic mentors are described here so you can recognize and avoid them. They do not assist you with your career and do not provide information to help you in making the transition from student to nurse. The four types of toxic mentors are avoiders, dumpers, blockers, and destroyers. As I describe each category, think back in your life and see if you recognize anyone who fits the description.

Avoiders are nonresponsive people who are unavailable or inaccessible. If you take an issue to them, they either do not get back to you or seem to vanish into thin air. *Dumpers* throw people into a new role or position and let them fail. They function on the "sink or swim motto," which produces a great deal of transition trauma. *Blockers* may refuse to help, withhold information needed to succeed, or stifle the development of the individual by hovering too closely. *Destroyers* tear down the individual by undermining in subtle or overt ways to destroy the novice nurse's confidence. They criticize you without regard for the quality of your work. "You're new, so you are wrong" is the destroyer's motto.

The nursing profession needs to find ways to deal with these negative behaviors to limit their impact. You personally need to recognize the characteristics and avoid people who demonstrate them.

Sometimes there is not a person available for you to ask to mentor you or who is willing to be a mentor. In that situation, you need to recognize that you still need mentoring. It may sound strange, but you are able to be your own mentor.

FOCUSED LEARNING CHART
How to Identify Toxic Mentors

Every novice nurse needs to be mentored. It is essential, however, that you recognize and avoid toxic mentors. Characteristics of toxic mentors include:

• Offering or agreeing to help but not following through.

• Avoiding you, as a new nurse, altogether.

• Behaving in a passive-aggressive manner.

• Demonstrating overt hostility.

• Giving criticism not based on fact.

• Complaining about you to others.

• Behaving in a way that destroys your confidence.

• Placing you in a new situation without providing support or adequate instruction.

• Embracing the mottos "Sink or swim" and "You're new, so you are wrong."

There are five self-mentoring strategies that can be used by all professionals making a transition:

• Interact with people. Ask questions, listen, and clarify what you know with others to enhance your understanding.

• Find and use references. Read books and journal articles.

• Observe people who are knowledgeable and who have insight.

• Enroll in educational programs, especially ones that include skill practices.

• Figure out solutions for yourself, reflect on them, and work them through on your own.

• Consider using the Internet as a mentoring resource. You can find critical information or contact experts in different geographic areas for information. There are chat rooms that can be helpful.

Use these self-mentoring techniques to assist you with every role transition. If you cannot find an experienced mentor, be proud to do it for yourself.

OTHER STRATEGIES

Three other strategies can help you make a successful transition to your new role or new job: networking, motivation, and commitment to lifelong learning. Transition happens not only when you move from student to nurse but also when you make major job changes. It is always a challenging time in a person's career.

Networking

One strategy to a smooth transition and continued professional success is networking. Similar to mentoring, networking is a skill that is not fully recognized or adopted by the nursing profession. I believe this is because nursing is predominantly female, and few women have mastered networking skills. However, networking is an effective method for informing people about your goals, concerns, or desires in an informal manner and is something you need to become comfortable doing.

Nurses can increase their power and influence personally and professionally by forming alliances with other groups and individuals. Alliances provide a mechanism for informal sharing of information, clarifying information, and making decisions. By being well networked, a person has "the edge" in terms of additional information and opinions of people with more experience or facts; it also allows people to get to know you. Remember the suggestion to make regular visits to the personnel director at the nursing home where you eventually want a job? That is another form of networking.

Having a well-networked mentor is a real bonus. A well-networked mentor can tell you about conferences to attend and how to get partial funding for them, job openings before they are posted, items of concern in your clinical practice, and how to resolve them before the concern makes it to your personnel file.

There are several ways a soon-to-be or a newly graduated LPN can start networking. One way to enhance your networking ability is to network with a faculty member. Consider the "take a faculty member to lunch" idea as your first step in building a network system. Faculty members know about jobs and application strategies and have an objective view of your strengths and areas of needed improvement. I think every student should have a "take a faculty person to lunch day" before graduation. First, by initiating the invitation and paying for the lunch, you have changed the role relationship between you and your faculty member; you are acting like a professional. You are assuming responsibility for the relationships you need to be successful and are being proactive in getting the information you need. The faculty person may be surprised by your invitation but should recognize the professional nature of what you are doing. At lunch, explain about your desire to develop a network in the area where you plan to be working and ask the questions you need answered. It is important to enjoy the time you spend together so that it can happen more naturally in the future.

Each member of the network has needs, and it is an accepted fact that each person should use the system to meet those needs. The other concept is that you cannot network successfully without being willing to meet someone else's needs. You need to have something to contribute. It may be your energy and enthusiasm, a contact with another person with whom you have networked, or your knowledge base. Everyone has to be willing to give and take for the system to be successful. You need to understand this before building your network.

Individuals in the network system must have a positive self-concept and believe that they can contribute to others' needs. Imagine what you have to offer to people because you understand paradigm shifts and their professional impact, use critical thinking, relate to people within the frameworks of Maslow's and Watson's theories, and know how to find the perfect job, identify and recruit a mentor, and network successfully. In my experience, LPNs in the past were not encouraged or taught how to incorporate many of these concepts into their practice, but you are the LPN of the future, and these concepts need to become part of you.

This is my personal example of networking: I have done a great deal of international travel as a nurse and as a tourist. Because I had done some personal traveling, someone at my state nurses' association gave my name and number to an international organization that wanted an experienced traveler to lead a group of physicians and nurses to the People's Republic of China. I was well networked with the nurses' association executive director, and my name was the first one to come to her mind. Because of that professional relationship, I had two wonderful, expense-paid trips to China. Then because I had that additional experience leading groups on international trips, I received other requests. I have been to several countries with expenses paid because of my informal network system. It is impossible to know ahead of time which networking contact will be your best reward. That is why you should form several alliances to promote your work as a nurse.

Most LPNs I know plan on working a long time. Most nursing careers are not short-term experiences. The nurses I see graduate have worked and sacrificed to obtain their education and licensure. They are proud of what they have done and plan on a career in nursing. That career can be rich in experience with others, information, and opportunity if you consciously decide to develop a network of people to complement what you are trying to do.

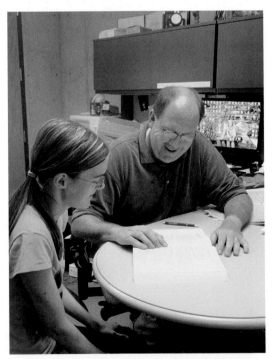

One way to enhance your networking ability is to network with a faculty member. Consider the "take a faculty member to lunch" idea as your first step in building a network system.

Motivation

When people decide to develop a network system, some basic concepts need to be understood. It is most important for you to have a desire to move ahead. Without that motivation, you do not need a network system, so why bother with it? If your goal is to be a nurse manager in the future, you are a person who has that desire.

Relate your future career as a nurse manager to Maslow's hierarchy. It is all about motivation. You need the "perfect job" so you will be motivated to come to work and do excellent work. You need to network so you will have the information that will motivate you to relate to others professionally. To be a leader you need to have a strong motivation to do excellent, caring, professional work as a nurse. That happens when you are well prepared with "knowing how" and "knowing that" knowledge and have a job that complements your career goals.

You cannot sit around and wait for motivation to come to you. Instead, you need to make a plan that takes into consideration the steps of Maslow's theory and the considerations discussed in this chapter. You must make for yourself a place and a way to be strongly motivated in what you do as a nurse to be successful.

This is a paradigm-shifting concept: Now is the time! Today's jobs for LPNs are different from LPN jobs in the past; this is the right time, and these are the right concepts for you to understand and use to meet the demands of the profession today.

Commitment to Lifelong Learning

The final strategy for your successful entry into the nursing profession is that of commitment to lifelong learning. I recognize that close to the graduation from a strenuous program such as yours is not the best time to introduce the idea that you aren't done. However, it is a concept that is important to your success in any LPN position and is crucial to your success as a nurse manager. Commitment to lifelong learning does not mean that you need an RN license, a master's degree, or a doctorate degree, although those options might be on your list of goals. It means that you do not allow the information you learned in nursing school to become stagnant.

The half-life of nursing knowledge is 5 years: In 5 years, 50% of what you learned in school is no longer usable. In 10 years, almost all of your current knowledge may be obsolete. I think this makes it clear why you should have a 5-year educational plan that complements your overall 5-year plan. If you don't, your education will become outdated.

Going back to school for an additional license or a degree in nursing is one option. Also valuable is conscientious attention to conferences and workshops to keep you on the cutting edge of the nursing practice. Professional journals and nursing organizations offer educational programs where you can earn continuing education units (CEUs). Some organizations offer CEUs via webinars or online courses you can complete when it is convenient for you. This is another way for you to maintain your nursing standards. CEUs also are required by many states to maintain your licensure. It is important for you to investigate what is necessary for renewal in your state and use CEUs and the learning that is offered.

Certifications

The modern LPN has the ability to enhance nursing practice with certifications. A certification is not an aspect of the LPN license. It is one way an LPN can expand practice without obtaining an RN license.

Most certifications come from two places. The most common for LPNs is the organization where the LPN is employed. The other is national certification given and managed by professional healthcare organizations. The most common employer certification for LPNs is an IV therapy certification in the states that do not have IV therapy as part of the practical nurse education. It is common for hospitals, nursing homes, and home health agencies to provide IV therapy certification for their LPN employees because it is cost effective for a facility to have an LPN rather than an RN provide IV treatment and administration. It makes the LPN more valuable and marketable if he or she has an IV certification.

Even though you, as an LPN, are certified in IV therapy, you cannot do all of the things an RN can do with an IV line. Learning what you legally can and cannot do with an IV is another reason you go to classes to become certified. There are some medications you cannot administer, and there are some types of IV lines you cannot work with at all. Your state board of nursing establishes these rules, and you are responsible for knowing them.

Some facilities require licensed personnel to become certified in such things as use of the glucometer, IV pumps, and other equipment. These are skills that might be taught in school that do not have an impact on your license. Because different health-care organizations have different equipment and ways of using the equipment, however, they require certification.

It is possible to become nationally certified in several areas. For a list of national certifications, see Box 8.2. These certifications are for your own skill development. They also can be used for CEU requirements if the different organizations offering the certification also offer CEUs. You may be wondering why you would want to spend more time and money to become certified in anything that is not required. First, you may want a certification in a specific aspect of nursing that holds your interest more strongly than others. You may see obtaining a specific certification as the avenue to a career change in which you are interested. There may be the need to maintain your license with CEUs. Finally, when you graduate, you are a licensed nurse who has a professional responsibility to be a lifelong learner. You would not want to be receiving care from a nurse who has not updated his or her knowledge for the past 10 years, and you do not want to be the nurse who is giving that same outdated care to someone else. You have

> ## Box 8.2 National Post-Licensure Certifications
>
> - National Association for Practical Nurse Education and Service, *napnes.org*—IV therapy, long-term care, and pharmacology
> - National Association of Licensed Practical Nurses, *http://nalpn.org/*—IV therapy and gerontology
> - American Board of Managed Care Nursing, *abmcn.org*—Managed care nursing
> - National Alliance of Wound Care and Ostomy, *nawccb.org*—Ostomy management specialist, wound care, diabetic wound, lymphedema lower extremity

a professional responsibility to keep learning all you can.

Career Ladder Learning

Many LPNs worked as certified nursing assistants (CNAs) before entering an LPN program. The nursing assistant certification is the first step in career ladder education. Many LPN and RN programs require CNA certification and experience before admission to their program. Some schools are established so that the student can come in as a CNA, earn the LPN licensure, move right on to the associate degree RN program and licensure, and then as an RN earn a baccalaureate degree in nursing. That type of program is called a *career ladder.*

The strongest point of career ladder education is that the student can be earning increasingly more money while going to school. Instead of being in a basic, baccalaureate nursing program where the student can work as a CNA only for the 4 years of school, a student in a career ladder program first can earn the CNA salary, then the LPN salary, and finally the RN salary. The increasing salary assists in paying for school and family expenses.

For students who eventually want to become an RN, the career ladder program is a reasonable way to proceed. If career ladder programs are not available in your community, you can design your own program. You can locate and become accepted to an associate degree nursing program at any time after you have become an LPN. You may be interested

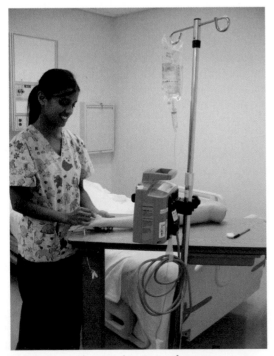

This LPN is working on her IV certification.

in earning your RN license immediately after you graduate with your LPN license, or you may want to wait for 10 years. Either way, you can locate qualified RN programs independently without the program being part of a career ladder system. When you look for an RN program, check to see whether it is accredited by a national nursing accreditation organization just in case the baccalaureate program you want to enter requires it. Some baccalaureate programs accept students from accredited schools only. It is a good idea to be aware of the requirements for the program to which you want admission.

An LPN does not need to feel anything but wonderful about being an LPN. It is not necessary to continue with formal school and earn an RN degree. It is an educational option, however. As you graduate, you will seek employment in a variety of settings and may find one in which you would like to work as an RN. If that is true, continue on with your formal education. Whatever your decision is about becoming an RN, it is your responsibility to maintain yourself as a lifelong learner in nursing. Read, attend conferences and workshops, obtain and maintain certification in an area of interest, and work diligently to maintain the high standards of your chosen profession.

You cannot afford to maintain a job without pursuing continuing learning opportunities. The obvious detriments are the danger to patients and the possibility of malpractice by you. Remember the need to feel safe from Maslow's point of view? Neither you nor the patient is safe if your knowledge is outdated.

One way to enhance your networking ability and lifelong learning goals is to belong to your professional organization, the National Association of Licensed Practical Nurses (NALPN) (http://www.nalpn.org). This is an experience that allows you to know and work with other LPNs and LPN leaders in your state and throughout the United States. One of the main purposes of the NFLPN is to sponsor continuing educational programs. The NFLPN provides you with a mechanism for meeting some of your goals.

The NFLPN was founded in 1949, and only LPNs can join. The activities of the association include defining ethical conduct, providing standards and scope of practice for LPNs, and offering educational programs (as mentioned earlier). Being an active member of the NFLPN is an important aspect of your transition into a nursing career.

Box 8.3 Professional Organizations

- National Association for Practical Nurse Education and Service, *www.napnes.org*
- National League for Nursing, *www.nln.org/*
- National Association of Licenses Practical Nurses, *http://nalpn.org/*
- Many clinically based professional organizations encourage LPN membership.

Becoming an active member of any professional organization is an important step in your career development. Membership provides you with an opportunity to network with other nurses interested in promoting the nursing profession and provides an opportunity to learn about current issues in nursing. A list of additional professional organizations available to LPNs is provided in Box 8.3.

As an LPN who is close to graduation, you will soon emerge into the world of nursing. Your roles, clients, and work environments may vary. Successful role transition now and in the future is crucial to your overall purpose of being a nurse. As you move from being a novice to an expert nurse, incorporate the strategies to assist you in being successful in this goal.

REAL-WORLD CASE STUDY

■ You are soon to be a graduate LPN who has worked the past 2 years as part of a nursing assistant and RN dyad team on the step-down intensive care unit (ICU) of a local hospital. You love your work and hope to be transferred to the ICU to work on one of the LPN and RN dyad teams there. While on the step-down unit, you have worked hard, attended educational programs when they were offered, and hoped that you someday could work in the ICU where the "action" is. You have recognized that the acuity of the ICU patient is a challenge that appeals to you. You are to graduate with your LPN license in 3 months.

1. What information should you gather to assist you in determining whether the ICU job is right for you as a new graduate? Discuss formal and informal mechanisms for gathering information.

Continued

**REAL-WORLD CASE
STUDY** *continued*

2. What strategies should you use to assist you in being considered for the job? Discuss how you would creatively apply the information shared in this chapter to a real situation such as this one.

Key Points

- "Knowing that" knowledge is developed during your nursing education. "Knowing how" knowledge is gained through clinical experience that increases your knowledge and skills.
- The nurse practice act is the law that governs your practice as a nurse and varies by state. The state board of nursing for each state is responsible for enforcing the nurse practice act for that state.
- When considering a job, you need to consider what the job is like on a day-to-day basis, what skills and experience you will need to learn, and whether there will be support systems available, such as orientation and a preceptorship.
- It is important to develop a 5-year career plan that allows for some flexibility.
- When selecting a mentor, you want to find someone who is interested in you as a person and is willing to support and guide you as you start your nursing career. It is important to avoid toxic mentors. A toxic mentor is an individual who demonstrates overt hostility toward a person, gives criticism that is not based in fact, behaves in a manner that destroys another person's confidence, or places someone in a situation without providing adequate support.
- Networking provides an opportunity to meet other nurses who share your interests. Individuals within your network can share job

opportunities and other information that can have a positive impact on your nursing career.
- The concept of lifelong learning is important to your career. Seek out workshops, conferences, and certifications that will keep your nursing knowledge current.
- Individuals transitioning from a student role to the role of an LPN may find themselves at the safety level on Maslow's hierarchy of needs. A student may feel vulnerable and unsafe in the new working environment until she or he makes a successful transition from student to nurse.
- Concepts to consider in developing your career plan are self-evaluation and self-monitoring of progress. When developing a career plan, you need to evaluate your own abilities and develop a plan that best fits those abilities. Self-monitoring is the process of looking at your career plan each year to see whether you have met your goals and making necessary changes to your plan if needed.
- Joining a professional organization is a good way to enhance networking opportunities and lifelong learning goals. Membership in professional organizations provides access to other nurses on local and national levels with similar interests. Professional organizations also provide access to certifications and other educational opportunities.

ANSWERS TO REAL-WORLD CASE STUDY

1. How should you gather information to assist you in deciding if you should apply for the job? First, let's discuss the information you need. The formal mechanism is to go to the human resources office and complete an application for the job. At that time it is appropriate to ask questions about the following:
   - Salary
   - Shifts available
   - Educational opportunities
   - Orientation and a preceptorship

   The employee in human resources may not know the answers to such specific questions. In addition, there may not be a job opening, and without a job opening no one can take your application.

2. The informal search for information can involve many strategies. You have 3 months before you can accept a job there. It is possible for you to get the information you need through an informal network system. You probably already have one established from working in your area for so long and possibly have not recognized it for what it is.

   You frequently take transfers from the ICU. The RNs exchange reports while you and the LPN assist the patient in getting comfortable and oriented to the room. A meaningful networking strategy may be to talk to the LPN about the job and its opportunities. Important, realistic day-to-day information about the job that you can glean this way includes the following:
   - Is it a good job for an LPN, especially for one who is a new graduate?
   - Is there an orientation program? You specifically need to know about this because you realize that the step-down unit and ICU are not the same.
   - Are educational programs available that can assist you in developing and maintaining the highly technical skills that are necessary for the ICU?

   If this information sounds positive to you, there is one more important piece of information you should gather: When does the LPN think a new opening may occur?

   Remember that networking means all parties have something to offer to the network. Before you talk to the LPNs in the ICU, you may need to define what you have to offer. Important aspects of being part of an informal network are to be alert to the opportunities that arise and to work with the people in your network. This lets people in the ICU know that you are interested in the job.

   Another strategy is to identify and recruit a mentor before you get the job. The mentor could assist you in refining skills such as charting or wound assessment that would not be contradictory to the nurse practice act. For example, as a nursing assistant, you should not be looking for a mentor for IV therapy or ventilator management skills.

   If you know the nurse manager for the ICU, you can make an appointment with the manager at a date close to your graduation. At this time, you should tell him or her what your goal is and how pleased you are with the information that you have identified about the job. Let the manager know about your mentorship and what you are learning there, and then share your 5-year plan. This information shows you are someone who is on his or her way to a meaningful career. Admit that your plan may change and that you are flexible in making it.

   None of these strategies should take on the appearance of what is commonly referred to as "brownnosing." Be sincere in what you are doing and show a commitment to what your future holds. Let your energy and enthusiasm show. Show to people that you are a lifelong learner and what you believe about being a nurse. Identifying and working with a mentor are important parts of successfully entering into nursing practice.

REVIEW QUESTIONS

1. Which statement best reflects the nurse with "knowing that" knowledge?
   1. The nurse has been working on the surgical unit for the past 5 years and feels comfortable taking care of the patient population.
   2. The nurse is a recent graduate and has the basic knowledge learned through her nursing classes.
   3. The nurse has worked on the surgical floor for several years and is now moving to the intensive care unit.
   4. The LPN just completed her RN program and will continue to work on the same unit.

2. When looking for a new job, which best describes the most important thing you should consider?
   1. The shifts you will be working
   2. The type of health insurance provided
   3. The process for orientation
   4. The salary you will be paid

3. Which of the following are examples of a toxic mentor? Select all that apply.
   1. Offers to help you but does not follow through
   2. Provides opportunities to learn new skills
   3. Places you in a new situation without providing support
   4. Provides positive feedback

4. You are looking for someone to mentor you. John has worked on the unit for several years and is respected by his peers. John would be a good mentor.
   1. True
   2. False

5. Which statement best describes the reason to join a professional organization?
   1. It is important to your employer.
   2. The other nurses you work with have joined an organization.
   3. You will have an opportunity to network with other nurses.
   4. It will look good on your résumé.

References

Benner, P. (2000). *From novice to expert: Excellence and power in clinical nursing practice, commemorative edition.* New York: Pearson Education.

Bozionelos, N., Konstantinos, K., Van der Heijden, B., Rousseau, D. M., Bozionelos, G., Hoyland, T., . . . Van der Heijdel, C. (2016). Employability and job performance as links in the relationship between mentoring receipt and career success: A study in SMEs. *Group & Organization Management, 41*(2), 135–171. doi:10.1177/1059601115617086

Web Resources

National Association for Practical Nurse Education and Service www.napnes.org

National Council of State Boards of Nursing www.ncsbn.org

National Association of Licensed Practical Nurses www.nalpn.org/

Registered Practical Nursing Association of Ontario www.rpnao.org

Employment Process

KEY TERMS

Cover letter
Interview
Letter of resignation
Résumé

CHAPTER CONCEPT

Professionalism

LEARNING OUTCOMES

1. Identify at least three crucial employer expectations.
2. List the three items that are essential in a cover letter.
3. Write a professional résumé.
4. Discuss three different types of interviews and the way to prepare for each of them.
5. List significant factors for terminating a job in a professional manner.

Let whoever is in charge keep this simple question in her head (not how can I always do this right thing myself, but) how can I provide for this right thing to always be done?

—Florence Nightingale

Florence Nightingale is one of my favorite historical figures. She was a great paradigm shifter, especially for her era. Her courage and commitment have yet to be matched in the nursing profession. I think it is important to consider what she is saying in the statement just given. Her question, "How can I provide for this right thing to always be done?" is an appropriate one for modern nursing. How can a nurse manager or an organization provide for the right thing to be done? The answer is simple: Hire the right personnel for the job and support them in doing their work.

At this point in your education, you are beginning to think about the job where you can "provide for [the] right thing to always be done." In Chapter 8, ideas were shared to assist you in identifying the perfect job for you and in doing well at that position through the use of mentoring and networking. Identifying your career track and developing mentors and a professional network are essential for you to be successful at the job you accept. You need, however, to understand and integrate into your professional personality additional aspects for securing the perfect job.

EMPLOYER EXPECTATIONS

Another aspect of securing the perfect job is to be clear about what your employer expects from you. In general, all employers have the right to expect a person to be well educated for the position being applied for and to have the skills and knowledge that represent that level of education, licensure, and experience. Other expectations are honesty, integrity, and a strong sense of responsibility. Employers expect licensed practical nurses (LPNs) to possess a professional level of communication skills, possess the ability to work on committees and other assignments that go beyond patient care, and ask for information or assistance when it is needed so that patients and other employees are not put into dangerous or compromising situations. An underlying expectation of every employer is for you to demonstrate loyalty to the institution and the people leading it.

It is hard to determine what expectations a new employer may have of you if you don't have a list of possible places to seek employment. There are several ways to identify where you might want to apply for a job. You can check with a local employment agency, read the newspaper want ads, check the Web site of an organization, search the Internet, or ask your friends, other nurses, and fellow students whether they know of job openings that fit your career plans. Connect with the people in your professional network system and talk to your mentor. Diverse, interesting, and challenging positions are available for LPNs. You need to identify the direction you want to take in your career and locate the appropriate employment position to match your goals.

Your understanding of the possible expectations of a future employer is helpful in preparing you for the job application and interview. One strategy is to take an informal tour of an organization you are interested in before submitting your application to the organization. This tour can give you an idea of some of the informal expectations of an employer. What is the dress code? Are people congregated around the desk talking when patient call lights are on, or are employees busily engaged in the process of giving quality care? What do the buildings and grounds look like? Are they clean, pleasant, and in good condition? What happens at mealtime for the patients? How do the patients look? Are they happy, do they have a "cared for" appearance, or do they look uncomfortable? This type of informal tour through a hospital or nursing home can give you information about the expectations of your potential employer and additional information for you regarding the desirability of the job. It can give you some insight into what the focus of your employment interview may be, and if you find positive things on your tour, you can make some informed comments during the interview. It is hard to take a tour if you are interested in applying at a home health agency or as an occupational health nurse. If that is the type of job you are seeking, you can use other strategies to determine the job expectations.

It is important to use your network system or some other mechanism for obtaining information regarding the philosophy and care priorities of the organization where you want to work. Some organizations provide this information on their Web sites. If your highest level skills are in acute care and you are applying for a job in an institution where chronic disease and rehabilitation are the priority, you need to be aware of those expectations

Finding the perfect job is a challenge for a new graduate. Having clear in your mind what you have to offer an employer and determining what the employer expects from you enhance your success in finding such a job.

before submitting your application. If the rehabilitation job is the one you want, you should share with the potential employer any preparation you have made for the position change and your willingness to be a lifelong learner. This preparation could be attending conferences aimed at your topic of interest, enrolling in a class at the local university, or reviewing textbooks. It would be unwise to apply for a job without knowing the personality of the organization and its priorities. When you have determined all you can about a potential employment situation and decided that you want to be seriously considered for the job, you need to use other professional-level skills to make the best application possible.

APPLICATION PROCESS

If you have identified several possible employers who meet your career goals and match your nursing philosophy, you need to make an application to each of them. It is appropriate to make several job applications at the same time. This makes the weeks following your application submissions busy and exciting.

Organizational Suggestions

To make this critical job-seeking time in your career organized and meaningful, consider several suggestions. First, when you have identified the organizations where you want to submit job applications, call the firm and obtain the name of the nurse recruiter. In the current job market, most companies prefer to have job applications submitted online. Be sure to check with the human resources office to determine the correct submission process.

When you start accumulating information about jobs that interest you, keep it in an organized list in a readily accessible place. It is best to keep a typed list of each institution with the phone number, address, and name of the nurse recruiter. This list should be accompanied by the information you gained from talking to others or going on the informal tour. To this list, add the date you sent your cover letter and résumé and notes on any information that the organization sends you.

After you send out your résumé and cover letter, make a follow-up phone call to ensure that they were received. A note to this effect should be added to your master list. It also is appropriate to make a phone call or send a short note to the people who have been helpful to you; for example, after the interview, a note would be appropriate. This simply adds another link to your networking chain.

Cover Letter

Not all employers require a cover letter, so include one only if it is requested (Connley, 2015). Be sure to address the information requested by the employer. If submitting a letter, remember this letter is a significant reflection of your professional personality and must be prepared thoughtfully. See a sample in Box 9.1. It is a business letter; consequently, it should be typed, free of errors, and formatted as a business letter. If you are not comfortable writing a business letter, consult someone who has experience in letter writing. This could be a friend or someone you hire specifically for the purpose of preparing your application.

Each letter should be individualized for the company to which you are applying. Do not use a form letter; instead, tailor what you write to fit the organization. Be sure to include key words from the job description because many employers use computer software to scan cover letters and résumés. Generally, the following three specific items need to be included in your cover letter:

• Statement of interest
• Statement of qualification
• Statement of availability to discuss the job

This letter should be only three or four paragraphs in length. The letter should not be longer than one page; conciseness is important in this communication.

Box 9.1 Sample Cover Letter

December 12, 2017
Mary Ellen Sylvester, Nursing Recruiter
Mountain View Home Health Agency
3571 South 125 East
Huntsville, Ohio 67801
Dear Ms. Sylvester:

I am writing in response to your advertisement in the *NAPNES* journal for the position of home health aide coordinator in the Mountain View Home Health Agency. I have a strong commitment to both home health and the aides who give such a vital service there.

I was employed as a home health aide while I was earning my LPN licensure and have worked the past year as an LPN caregiver. I have experience with computerized charting, personalizing care for a diverse population, planning educational programs, and the staffing process.

I am interested in working for your organization because of your strong reputation for quality, individualized care and the opportunity to use and further develop my management and organizational skills as an LPN.

I will telephone you next week to schedule an interview. If you need to contact me, please call (415) 555–6863 after 2 p.m.
Sincerely,
Elizabeth Haggen, LPN

Address the letter to an individual; this often is the nurse recruiter. Be specific in what you write; state the job you are applying for, request an interview with dates and times that are convenient for you, and provide your telephone number so that you can be reached easily to make the appointment. Do not give a number or time to call that results in an unanswered telephone. That is frustrating to the human resources department and can result in the person who is calling deciding to stop trying to reach you. It also is important to say in the letter that if you do not hear from them within a week, you plan to call to schedule an interview with the appropriate person.

Preparing a Résumé

Preparing a résumé is important in your search for the perfect job. A résumé is a summary of who you are as a professional person and often determines whether you receive further consideration for the position in which you have an interest. It is best to be succinct in preparing your résumé; ideally, it should be only one page. This may be a relief when you prepare your first résumé; however, after you have been a licensed nurse for 5 or more years, you may find it a challenge to condense your career into one page. If the information is crucial to presenting a complete picture of who you are professionally, you may extend the résumé to two or more pages. Keep in mind that a résumé longer than two pages may seem too long to some nurse recruiters. Be careful not to "pad" your résumé with items that do not relate to the job for which you are applying. Focus on the information that matches the job description.

The résumé is another aspect of the application process for which you may need assistance. The same rules apply to this document as to the cover letter. It must be typed, must be free of errors, and must have only significant information on it. Use short, bulleted statements that include key words from the job description. When you have the first or second draft of your résumé on paper, it may be helpful to have someone review it for you. If you have a mentor, it would be appropriate for that person to critique your work. If you do not ask a mentor, ask an experienced nurse or a current or previous faculty member. Your résumé is the vital first impression you make on your future employer. It may be circulated from the human resources office to the nurse manager and, in some organizations, to staff nurses who take part in the interview process. This document is crucial to the employment process and is one that you need to take seriously. The objective is for your résumé to represent you honestly and professionally.

It should be fun to prepare your résumé, unless it has been left as a last-minute project and you are working under a time constraint to complete it. It is an opportunity to review your career goals and to see where you are on your 5-year timeline. In the beginning, write everything that you can remember about what you have done or are doing as part of your career as an LPN. Then begin sorting the information into sections that make sense. Generally, these sections include the following:

• *Personal information*—including name and contact information, both phone number and e-mail address

• **Professional summary**—include your strengths and experiences
• **Experience**—names of employers, dates of employment, positions held, and job tasks
• **Educational background**—degrees, institutions, graduation dates (actual or expected)
• **License and certifications**
• **References**—names of individuals who can give specific information about your prior job performance

It generally takes time and creativity to arrange this information in an easily readable style on one page. Several resources, including résumé templates, are available online for your use. Word processing software such as Word provides résumé templates. It is also wise to check with the human resources office to see whether they have a preferred format for résumés. The appearance and the content of your résumé are crucial, so do not leave it until the last minute in your job search. Box 9.2 shows a sample résumé.

Box 9.2 Sample Résumé

Eliria Rodriguez

Address

462 North 275 East
Tremonton, North Carolina 47635
(612) 555–3941
erodriguez@email.com

Professional Summary

Medical-surgical experience, hardworking, Spanish speaking, available any shift, provide patient-centered care, computerized charting experience, IV certified

Education

Place	Level of Education	Year
Community College of Tremonton	LPN Diploma	2011
Community College of Tremonton	Enrolled in ADN Program	2013

Professional Experience

| Home Health Aide | Fruit Heights Home Health Agency | 2007–2011 |

• Gave personal care to diverse population
• Provided bathing, feeding, and other activities of daily living support
• Measured vital signs

| Staff Nurse, Fruit Heights Home Health Agency | 2011 to present |

• Work with a wide variety of clients in the home
• Dress wounds, administer medications, and work closely with aides and RNs
• Orient aides and provide educational experiences for the aides
• Develop monthly staffing schedule

License/Certifications

Colorado State Board of Nursing to present	LPN License	2011
Williams Hospital	Certified in IV Therapy	2012
Fruit Heights Home Health Agency	Basic Management Techniques	2012

References

John Reed 555-555-4545
Phyllis Ashurst 555-555-9824

PREPARING FOR THE INTERVIEW

A job interview is one of the real adventures in one's professional life. It is never easy unless going through the interview is just a formality for a job that already has been promised to you. Few of us have that type of promise. Current job interviews vary in format depending on the management style of the person responsible for the interview process or the policies of the organization. Because of this diversity, you need to be prepared for whatever the interview may bring.

An interview should not be viewed as a casual step in the employment process. At this point, you have made your decision about where you would like to work; submitted your cover letter, application, and résumé; and kept records of each organization where you have made an application. When you get a phone call inviting you for an interview, it means that you have successfully passed the first step in your prospective employer's scrutiny of you. The interview often is "round two" of the process.

Be prepared for the interview. More specific details on the types of interviews you may be asked to participate in are given later in this chapter. To start with, however, consider the following tried-and-true "shoulds" of participating in a job interview:

• Arrive 5 minutes early for the interview. I remember one of my first job interviews. I wasn't sure how to get to the facility, and I didn't know where the personnel office was located. In my effort not to take anything for granted, I spent 35 minutes waiting in my car in the parking lot because I was too early. This was after I went into the building and located the office where the interview was scheduled. My point is that there is seldom a satisfactory excuse for being late, and being too early makes you look unsophisticated and insecure.
• The clothing you wear to an interview is crucial to your success. You should dress in a manner that tells anyone who sees you that you have pride in yourself and in your profession. Anticipate what the interviewer might be wearing and dress accordingly. In most cases, you want to dress one or two levels up from the job for which you are applying but you don't want to overdress. You may also want to ask the personnel in the human resources office the appropriate level of dress. As a nurse, you will most

likely be wearing scrubs when you work, so a nice pair of dress slacks with a collared shirt and jacket would be appropriate for men; women should wear nice dress slacks or a dress. For more suggestions on how to dress for an interview, see Box 9.3.
• Take a file to the interview that contains your LPN license, cardiopulmonary resuscitation card, hepatitis B and tetanus vaccinations, and tuberculosis skin test results that are less than 12 months old. If you have additional education, such as intravenous certification, also include that information.
• Prepare several questions you can ask during the interview. The questions might include the type of charting used in the organization, how staffing is determined, and resources available to support you in your new job.
• Bring a copy of the résumé you sent so that you have in your hand the same document that your interviewer has.

The applicant's erect posture when entering the room, smile, and firm handshake generally attract positive attention from the interviewer. I was involved in conducting numerous job interviews during one of my nurse management positions. I loved to interview the person who came in smiling, looked polished, dressed professionally, and directly approached me with a hand extended to shake mine. I thought, "This is a real person! Someone who is both interesting and interested in this job. It means something for her or him to be here!" If you are uncomfortable with your

Box 9.3 Dressing for an Interview

• Clothing should be clean and pressed.
• Hair should be neat, clean, and styled conservatively.
• Jewelry should be kept to a minimum and should be tasteful.
• Makeup and nail polish should be applied conservatively.
• Men should be clean shaven or have a healthy-looking beard or moustache.
• Remove facial piercings and cover tattoos when possible.
• Avoid using aftershave and perfume.

"entrance" skills, you need to practice them so that you are comfortable and confident using them. I suggest finding a friend to practice with who will offer a gentle critique of your entrance. When you are comfortable with this, you need to prepare for the types of interviews that are possible.

Many organizations have leveled interviews. Your initial interview may be the first of several. Some organizations have someone in the human resources department conduct the initial interview. If that goes well, the applicant may be called back to interview with the nurse manager.

A third interview may take place with members of the nursing staff. This type of leveled process is rigorous and often tests the applicant's desire for the job. That testing is still another aspect of the process. The prospective employer wants to see whether you have the stamina and commitment to continue through the process. Another reason for leveled interviews is to give numerous people, who could be your fellow workers, an opportunity to meet you and learn more about you. It gives you the opportunity to interact with several of your potential colleagues and should assist you in determining whether this job is really the one you desire. The committee interview is common and one you should be psychologically prepared for. This process is a great opportunity.

Most interviews follow a general format. You must be prepared, however, in case your interviewer does not follow an outline. Usually the first few minutes of an interview allow both people to become comfortable with each other. It is an "ice-breaking" time that allows for casual conversation and generally assists in the goal of having an effective interview because both people are relaxed.

When a comfort level has been established, the experienced interviewer becomes specific in obtaining information from you. It is important for you to be prepared for the following types of questions:

- *Motivation.* Why did you apply with this company? Why do you think you are right for this position? What do you see yourself doing next?
- *Present employer.* What do you do in your current position? Tell me about your success at your job. What do you like most about your current position? What do you like least? Why do you want to change jobs?
- *Professional.* What is your philosophy of nursing? Do you belong to professional

organizations? If you do, what advantage do you see to your membership? What are your career goals? Tell me your 5-year career plan.
- *Contribution to the organization.* What can you offer this organization?
- *Scenarios or case studies.* You may be read a case study or scenario and asked to respond to it. This is a test of your knowledge base and your ability to make decisions and to think under pressure. Some of the scenarios could involve ethical issues, and others could involve clinical situations. It is difficult to prepare for these except to have studied hard as a student with the goal of integrating the information shared in class.

There are some legal aspects of a job interview that are important for you to know. It is illegal for an interviewer to ask you any questions about your age, ethnic background, birthplace, religion, credit rating, sexual preference, number of dependents and their ages, reasons for any previous arrests, or pregnancy or childcare arrangements. If one of these questions is asked and you think answering it would affect your interview positively, you may answer it. Nevertheless, the laws were written to protect you from discrimination, and you are encouraged to use those laws for your own benefit if you feel you need to do so.

You now have been exposed to more information about job interviews than most people have been. It will not be meaningful information for you unless you work to integrate it into your professional self. You need to study and review this information until it seems to be a natural part of you. Find a friend, a more experienced nurse, or a mentor who can practice interviewing with you so that you become comfortable with the process. It may be necessary for you to talk

The interviewing process is often a rigorous one. Going to the interview organized and prepared enhances your ability to manage it successfully.

to someone with more experience to help you identify and verbalize your nursing philosophy and your 5-year career plan. You should become adept at responding to scenarios and case studies. As you practice, you gain confidence in responding to these types of questions and become good at "thinking on your feet."

After you have completed the interview, it is appropriate to send an e-mail thank-you note within 24 hours and follow it up with a written thank-you note mailed the day after the interview. This demonstrates to the interviewer that you are a conscientious applicant (Lawlor, 2015).

Don't let the work of an interview prevent you from seeking another job. There are new and exciting jobs available to LPNs. You should not miss participating in the adventures being professionally carved out for you as an LPN. Just take a deep breath and remember something that used to be really difficult for you, such as giving your first intramuscular injection or inserting a bladder catheter. They were difficult tasks and presented real challenges for the novice student. Now they are a part of what you know and are able to do. The same can be true of job application and interviewing skills if you study them and practice them as you have done with many of your clinical skills.

There are many exciting and interesting jobs available for LPNs. If you are ready for a new position, take the experience you have gained from applying for your first job and locate another one. The newspaper is often a great place to start.

REFLECTIVE THINKING

The process of an interview can have unexpected aspects. Preparing for an interview in general cannot always prepare you for a question such as the one listed here. It is a question a nurse recruiter I know commonly uses in interviews when he cannot make the decision between two qualified candidates. To answer the question effectively, the respondent must show knowledge and personality. Read the question and write your response in your class notebook. Then compare your response with the one written here. The question is: You are being interviewed by the owner of a circus, and he has offered you your choice of three jobs: (1) clown, (2) ringmaster, or (3) juggler. Which job would you choose and why?

- The nurse recruiter who designed this question would never hire people who responded that they wanted the position of the clown. Most organizations need someone who is more focused on work than on having fun.
- If the response was ringmaster, the applicant was eliminated from the process as well. Why? Unless the position was an upper management position, another "boss" or even "bossy" person was not needed.
- When the applicant answered juggler, the interview process continued. Every organization needs people who are willing to try juggling more than one need of the organization. Cheers for the jugglers!

LETTER OF RESIGNATION

It has been explained in previous chapters and earlier in this one that one expectation of employment is loyalty. This loyalty can be expressed in many ways. One of the most telling is the manner in which an employee terminates employment. Is it done without consideration of the organization, other employees, or the clients who need continuous care? Disregard for others is not an acceptable professional behavior. This section of the chapter outlines for you the proper way to terminate employment.

Do you remember how challenging it was to get the job you may now be considering leaving? There was the résumé, cover letter, many telephone calls, and the arduous interviews. You really wanted that job, or you would not have put so much effort into obtaining it. Now it is time for you to leave your current employment situation. The reasons may be simple or complex. Perhaps you are moving to be closer to your extended family, or the management style of the organization has changed and you have not found it to be compatible with your style. Perhaps it is time to move on because of your career plans. Maybe it is time to identify another goal for yourself. The reasons for seeking the job and the reasons for leaving it all need to be treated with respect.

Unless you are experiencing a dreadful emergency, you need to allow your existing employer 2 weeks' notice of your leaving. This is the minimum requirement of professional courtesy. Your resignation should be in the form of a professional letter with the same characteristics discussed for the cover letter. The information in the letter should state your plan to terminate your association with your employer, the last day you plan to work, and (if it is sincere) your appreciation of the job you are leaving. You could list some of the advantages you received while in your current position. The letter should be hand delivered to your immediate employer or nurse manager, and you should explain verbally what you are doing. It is inappropriate for you to tell other employees of your decision to terminate until you have notified your immediate supervisor. After the letter of resignation has been submitted, you can inform anyone you wish about your decision. Terminating in this manner is the professional way to do it. It also is the best method for building a strong set of employment references for future use.

After you leave your job and go to your new position, you still owe loyalty to your previous employer. This specifically means that you do not share negative or "in-house" information about your old job with people from your new job. To do so is to betray the trust you have developed with your previous employer, and it is not the way to develop trust with the new people with whom you are working.

Again, I refer to the statement by Nightingale at the beginning of this chapter. How can you provide for the right things to always be done? You prepare yourself for doing the most effective job you can, seek that job out, and do it with polish and commitment. Nightingale was a thinking woman, and I believe it should not be difficult for any of us, as licensed nurses, to follow our quest for the right things to happen.

REAL-WORLD CASE STUDY

■ You are 3 months from graduating from an accredited LPN program, and you are excited about your upcoming role as an LPN. You have decided that you want to work in a hospital for 1 or 2 years to polish your clinical skills and have role models and mentors available to you. You have had clinical experience in a local 300-bed hospital and that setting is appealing to you as a place of employment.

1. Describe how you may determine in which area of the hospital you want to work and how you are going to make an application at the hospital.
2. Write a cover letter and prepare a résumé.
3. Prepare a filing system for three hospital applications and submit it to your faculty person with your letter and résumé

Key Points

■ Employers expect employees to have the appropriate skills and knowledge for the job. Other expectations for employees include good communication skills and the willingness to work on committees and other projects beyond patient care. An underlying expectation of every employer is for an employee to demonstrate loyalty to the organization and its leaders.
■ There are several ways to find a potential job. They include searching for organization Web sites and newspaper want ads and asking friends, colleagues, and other students about current job openings. Most organizations prefer to have applicants apply for jobs online. Always check with the human resources department for their preference.
■ Cover letters should include your statement of interest for the job, a list of your qualifications, and your availability for the job. Not all organizations require a cover letter, so check for preferences.

- A résumé is a brief outline of your qualifications, job experience, and education. The résumé should be well organized and easy to read. The length of the résumé will depend on your experience and the job for which you are applying.
- When dressing for an interview, dress one or two levels above the job for which you are applying. Do not overdress. Make sure your clothing is clean and you are well groomed. Remove facial piercings and cover tattoos.
- When interviewing for a job, an applicant may have several interviews as part of the process. The applicant may interview with the human resources director, the nurse manager, and members of the nursing unit for which the applicant is applying. For each level of interviews the applicant should be ready to answer questions regarding prior experience, motivation for the job, and what the applicant will contribute to the organization.
- Prior to an interview, prepare responses to possible questions about your motivation for applying for the job, what you do in your current position, your philosophy of nursing, what you will contribute to the organization, and possible clinically based work-related scenarios.
- During the interview, be sure to address questions concisely. Prepare questions you can ask during the interview.
- After the interview, send a thank-you letter.
- There are several factors that may require someone to terminate a job. The reasons to terminate may have something to do with a change in management that is not compatible with an individual's needs or it is time for the person to move on because of career plans. It may be that the individual simply needs to move to live closer to extended family. When terminating a job, it is important to provide the current employer with 2 weeks' notice in the form of a professionally written letter of resignation.

ANSWERS TO REAL-WORLD CASE STUDY

1. The area in which you choose to apply for a position depends on your career goals. It is a reasonable consideration to want to work in an area where you may have many opportunities to improve on your clinical skills, but you need to ask yourself, Which skills? Do you want to be great at care of adults, children, or families? Your career plan determines your optimal place to work. After you have identified which area is for you, be alert to available positions on that unit. Do you know anyone who works there and who could serve as part of your network? If you do, take the person to lunch or to the cafeteria for a quiet moment to discuss the possibilities for you and your wish to be employed there.

2. Use the information in this chapter to write your cover letter and prepare your résumé. Use classmates, faculty, and appropriate other persons and their ideas to make this exercise meaningful. Have someone review your work and give you feedback. Submit your work to your faculty person for evaluation.

3. The creation of a filing system should be a pleasant experience. Make it user friendly, and let it reflect your personality. Be creative and original just for the fun of it! This can help when job searching is tedious.

REVIEW QUESTIONS

1. Maria is looking for a job as an LPN. She is not sure how to decide which job will be best for her. Which best describes what she needs to know about the organization?
   1. The philosophy and care priorities of the organization
   2. The number of hours she will be working
   3. The nurse-to-patient ratio
   4. The organization's patient satisfaction scores

2. Which best describes the information you should include in a cover letter?
   1. The number of hours you are willing to work
   2. The shifts you are willing to work
   3. The job for which you are applying
   4. The name of your current employer

3. What information should be included in a résumé?
   1. Work experience
   2. Summary of qualifications
   3. Education
   4. All of the above

4. Which best describes how to submit your résumé?
   1. Mail it directly to the organization.
   2. Hand deliver it to the human resources office.
   3. Contact the human resources office to identify the correct process.
   4. E-mail a copy to the human resources office.

5. What best describes how you should terminate a job?
   1. Let your coworkers know as soon as you decide to quit.
   2. E-mail a letter of resignation to your immediate supervisor.
   3. Directly contact the human resources department.
   4. Discuss it with your immediate supervisor.

References

Connley, C. (2015). Resume myths to debunk in 2015. *Black Enterprise, 45*(6), 46.

Lawlor, J. (2015). Land that next job: Tips for new pros seeking new opportunities. *Public Relations Tactics, 22*(11), 8.

Web Resources

The Complete Guide to Resume Writing for Nursing Students and Alumni http://nursing.jhu.edu/life_at_hopkins/student_resources/center/documents/resume_guide.pdf

10

Leadership and Management as a Professional Concept

KEY TERMS

Autocratic leader
Democratic leader
Emotional intelligence
Formal leader
Informal leader
Laissez-faire leader
Leadership
Management
Multicratic or participative leader
Transformational leader

CHAPTER CONCEPTS

Leadership and Management
Collaboration

LEARNING OUTCOMES

1. Compare the concepts of leadership and management regarding purpose and function.
2. Identify the importance of an informal leader in an organization.
3. Describe how people become aware of and develop leadership and management traits.
4. Clarify the current role of an LPN in leadership and management from a historical perspective.
5. Describe common leadership styles and how they relate to Dr. Abraham Maslow's hierarchy of needs and Dr. Jean Watson's science of human caring.

What lies behind us and what lies before us are tiny matters compared to what lies within us.

—Oliver Wendell Holmes

I would like you to take a few minutes to sit and think before you go too far into this chapter. I want you to consider the "scripts" that each person has in his or her mind. For example, consider how you did your gift shopping for the last holiday season: (1) Did you write a list, check the ads, and shop early, or (2) did you wait until mid-December, charge many items, and wait in long, noisy lines? Some of you answer with a resounding "yes" to the first description, and others think it sounds boring and devoid of the fun of the holidays. The same is true of the second description: For some of you, it sounds like "what makes the holiday season fun," and for others it seems too stressful and disorganized. For you to understand and use leadership and management principles effectively, you need a clear understanding of yourself. That is what Oliver Wendell Holmes is referring to when he talks about the importance of knowing what lies within each of us.

The concept of personal scripts within us is based on transactional analysis techniques. The scripts come from a lifetime of learning and have a significant impact on the activities we, as nurses, participate in every day. They are like "tape recordings" of our lives. We don't have every second of our lives readily available to us on these mental tapes, but many segments play over and over again and in that way influence our basic personalities.

I clearly remember my mother standing with her hands on her hips, raising her voice at me, and saying, "Go clean your room!" There was no negotiation, no appropriate response from me, only the direct command given. I didn't like my mother talking to me that way, and I didn't like cleaning my room. I found it difficult to make my bed because it was against the wall, and it was hard to make it look pretty. Also, I never knew where to put my toys. Should I leave them out where I would be playing with them next, or should I put them away? This picture of frustration and dissatisfaction is one of my tapes. I didn't realize how well "filmed" it was until I found myself standing in my daughter's doorway with my hands on my hips, raising my voice, and saying, "Go clean your

room!" I was replaying a tape from my childhood. It was a tape I didn't like; nevertheless, it had been powerfully planted into my brain, and there I was playing it.

All people have tapes in their mind filed under multiple categories. I have talked about a parenting tape; we also have leadership tapes, management tapes, and communication-style tapes. Whatever you read in this book about leadership and management, you may integrate it with what already exists in your mind. This happens without you thinking about the process of integration; it is a natural phenomenon of learning. What emerges is a leadership and management style that is an integration of the new and the old information and is uniquely you. That is why I want you to spend some time thinking about what already exists on your tapes.

Do you have tapes of terrific managers and strong, independent leaders? Are some of your leadership and management tapes of dysfunctional people who abused their power in an organization? Without thinking of specific tapes, what is your general approach to other people? Are you caring and patient, brusque and harried, or passive and barely responsive? You know best what is within yourself, and you need to spend some time identifying those previously learned patterns of leading and managing. After you have identified them, you should consider which ones you like and which ones you want to change. Only through this introspective process can you emerge with the leadership and management style that is genuinely you.

REFLECTIVE THINKING

Consider your most predominant "tapes" on the following issues, and write a brief summary of what the tapes contain that is pertinent to developing your personal leadership and management style. Record your thinking in your classroom notebook.

1. My communication-style tape contains:
2. The tape about my favorite leadership role model contains:
3. My "greatest fears about becoming a leader" tape contains:
4. The most important tape I can develop for me as a leader/manager would contain:

LEADERSHIP VERSUS MANAGEMENT

Many people do not consider the differences between the terms *leadership* and *management.* They are terms that often blend in a person's mind without a clear concept of their unique and powerful differences. You need to understand these concepts, and through understanding them, you can integrate them into your system of tapes.

Leadership comes first; management is second. In the words of the late Stephen R. Covey (2013), a great man in the leadership and management arena: "Management is doing things right; leadership is doing the right thing." Covey continues by saying that management is efficiency in climbing the ladder of success, and leadership determines whether the ladder is leaning against the right wall.

Covey extends this thought with an amusing analogy. Suppose the goal of your organization was to make a trail in a dense and dangerous jungle. What would be the role of the managers? They would be directing the people who were working the machetes. They would have the job descriptions written, have the machinery available for sharpening the machetes, and provide food and water. All these activities seem to be effective. The goal of the managers is to get the work done through others—they are the "hands-on" type of people. Meanwhile, where are the leaders? They are the people who have the jungle maps in hand and are responsible for climbing the tallest tree and saying, "Oh, no! This is the wrong jungle!" Preferably, they would climb that tree and say, "Good work! This is the right jungle and we're moving in the right direction!"

More concrete definitions of leadership and management follow:

- *Leadership:* The personal traits necessary to establish vision and goals for an organization and the ability to influence others to willingly meet the goals.
- *Management:* The personal traits necessary to plan, organize, motivate, and direct the personnel and material resources of an organization.

These definitions complement the analogy of the jungle and should clarify the differences between the two roles. Nevertheless, something this complex is never simple. Additional information about each concept follows.

Formal Leader

There is a great deal of material written about the concept of leadership. It is strongly desirable to have an effective leader in an organization, and it is generally distressing when the organization's formal leader is not effective at the job of leading. This person is the boss, the one whose directions are followed with minimal challenges. In health care, this person may have the title of the administrator, president, or chief executive officer.

This top-line leader often does not interact with patients or give them care, and in some settings the formal leader does not interact frequently with the staff. The responsibility of the assigned leader is to anticipate the changes in health-care systems and to lead the organization to a comfortable or successful place in that future awareness or vision. This is the person who should know when to expand an organization and when to cut the caseload. On the one hand, the risk is great in such a job because a mistake can have serious consequences. There is no room for even a tiny error when making decisions for the multimillion-dollar concerns that deliver health care in the United States today. On the other hand, when a decision has been made that demonstrates the leader's ability to foresee the needs of the organization, the value of that person increases, as does the value of the organization.

Most organizations have leaders on another level. This could be a nurse manager in a hospital or nursing home or a case manager in a home health agency. These leaders are accountable to the higher-level administrator but have their own domain in which to lead. This also is a formal leader: someone who has a title and generally an office. This formal leader does not often give patient care but frequently interacts with the staff.

Informal Leader

Another type of leader is the informal leader. This is a person without an official title or office. It is the person on the care team who is respected because of personal wisdom and the willingness to share it and who is a role model for excellent leadership on a day-to-day basis. This person does not prepare the schedule or determine the raises but instead works within the assigned workload while quietly leading the care team to a higher standard of performance or a successful change in a modality of care. This is the person to whom everyone

FOCUSED LEARNING CHART

Basic Principles of Leadership and Management

LEADERSHIP	MANAGEMENT
Comes first, before management	Follows the vision and goals of leadership
Requires the ability to develop vision and goals	Requires the ability to plan, organize, motivate, and direct
"Doing the right thing"	"Doing things right"

goes for expert assistance in changing a dressing, starting an intravenous line, or comforting a dying person and the family. Often the leadership skills of this person are associated with expertise in the art of nursing.

REFLECTIVE THINKING

Identify the highest level formal leader in the organization of your choice (e.g., work, school, church, family). Then list:

1. Positive characteristics of this person:
2. Less desirable characteristics of this person:

Identify an informal leader in the organization of your choice (e.g., work, school, church, family). Then list:

1. Reasons I perceive this person as an informal leader:
2. Positive characteristics of this person:

The informal leader is easily identified within the group. It is the individual to whom everyone looks when a decision has to be made or when a controversial topic is discussed. This person has power among the group members that has been earned through competent work and caring attitudes toward colleagues and patients.

An effective formal leader looks for, identifies, and respects informal leaders because informal leaders have power with the group, expertise in patient care, and ability to lead the group in the direction of the formal leader's choice. A wise formal leader quickly develops a positive working relationship with the informal leaders in the organization. Unwise leaders engage in power struggles with informal leaders. These power struggles do not complement the work of the team and diminish the effectiveness of the formal leader. Also, an important leadership concept you need to know is

that every time, always, no exception, there are no winners in a power struggle! Never! So, avoid them, teach your staff to avoid them, and be a role model in developing more positive ways to resolve differences.

An example of an informal leader in my former organization, a statewide university, is the departmental administrative assistant. She has the power to determine when a person is paid for overload teaching, when books are ordered, and when an issue from a faculty person is quietly and appropriately shared with the administrator of the organization. This person never manipulates people with her power and is careful concerning the issues she supports with the administrator. It is a clear power line and one that a wise faculty person should use with respect.

How can an informal leader be this powerful? I have spent a great deal of my career in nursing homes, and many times the strongest informal leader was a nursing assistant. As a novice nurse, I would try to understand how someone with the least education in leadership and management could be the most powerful person in the facility. It took me a while, but I finally determined how that happened. Leadership as well as management can be a natural characteristic of a person. You have heard the phrase, "He is a natural born leader." It is true. Some of that comes from the personal tapes the person has playing. Perhaps this person was raised in a family in which strong leadership traits were exhibited or has worked in places where the leadership examples were excellent. For some people, leadership is a natural ability, an instinct, or a trait the person has learned through trial and error. Leadership skills are apparent on any educational level and in any job description.

Can you identify the formal and informal leaders in your organization? For some readers, that is in a school system, and for others that is at a job.

Whatever role you have in the organization, it is important to identify the formal and informal leaders for future reference. You also should watch them and observe how they perform their responsibilities. Identify the skills they use and determine what you think about the results of their work.

Management

Management is the ability to organize details so that the leader's vision and goals can be achieved successfully. If the leadership is ineffective, it does not matter how great the managers are; no one can be successful when working for a poor-quality leader. Covey (2013), a man with a great sense of humor, says that efficient management without effective leadership is like straightening deck chairs on the *Titanic.* No amount of good management can compensate for poor leadership.

The manager often is seen as the person who is responsible for getting work done through others. This responsibility requires excellent interpersonal relationship skills; broad understanding of the organization and how it works; and the ability to perceive the organization as client focused, to establish goals and objectives, to use person power and physical resources, and to act as an agent of change. As you review this list of qualifications, it is easy to identify that each one is essential to "getting the job done."

A serious leadership and management problem occurs when the leader spends a large amount of time doing the managing. This may seem helpful to the manager at first, but soon someone may notice that there is no leadership, no vision, and no goals; in short, there is no direction in which the organization should go. This situation occurs because the leader is sinking in the details required of the manager and is unable to do the leading. The roles of leader and manager are different and need to be recognized as such.

Similar to leadership, management is a trait that can be a natural behavior for a person. Management can be done by instinct or learned and filed on one's personal tapes. The point of learning more about leadership and management is to add your natural instincts and abilities to the tapes. The challenge is for you to integrate who you are with the new ideas that are shared throughout this book. Some people have a natural ability to lead or manage or to do both, but everyone can become a better leader or manager by studying and practicing these skills.

Managers generally work closely with the caregivers and provide them with guidance, information, and actual assistance with the day-to-day work.

HISTORICAL OVERVIEW OF NURSING LEADERSHIP AND MANAGEMENT ROLES

In nursing's long history, there have been many leaders and managers. Discussed here are Florence Nightingale, Lillian Wald, Mary Brewster, and Dr. Jean Watson.

Florence Nightingale

Florence Nightingale is an excellent example of a nursing leader. I classify her as a leader and not a manager because of her vision. She had a vision for nurses in her century, and although she did much of the management in the beginning, she soon hired managers to get the work of the profession done. This work happened in her schools of nursing and in the foundling homes she started.

My favorite story about Nightingale is her approach to the situation she faced during the Crimean War. She went with a sack of gold tied under her skirt and accompanied by 38 women who expressed a desire to be nurses (there was no education available for nurses at that time in England). When they reached Crimea, she and her nurses were asked to live together in a one-room apartment and were forbidden to work on the wards with the wounded soldiers. Because she had a vision of what she and her nurses could do, she waited. They made no complaints about the extremely cramped living space (they had to sleep in shifts), and they busied themselves by making bandages and cleaning instead of protesting because they were not allowed to work with the wounded. Nightingale had a goal, and she meant to achieve it. One day there were 1,300 soldiers brought by boat to the hospital where she and the other nurses were assigned. The chief surgeon of the hospital went quietly to her and asked whether she and her nurses could "help out in the wards." They did, and once they were admitted, they did not leave.

Nightingale could have "thrown a tantrum" over the living conditions, stomped about, and taken her nurses back to England. She could have been aggressive and uncompromising to the chief surgeon about working in the wards until he ordered her and her nurses back to England. None of those things happened because she was a leader with a vision and goals. Her goal was to work in the wards with the soldiers, and she patiently bided her time until she was invited into that care setting. These actions demonstrate the attributes of a leader.

Lillian Wald

Lillian Wald and Mary Brewster established the first visiting nurse service in the United States and the Henry Street Settlement House on the Lower East Side of New York City. Wald, the daughter of a wealthy man, was giving a lecture on how to make a bed to a group of immigrant women in that part of the city when a child entered the room, asking for help. Wald and Brewster went with the child and found a foul tenement where nine pitifully undernourished people were sleeping, most of them on the floor. Wald had never been aware that such suffering existed. Despite her wealthy background, she went to work, recruited others to come to work, and contacted physicians. By the end of the day, the room was clean (she did much of the cleaning herself), each person had bedding and clean clothes, and each one had been seen by the physician. The apartment also was stocked with nourishing food. To accomplish so much in part of a day required management skills, and Wald had them. She was able to get work done through others. The establishment of the Henry Street Settlement House required leadership skills, and she had those too. Our nursing history is rich with examples of leadership and management in nursing practice.

Dr. Jean Watson

During a time when nursing was striving to be more like the medical model or paradigm of care, Watson's work with the science of human caring pioneered the effort to establish creditability for nurses who adopt the nursing paradigm instead of the medical paradigm.

An understanding of these two paradigms is crucial for your understanding of Watson's work and as a background for your own career in leadership and management positions. The medical model paradigm has a great deal to do with the role of women in society and the fact that nursing previously was an all-female profession. At the present time, less than 8% of nurses in the United States are men, but the number is growing.

As a student nurse (40+ years ago), I was required to stand when a physician came on the floor and was evaluated on how tolerant I was of physician tantrums. (I have had charts thrown at me, have had telephones hung up in my ear, and have received inappropriate criticism from physicians in front of patients and their families.) This is how many nurses were treated. It was with an unrealistic

Dr. Jean Watson, distinguished professor, nurse theorist, and humanitarian. (Source: *Anderson, M. A. [2000]. To be a nurse [p. 222]. Philadelphia: F. A. Davis.)*

valuing of the physician's role because of gender and power. This was the accepted paradigm.

Since then, nurses have sought more respect and creditability, initially by acting more like physicians. This has brought about a positive change in the development of the nurse practitioner role. In this role, a nurse initially was referred to as a "mini-doctor." This role eventually gave the nurse practitioner prescriptive practice (previously a physician's activity) and autonomy in making physical assessments and engaging in a wide variety of other clinically focused behaviors. These nurses worked as a team member with physicians and eventually changed the manner in which nursing was viewed. (I am proud of the nurse practitioners in our profession and salute them for their courage in altering the role of nurses.) For some people in some situations, however, the role looked like the mini-doctor role, and some of the basic tenets of nursing were being threatened.

Watson introduced her caring theory at this point in nursing history. This theory gave back to nurses the vision of holistic nursing and personal caring. These concepts generally have not been the paradigm of medicine and work well with the nursing paradigm of care. Watson's caring theory brought back to the nursing profession a legitimate framework for co-participating in care with clients and focusing on human individuality and the soul. This is an example of leadership with vision and goals in that Watson brought about a change and an awareness that was in jeopardy of being lost to the profession.

WHERE IS THE LICENSED PRACTICAL NURSE IN THIS HISTORICAL PICTURE?

Chapter 1 provides an excellent overview of the history of the licensed practical nurse (LPN). The emphasis of this chapter is on the caregiver of today. Many people in the health-care environment argue that leadership and management are not appropriate roles for the LPN. It already has been discussed in this book that LPNs are managers of care for the clients to whom they are assigned. You are managers, and in many settings you also are leaders. These roles should never preclude the laws of your state's nurse practice act or alter the fact that an LPN is required to practice under the supervision of a registered nurse (RN) or physician.

Anyone who questions the need for leadership and management skills in the LPN domain of practice should walk down the hallway of any nursing home or hospital in the United States. A tour of such facilities verifies not whether that role should be taken by LPNs, but that it already has been taken by LPNs. The least the profession can and should do is to educate LPNs for the role that they will play in health care.

One factor that has brought about this role identification is the work redesign of many health-care organizations. In 1994, when the idea of health-care reform was introduced by the Clinton administration, most health-care organizations moved quickly into a mode of cost saving as a way of preparing for the changes that were expected. Health-care reform did not materialize in the way that was anticipated, but after the cost-cutting measures were initiated, most administrators were not willing to alter them.

One of the most significant changes was the laying off or loss by attrition of large numbers of RNs and hiring LPNs as their replacements. This was a natural picture of change that dramatically affected the delivery of care for all nurses. LPNs found they were required to assume more management responsibility in terms of working as the manager of other LPNs and multiskilled paraprofessional workers. Historically, LPNs have been managers and leaders in long-term care facilities. Many LPNs have been employed in leadership roles as directors of nursing. Additionally, LPNs frequently are charge nurses in long-term care facilities; this has been the case since the 1990s and for even longer in some parts of the United States. LPNs have opportunities to assume the role of leader and manager in today's health-care paradigm. These roles have been outlined by leaders with vision and goals and have been supported by other nurses and clients. I do not think this is an issue to question at this point in nursing history.

LEADERSHIP STYLES

There are many leadership styles, and it is important for the LPN to know and understand them (Box 10.1). You need to understand your own predominant style and reinforce it or alter it depending on its effectiveness. It also is important to be able to understand the styles and the approaches of others in these roles. Remember the importance

Box 10.1 Leadership Styles

- Autocratic—task oriented; makes decisions independently
- Democratic—focuses on the abilities of each individual; uses group process to make decisions
- Laissez-faire—does not assume leadership responsibilities; leaves employees to make their own decisions
- Multicratic or participative—seeks input from others then makes final decisions; able to empower employees
- Transformational—encourages people to look at issues from different perspectives and become more involved in the process of change; empowerment of others is more important than their own power

of knowing what lies within yourself? This is part of what determines your preferred type of leadership. What you gain from this book, other learning experiences, and the leaders and managers you have worked with and are going to work with throughout your career should contribute to your leadership style. Research has identified five styles of leadership from various fields, not just nursing or health care.

Autocratic Leader

An autocratic leader tends to have traits that are not appealing to most workers. This person is task oriented; makes decisions independently instead of using input from the group; and motivates employees through praise, blame, and reward. This type of leader is more likely to issue disruptive commands to subordinates than are other leadership types. These commands, as opposed to requests, often interfere with the worker's expressed wishes and ongoing activities.

Many workers avoid autocratic leaders because working with them is too uncomfortable. This type of leader often says, "My employees never have to wonder where they stand with me because I just tell them." In contrast, the employees may say, "I avoid being around my boss because I never know when he or she is going to blast me!"

When an autocratic leader hires a manager who also is autocratic, the result often is a power

struggle between them. This type of emotional activity does not allow either the leader or the manager to focus on the needs of the organization. The leader's vision is lost in the struggle to come out the victor when interacting with the autocratic manager. The same is true of the manager. Too often this person's time is spent planning how to survive the next power struggle with the leader instead of how to work toward the goals of the organization.

There is a basic rule about power struggles as mentioned earlier in the chapter: No one wins in a power struggle! The leader and manager who participate in this type of autocratic activity are disabling the organization and often are not aware of what they are doing.

There are advantages in having an autocratic leader, and it is one I explain every semester to my management students. The classic example of when an autocratic leader really is the best person for the situation is in an emergency. When I am making this point in the classroom, I become dramatic and let the students know that if I were to fall over with a cardiac arrest, I would want the most autocratic person in the room to take over, order people around without regard for their feelings, and save my life! In this scenario, I see a powerful need for an autocratic leader, don't you?

The point of gaining some understanding into the different types of leadership styles is to "know one when you see one" and to know how to work most effectively with that person. What have you learned about working with an autocratic leader?

- Expect praise and criticism; both are energetically given. You always know where you stand with this type of person.
- The instructions you receive from an autocratic leader are not hidden or subtle.
- Never get into a power struggle with this type of person. You and the organization will be the losers.
- Trust this type of leader in an emergency.
- Do not expect to participate in group decision making when you have an autocratic leader.
- People who work under an autocratic leader seldom move beyond Maslow's level of safety while in the work setting.
- Autocratic leaders generally do not show the qualities of the science of human caring in their work with their subordinates.

Democratic Leader

The term *democratic* causes most people to think of the founding fathers of the United States and the positive governmental innovations they instituted. Most people don't recognize the length of time it took to get the Declaration of Independence and the Bill of Rights written and agreed upon.

A democratic leader is focused on the individual characteristics and abilities of each subordinate. This is a plus for employees who are in school or have family problems that require a specialized schedule. This type of leader uses personal and positional power to achieve the desirable outcomes and never loses the overall commitment to whatever is best for the group.

A democratic leader uses the group process to make all major decisions. This person provides an empowering environment for the people being led, encouraging them to establish their own goals and to make plans to achieve their goals. These traits are appealing to most employees because the individual person is well represented in all activities of the organization.

Democratic leaders are more likely than autocratic leaders to give suggestions and more willing to share information. This style of leadership encourages the process of group mindedness and requires a strong commitment of time to make decisions through the process of the group. (Remember it took a long time to achieve an agreement on the Declaration of Independence!)

Most people are initially drawn to the democratic leader. They like the individualized attention this type of leader gives to subordinates and enjoy being part of a team. Sometimes members of the group choose to leave this type of leader because of the time-consuming process of making decisions. Group decision making is challenging and requires a commitment from each employee to spend the time necessary to accomplish the goals of the group. This type of leader would not participate in a power struggle, but instead the problem would be turned over to the group to manage.

Democratic leaders are pleasant people to work with, and generally the work environment is equally pleasant. The problem occurs when there is an emergency in the organization and there isn't time for the group to process the solution. This is a serious problem for a manager who is unaccustomed to solving problems without the input of the group.

What have you learned about working with a democratic leader?

- Your individual needs generally will be met if they do not interfere with the larger needs of the group.
- You need to make a time commitment to work with the group process.
- No secrets or information are kept from individuals who work with a democratic leader.
- Within the group, each person is seen as a unique individual.
- Emergencies within this leadership environment are stressful, especially if a decision needs to be made quickly.
- People who work for a democratic leader often can move to social and even self-esteem needs on Maslow's hierarchy of needs scale.
- This leader often works within the science of human caring framework.

Laissez-Faire Leader

The laissez-faire leader is often referred to as the "let alone" leader. This person refuses to assume the leadership responsibilities that accompany the job, leaving the workers without direction, supervision, or coordination in their projects. It also gives the workers the opportunity to plan, perform, and evaluate their work in any manner they desire.

Laissez-faire leaders do not give praise, criticism, feedback, or information. The level of satisfaction with this type of arrangement depends on the individual worker. Because there is no leader to organize and manage group work, the workers decide on the presence or absence of group work. Without a leader, some members want to work as a group and others refuse to do so. Generally, this is a frustrating situation even for the most autonomous employees because there is a tendency for people not to work together.

Many people avoid working with a laissez-faire leader because of the high level of dissatisfaction caused by the lack of guidance, caring, and instructions. People who work on a laissez-faire unit usually are out of synchrony with the rest of the organization because information from other segments of the organization has not been channeled to them by the laissez-faire leader.

What have you learned about a laissez-faire leader?

- This type of leader does not give you guidance, information, or individualized attention.

- This work environment provides a great deal of autonomy.
- There is chaos in the system because of the lack of information.
- You are usually out of synchrony with the rest of the organization because of the lack of information being channeled to you.
- Feelings of resentment toward the leader often exist.
- This leader generally does not provide mechanisms for the workers to move beyond the safety level of Maslow's hierarchy of needs.
- Generally, this type of leader probably hasn't heard of the science of human caring and doesn't practice it professionally.

Multicratic or Participative Leader

The multicratic or participative leader is a compromise between the autocratic and democratic leader. This person develops a personal analysis of all problems, makes proposals to the group based on this analysis, and invites the group members to give their criticism and comments. This leader personally processes the feedback from the group and then makes all final decisions. This person works well within the group and in an emergency when matters must be handled immediately.

The participative leader has the best attributes of the autocratic and democratic leadership styles. This type of leader provides many advantages for workers and managers. Confidence emanates from the leader to the managers and workers, which is empowering; most employees enjoy this type of interaction. It allows the employees to share their ideas freely with the leader and contribute to the goal-setting process in a significant manner. Control and power are widely spread throughout the group because of this style of leadership.

What have you learned about a participative leader?

- The leader plays an active role in making decisions for the work group.
- The leader provides an empowering environment.
- No secrets or information are kept from members of the group.
- Group members have a free exchange of ideas.
- The participative leader encourages people to function on the social and self-esteem levels of Maslow's hierarchy of needs.

Participative managers listen carefully to all that the other team members have to say and value their input.

- This type of leader generally functions within the science of human caring framework.

Transformational Leader

A more contemporary leadership style is transformational leadership. A transformational leader focuses on a clear vision and working toward that vision. This person accepts change and is willing to make the most of it. This leader recognizes the uncertainty of the current healthcare environment and encourages individuals to question the established views of the organization as well as the views of the leader. This allows everyone the opportunity to look at issues from different perspectives and to come up with a better approach to meet identified goals. Transformational leaders develop their followers' interests and commitment to the mission of the group by encouraging problem solving and supporting them in becoming more involved in the change process. This leader believes the empowerment of others is more important than their own sense of power (Roussel, Harris, & Thomas, 2016).

What have you learned about a transformational leader?

- The transformational leader develops a clear vision and shares it with the group.
- Group members are allowed to question the leader.
- This type of leader understands the importance of interpersonal relationships.
- Empowerment of others is encouraged.
- This leader encourages people to function on the social and self-esteem levels of Maslow's hierarchy of needs.

• This person works within the science of human caring framework.

Emotional Intelligence and Leadership

Leaders, no matter what their style, must be able to manage their emotions when interacting with others. The ability to perceive and express your emotions is referred to as emotional intelligence (EI) or emotional competence (Northhouse, 2015). Some experts say that in most situations EI is more important than cognitive intelligence when dealing with individuals, and that it is a leadership trait that can be developed over time. A key component of EI is self-awareness (Tyczkowski et al., 2015). Self-awareness is the ability to recognize your own emotions and how you behave related to those emotions. As a leader, it is important to understand how your emotions impact your behavior toward others so you can change undesirable behaviors. Refer to Chapter 11 for suggestions on controlling your emotions.

Other components of EI include self-regulation, motivation, empathy, and social skills (MindTools, n.d.). Individuals who exercise self-regulation keep their emotions in check and do not make quick decisions based on the emotion they are experiencing at the time. Individuals with a high EI are usually highly motivated to accomplish tasks and enjoy a challenge. They are also empathetic toward others and recognize their coworkers' feelings and needs, often before they are expressed. Finally, individuals with a high EI have the ability to interact well with others and maintain good relationships. These EI components are all good traits that a leader should possess.

Leaders with high EI bring out the best and build stronger relationships with their staff, which improves collaboration and teamwork. When leaders are aware of their emotions and the impact of their emotions on others, they will be more successful leaders. There are several EI tests available on the Internet if you are interested in determining your level of emotional intelligence.

WHAT TYPE OF LEADER ARE YOU?

If you were to categorize the type of leadership that allows you to do your best work, which one would it be? Do you seek the honesty and directness of the autocratic leader, thrive on the group discussions of the democratic leader, need the autonomy of the laissez-faire leader, or gain confidence and professional strength working with a participative or transformational leader? Each leadership style has inherent advantages and disadvantages, and you need to identify the ones that support you in being the best LPN you can become.

If you are offered a management position, you should look closely at the leader and determine whether you can work with the leadership style predominantly used by that person. None of this happens unless you carefully examine yourself. One way of defining your best leadership style is to take the Leadership and Followership Style Test (Box 10.2) (Frew, 1977). This test helps you identify your ideal image of leadership by rating 20 statements according to your level of agreement. It is not necessary to have experience as a leader to benefit from taking the test.

It is important for you to take the necessary time to review your Leadership and Followership Style Test results and relate them to the personal tapes in your mind that you have on leadership and management and the exercises you have done in this chapter. Then combine all of the information with what you have learned and the experience you have had in leadership and management roles; this should give you accurate and timely information about yourself, your abilities, and your understanding of leadership and management techniques. Additional information regarding the skills of leadership and management are presented later in this textbook. Give yourself the time and opportunity to examine these features as they are presented so that you can integrate them into your inner person.

It is crucial that you identify where you are comfortable working and the type of people with whom you do your best work. This information should assist you in making meaningful 1-, 3-, and 5-year goals for your career based on accurate information. The leadership and management skills and personality you are developing become the future tapes for your career. Be sure you are putting valuable and useful information into those tapes.

Box 10.2 Leadership and Followership Style Test

Structural Leadership Profile

The following 20 statements relate to your ideal image of leadership. We ask that as you respond to them, you imagine yourself to be a leader and then rate them in a way that would reflect your particular style of leadership. It makes no difference what kind of leadership experience, if any, you have had or are currently involved in. The purpose here is to establish your ideal preference for relating with subordinates.

The format includes a five-point scale ranging from *strongly agree* to *strongly disagree* for each statement. Please select one point on each scale and mark it as you read the 20 statements relating to leadership. You may omit rating any that are confusing or that you feel you cannot rate.

	Strongly Agree	Agree	Mixed Feelings	Disagree	Strongly Disagree
1. When I tell a subordinate to do something, I expect him or her to do it with no questions asked. After all, I am responsible for what he or she does, not the subordinate.	1	2	3	4	5
2. Tight control by a leader usually does more harm than good. People generally do the best job when they are allowed to exercise self-control.	5	4	3	2	1
3. Although discipline is important in an organization, the effective leader should mediate the use of disciplinary procedures with his or her knowledge of the people and the situation.	1	2	3	4	5
4. A leader must make every effort to subdivide the tasks of the people to the greatest possible extent.	1	2	3	4	5
5. Shared leadership or truly democratic process in a group can work only when there is a recognized leader who assists the process.	1	2	3	4	5
6. As a leader, I am ultimately responsible for all of the actions of my group. If our activities result in benefits for the organization, I should be rewarded accordingly.	1	2	3	4	5
7. Most persons require only minimum direction on the part of their leader to do a good job.	5	4	3	2	1
8. One's subordinates usually require the control of a strict leader.	1	2	3	4	5
9. Leadership might be shared among participants of a group so that at any one time there could be two or more leaders.	5	4	3	2	1

Continued

Box 10.2 Leadership and Followership Style Test—cont'd

	Strongly Agree	Agree	Mixed Feelings	Disagree	Strongly Disagree
10. Leadership should generally come from the top, but there are some logical exceptions to this rule.	5	4	3	2	1
11. The disciplinary function of the leader is simply to seek democratic opinions regarding problems as they arise.	5	4	3	2	1
12. The engineering problems, the management time, and the worker frustration caused by the division of labor are hardly ever worth the savings. In most cases, workers could do the best job of determining their own job content.	5	4	3	2	1
13. The leader ought to be the group member whom the other members elect to coordinate their activities and to represent the group to the rest of the organization.	5	4	3	2	1
14. A leader needs to exercise some control over his or her people.	1	2	3	4	5
15. There must be one and only one recognized leader in a group.	1	2	3	4	5
16. A good leader must establish and strictly enforce an impersonal system of discipline.	1	2	3	4	5
17. Discipline codes should be flexible, and they should allow for individual decisions by the leader, given each particular situation.	5	4	3	2	1
18. Basically, people are responsible for themselves and no one else; thus, a leader cannot be blamed for or take credit for the work of subordinates.	5	4	3	2	1
19. The job of the leader is to relate to subordinates the task to be done, to ask them for the ways in which it can best be accomplished, and then to help arrive at a consensus plan of attack.	5	4	3	2	1
20. A position of leadership implies the general superiority of its incumbent over his or her workers.	1	2	3	4	5

Box 10.2 Leadership and Followership Style Test—cont'd

Structural Followership Profile

This section of the questionnaire includes statements about the type of boss you prefer. Imagine yourself to be in a subordinate position of some kind and use your responses to indicate your preference for the way in which a leader might relate to you. The format is identical to that in the previous section.

	Strongly Agree	Agree	Mixed Feelings	Disagree	Strongly Disagree
1. I expect my job to be very explicitly outlined for me.	1	2	3	4	5
2. When the boss says to do something, I do it. After all, he or she is the boss.	1	2	3	4	5
3. Rigid rules and regulations usually cause me to become frustrated and inefficient.	5	4	3	2	1
4. I am ultimately responsible for and capable of self-discipline based on my contacts with the people around me.	1	2	3	4	5
5. My jobs should be made as short in duration as possible, so that I can achieve efficiency through repetition.	1	2	3	4	5
6. Within reasonable limits I try to accommodate requests from persons who are not my boss because these requests are typically in the best interest of the company.	5	4	3	2	1
7. When the boss tells me to do something that is the wrong thing to do, it is his or her fault, not mine, when I do it.	1	2	3	4	5
8. It is up to my leader to provide a set of rules by which I can measure my performance.	1	2	3	4	5
9. The boss is the boss. The fact of that promotion suggests that he or she has something on the ball.	1	2	3	4	5
10. I only accept orders from my boss.	1	2	3	4	5
11. I would prefer for my boss to give me general objectives and guidelines and then allow me to do the job my way.	5	4	3	2	1
12. If I do something that is not right, it is my own fault, even if my supervisor told me to do it.	5	4	3	2	1
13. I prefer jobs that are not repetitious, the kind of task that is new and different each time.	5	4	3	2	1

Continued

Box 10.2 Leadership and Followership Style Test—cont'd

	Strongly Agree	Agree	Mixed Feelings	Disagree	Strongly Disagree
14. My supervisor is in no way superior to me by virtue of position. He or she does a different kind of job, one that includes a lot of managing and coordinating.	5	4	3	2	1
15. I expect my leader to give me disciplinary guidelines.	1	2	3	4	5
16. I prefer to tell my supervisor what I can or at least should be doing. I am ultimately responsible for my own work.	5	4	3	2	1

Scoring Interpretation

You may score your own leadership and followership styles by averaging the numbers below your answers to the individual items. For example, if you scored item number one *Strongly agree,* you will find the point value of "1" below that answer (Leadership Profile). To obtain your overall leadership style, add all the numerical values that are associated with the 20 leadership items and divide by 20. The resulting average is your leadership style.

Interpretations

Score	Description	Leadership Style	Followership Style
Less than 1.9	Very autocratic	Boss decides and announces decisions, rules, orientation	Cannot function well without programs and procedures; needs feedback
2.0–2.4	Moderately autocratic	Announces decisions but asks for questions; makes exceptions to rules	Needs solid structure and feedback but can also carry on independently
2.5–3.4	Mixed	Boss suggests ideas and consults groups; many exceptions to regulations	Mixture of above and below
3.5–4.0	Moderately participative	Group decides on basis of boss's suggestions; rules are few; group proceeds as they see fit	Independent worker, doesn't need close supervision, just a bit of feedback
Greater than 4.1	Very democratic	Group is in charge of decisions; boss is coordinator, group makes any rules	Self-starter, likes to challenge new things by him- or herself

Scores on this instrument vary depending on mood and circumstances. Your leadership or followership style is best described by the range of scores from several different test times.

Source: Frew, D. R. (1977). Leadership and followership. *Personnel Journal, 56*(2), 90–97, with permission.

REAL-WORLD CASE STUDY

■ You have been offered the job of nurse manager for a 40-bed unit in a long-term care facility. You are excited about the opportunity to use the leadership and management content you have learned in school and to determine for yourself what really works in your leadership style. You are a novice leader and manager and want to be sure the position is right for you.

1. What aspects of the position and yourself are you going to examine before deciding whether the job is right for you?

2. If your search for information indicates that the job is one you should apply for, what questions are important for you to ask during interviews as a check to see whether your initial analysis was correct or to gain additional information?
3. Assuming you take the job, what is an important aspect for you to identify quickly on your unit?
4. Write a summary of the information you have about your personal leadership and management style at this point in your career. Include all of the information you can gather.

Key Points

- Although the terms are often used interchangeably, there is a difference between leadership and management. Leadership is the ability to establish a vision for an organization and influence others to willingly meet the goals. Management is the ability to plan, organize, motivate, and direct the personnel and resources of an organization.
- Informal leaders often have more power than do formal leaders. An informal leader is a respected individual without a formal title that people *choose* to follow. Informal leaders are important to an organization because they have power within the group, expertise in patient care, and the ability to lead the group in the direction of the formal leader's choice.
- Historically, LPNs have been managers and leaders in long-term care facilities. In more recent years, manager roles for LPNs have expanded into other health-care organizations. LPNs are also managers of care for their patients and, as expert nurses, provide leadership for unlicensed personnel.
- Some of the most common leadership styles are autocratic, democratic, laissez-faire, multicratic or participative, and transformational.

- The multicratic or participative and transformational leadership styles are supported by Watson's science of human caring because they focus on the needs of the individuals being led and not just the needs of the leader or the tasks that need to be accomplished. Leaders who use the multicratic or participative or transformational styles are also supported by Maslow's hierarchy of needs, because this type of leader meets the basic needs of employees and provides them with the necessary resources and support to move to the higher levels on the hierarchy.
- Individual leadership styles may change, depending on the situation and the work that needs to be done. Most people develop their own leadership style by having an understanding of their own predominate style of working with people. Learning opportunities and working with other leaders who demonstrate quality leadership skills can also play a role in developing a leadership style.
- If a person has emotional intelligence, she or he is aware of how her or his emotions and behaviors impact others. Every nurse should understand the concept of emotional intelligence, especially nurse leaders.

ANSWERS TO REAL-WORLD CASE STUDY

1. You should spend time doing the following:
   - Review your personal tapes to see what is already in your leadership and management personality.
   - Take the Leadership and Followership Style Test and personally analyze the results.
   - Ask people with whom you have recently worked or recent faculty members to give you feedback about what they have observed about your leadership and management style and skills.
   - Use your network system at the nursing home where you have been offered the job to:
     ○ Determine the leadership style of the administrator. Then compare it with what you know about yourself.
     ○ Determine the management style of the previous nurse manager on the unit where you are considering going to work. Try to determine whether it was a satisfactory style for the people who worked there. Compare what you discover with what you know about yourself.

2. You should consider asking about the following during the interview:
   - What is the formal organizational structure, and where do you fit into it?
   - How does the interviewer perceive the management style of the previous nurse manager? Was it effective?
   - How does the administrator prefer resolving problems?
   - Is there a management team that you are to be expected to work with in this position?
   - Is there a mentor assigned to you or available to you during your orientation period?
   - Will there be an opportunity for continuing education in nursing management while you are in this job position?

3. Who are the informal leaders of the unit?

4. Keep this summary for future reference when applying for a leadership or management job or when comparing it with your situation in 3 to 5 years.

REVIEW QUESTIONS

1. Which qualities best describe informal leaders? Select all that apply.
   1. The individual is competent in their nursing care.
   2. Other staff members seek their assistance.
   3. They do not have a formal title.
   4. The nurse manager always asks for their advice.

2. The LPN is working as a charge nurse in a rehabilitation facility. He has concerns about the manner in which staff are providing care to the patients. Which sentence best describes a participative leadership style?
   1. He independently decides how to address the problem with no input from the staff.
   2. He sets up a meeting with the staff to obtain their input and then makes the decision about how to proceed.
   3. He seeks input from the staff and works with the group to determine a plan.
   4. He doesn't do anything and waits for the staff to figure out things on their own.

3. The nurse manager needs to change the process for scheduling. She has some ideas about how to make the change but is concerned about the impact of the change on individual staff members. As a leader, she invites input and suggestions from the staff and encourages them to ask questions. Which type of leadership does this best describe?
   1. Laissez-faire
   2. Democratic
   3. Transformational
   4. Multicratic or participative

4. The concepts of leadership and management are different.
   1. True
   2. False

5. The LPN is concerned about a resident's blood sugar. She mentioned her concerns to the physician but was not happy with the physician's response. If the LPN is demonstrating high emotional intelligence, she will:
   1. Immediately tell the physician she does not agree with him.
   2. Tell the nurse manager that the physician will not listen to her regarding her concern.
   3. Wait for the nurse practitioner to visit the patient to voice her concerns.
   4. Take some time to process the conversation and then discuss the matter again with the physician.

References

Covey, S. R. (2013). *The 7 habits of highly successful people: Powerful lessons in personal change.* New York: Simon & Schuster.

Frew, D. R. (1977). Leadership and followership. *Personnel Journal, 54*(2), 90–97.

MindTools. (n.d.). Emotional intelligence: Developing strong people skills. Retrieved from https://www.mindtools.com/pages/article/newCDV_59.htm

Northhouse, P. G. (2015). *Leadership: Theory and practice* (7th ed.). Los Angeles: Sage.

Roussel, L., Harris, J. L., & Thomas, T. (2016). *Management and leadership for nurse administrators* (7th ed.). Sudbury, MA: Jones & Bartlett.

Tyczkowski, B., Vandenhouten, C., Reilly, J., Bansal, G., Kubsch, S. M., & Jakkola, R. (2015). Emotional intelligence (EI) and nursing leadership styles among nurse managers. *Nursing Administration Quarterly, 39*(2), 172–180.

Web Resources

American Organization of Nurse Executives www.aone.org/

Mindtools www.mindtools.com/

11 Communication Skills in Leadership and Management

KEY TERMS

Active listening
Aggressive communication
Assertive communication
Communication
Communication block
CUS
Feedback
Nonassertive communication
Nonverbal communication
Passive-aggressive
    communication
SBAR
Two-Challenge Rule

CHAPTER CONCEPT

Communication

LEARNING OUTCOMES

1. Define effective communication.
2. Discuss four basic communication skills that can be used successfully in the classroom.
3. List seven communication principles appropriate for the clinical setting.
4. Define failed communication.
5. Compare and contrast assertive, nonassertive, aggressive, and passive-aggressive communication.
6. Use three effective communication tools.

We have committed the Golden Rule to memory.
Now let's commit it to life.

—Edwin Markham

In the busy world of school, work, and family, you must hear a billion words a week. Words, sentences, and the ability to think are crucial to your very survival, and they enhance the quality of your life. Your use of words also has a significant impact on the survival and quality of life of the patients to whom you give care.

Imagine not speaking for a day. If it were a school day, you would miss out on the opportunity to study effectively with others or to ask questions. If you were working in a hospital or nursing home, you simply could not do your job without being able to talk to others. Speaking is important, but it is only one aspect of communication. Speaking is the physical act of saying words. Communication is the effective use of words to share ideas, meaning, and emotion with others. It is the ability to think critically and put together thoughts so that they have meaning for another person. Communication occurs when the sender and the receiver of the message have understood its meaning.

To be an educated person and a nurse who provides meaningful nursing care, you must learn how to communicate in the classroom and in clinical settings, and after you graduate, you need to be able to communicate as a nurse manager. It takes awareness, work, and study. It is a process that must continue as you mature as a nurse. This chapter covers material about communication in the classroom and the clinical area as a student. We begin by discussing communication skills in the academic setting.

COMMUNICATION IN THE ACADEMIC SETTING

It may seem strange to say you need different communication skills for your roles as a student and a nurse, but it is true. Let's look at two student situations. One student, George, is straight out of high school and has been admitted into the licensed practical nurse (LPN) program at the local community college. George worked hard all summer to earn enough money to pay tuition and buy books for his first semester. He is on campus for the first time when he comes to his 8 a.m. nursing class. It took him more time than he anticipated to find a parking place, and now he is worried about getting to the classroom on time. It is 8 a.m. exactly when he walks into a room with 32 other students.

Following George is Helena, a 34-year-old woman who has three children and an alcoholic husband who left her 1 year ago. She was frustrated with her life and minimum wage job, so she went to job counseling. Eventually Helena was advised to apply for the LPN program. She is the first person in her family to graduate from high school, and now she is going to college. She is almost late for class because the new babysitter was a few minutes late.

Listening Skills

What communications skills do these two people need to get through their first day of school? They need listening skills, questioning skills, and friendly communication skills. I think listening is the most challenging, but it is one of the strongest communication skills a person can have in any setting. When high-level communication skills are needed, the smart person does not say a word and simply listens. George and Helena, in the classroom situation just described, need to listen to see whether class has started, whether anyone invites them to sit beside them, or whether the instructor has something to say, such as, "There are seats over here."

Listening allows you to get the right instructions for the overnight assignment, the right directions for studying for a test, or the information needed to locate a study group and to get there at the right time. Listening also is crucial to identify the emotions of another person so that you can respond to the person appropriately. If you are in doubt about a situation, stop and listen to what is being said by others until you get an accurate picture.

How can you tell whether you are a good listener? Simply stop and think about your relationships with people. Are you sought out for advice? Do people bring puzzling questions to you? If so, you are a good listener. People who come to you for your advice and knowledge seek you out because you listen to them. If people are constantly avoiding you or working around you and through others, perhaps you're not a good listener, and that is something you need to correct. Being a good listener takes practice. There are also several barriers to effective listening, including the following:

• A confusing message being sent
• Anxiety and stress
• Fatigue and hunger
• Too many interruptions
• Too many tasks to complete

Do any of these have an impact on your ability to listen?

Nonverbal Communication

Most people relate listening to something that is done only with the ears. Hearing is just one aspect of the skill of listening. The person who really wants to know what is happening in an interaction needs to "listen" visually as well, which means that while you are listening, you also are observing the behavior, facial expressions, posture, and gestures of the person with whom you are speaking. Is the person speaking and shaking a clenched fist? Is the person trying not to laugh while pretending to be serious? What is the posture, attire, or overall appearance (pale, clean, dirty) of the person to whom you are speaking? Does the person keep moving away from you or moving closer to you?

According to psychologists, the most honest communication is made through nonverbal channels. It is important for you to look carefully at the person, group, or environment that relates to the conversation to pick up on clues about what is happening in the interaction. The nonverbal clues are honest and generally reliable.

Nonverbal communication is nonspecific communication that transmits information. It could include the movements of a person (fast, slow, normal, purposeful, meaningless), the spatial relationships (how far away or how close the person is to you and others), the type of language used (slang, profanity, scientific, humorous), and the cultural attributes and appearance of the person. Each of these information-transmitting mechanisms needs to be considered so that you understand the entire message of the communication.

Negative or Hostile Communication

The normal physiological reaction to having someone behave in an aggressive or critical manner (yelling or physically threatening) is referred to as "fight or flight." When we feel threatened, our bodies release larger than normal amounts of adrenaline in response to increased stress levels. This response can be lifesaving if you're in danger, but it needs to be controlled if you're trying to communicate effectively. If someone is "yelling" at you, leaving the interaction (flight) means the problem cannot be resolved. There is no communication if you're not there. Fighting does no more than leaving. The objective of communication is to be successful in sending and receiving messages. You can avoid both natural reactions by listening.

If you can discipline yourself to think proactively (to anticipate and plan ahead) and listen to what the other person is saying, you are treating yourself and the other person with respect. As you are listening, focus your attention on the other person. Suppose you are George, from the introductory scenario for this chapter, and you are trying to schedule a study group with Helena from your fundamentals nursing class. She is being uncooperative in scheduling a time, and her voice is getting louder and louder as the two of you talk. You stop reacting to the negative things she has to say and start paying attention to her. What you find is that she is "yelling" and being uncooperative, but she also looks exhausted and ready to cry. When you start really listening to what she is saying, you understand that the problem is child care. (Remember Helena is a single parent.) Does this realization help you understand Helena's behavior?

The secret to effective communication is to observe nonverbal cues and to listen until the person has finished speaking. It is important to give the speaker your full attention. This is called *active listening.*

Some people decide they know what the "yelling" person is trying to say, then they interrupt and say what they think is important. Never do that if you want a successful outcome. Stop and listen. In our example, when Helena has finished speaking, George could say, "I think I understand what you are saying. Is the problem getting a reliable babysitter for your kids?" When the problem has been identified, it generally can be resolved. Perhaps the study group could meet at Helena's house after her children have gone to bed. Or maybe someone in the study group has a teenager who would babysit for Helena while the group meets.

Neither people nor situations can be understood if no one listens to discern the problem. This is true even if the information comes to you in a hostile manner. So, remember, *no* running away and *no* fighting. Instead, listen.

When a conversation becomes negative or hostile, it is always best to stop and listen rather than respond to what is being said. I have observed that educated people tend to control their emotions and react less to negative comments from others. You are embarking on an educational track; you need to learn this behavior. Don't react to negative things in a negative way. Be proactive. A *proactive* person anticipates what could happen in a situation and mentally prepares to deal with potential outcomes. For example, I made a commitment to myself that I would not lose my temper in public. In order not to lose my temper, I smile when something happens that angers me. I feel the anger and sense my temper rising, and then I smile. My anger is dissipated, and the person who is upset with me is often disarmed because what I am doing is so out of context with the situation. I plan and practice for when I might lose my temper, which allows me to keep it under control.

The opposite of proactive is reactive. A *reactive* person simply reacts to whatever happens in life. If someone is angry, the reactive person gets angry as well. There is no forethought or consideration of long-term consequences for the behavior. If a person generally loses control of his or her temper when others are critical, the person needs to (1) recognize his or her reactionary response and (2) determine proactively a way to control the negative behavior. The person might decide to clasp both hands in front whenever he or she senses feelings of anger. Clasping hands should help the person recognize the anger, with the idea being that if the anger is recognized, it can be stopped. It also occupies the person's hands so that he or she doesn't hit or shove someone in anger. This level of awareness helps a person really listen to what is happening in a conversation.

REFLECTIVE THINKING

What are some of the hostile or negative things that can occur in a conversation that cause you to react? It could be name-calling, pushing, or making insulting or cutting remarks. Identify and record in your class notebook three behaviors that tend to cause you to react negatively. Then list a thought or behavior that would assist you in listening rather than reacting. Be prepared to share these in class.

Questioning Skills

Helena and George are now in their third week of class, and things are going quite well. George has cut back on the number of hours he works so that he can study more, and he is dating less as well. He recognizes these as normal transition behaviors and isn't upset about the adjustments he has had to make. Helena has located a reliable babysitter and received financial aid that will pay for her tuition and books, so she too is feeling better about being in school. Now Helena and George need to focus their attention on being great students. Both of them find it difficult to ask questions, however. Helena and George don't want to ask "dumb" questions, and because of that fear they simply do not ask any questions. Because of this behavior, Helena was late with an assignment and George did an entire assignment incorrectly because he didn't clarify the purpose of it with the instructor.

There is a rule about questions in the classroom: There are *no* "dumb" questions. Generally, when a student has a question, it is one that several others in the class wanted to ask but were afraid to do so. So remember, there are no "dumb" questions, simply questions that need to be answered. I have mentioned this information previously, but here it is again!

If your question is about an assignment or test, be sure you review the syllabus first to see whether the information you need is there. Do not go to the instructor with a question that he or she has carefully spelled out in the syllabus. But if you have questions after reviewing the syllabus, go to the instructor. You should be confident and pleasant. You should be empowered enough not to preface your question with, "This is a dumb question, but . . ." You should be clear on what you want to ask and not leave the conversation without getting the information you need. When all involved participants achieve their goals, communication is successful.

Most faculty members I know enjoy students with questioning minds. I encourage you to ask questions and explore options. Don't limit yourself to asking only about assignments and tests; ask for clarification about concepts as well. This type of questioning should be a collegial exchange of thoughts and ideas. For the instructor, challenging questions are part of the fun of teaching. Learning is fun, and sharing your thinking with others is a scholarly activity. As we have been discussing, make sure you listen to the response.

Successful communication occurs when both the sender and the receiver exchange and understand information.

Friendly Conversation

Friendly conversation is a significant aspect of what makes school fun. It is the ability to talk to others about school-related and other issues. Being able to make friendly conversation with all types of people on campus not only contributes to your enjoyment of school, it also improves your social skills, which are an important part of effective nursing.

You need three things to be good at making conversation. First, you need a desire to make friendly conversation; second, you need to be able to ask questions; and third, you need to listen to the answers. The key is to ask questions that express an interest in another person but are not invasive. For example, ask about books, movies, and hobbies.

COMMUNICATION IN THE CLINICAL SETTING

When you are working in the clinical area as a student nurse, you are working under the licensure of a registered nurse (RN) who is acting as your clinical preceptor. You are given this privilege so that you can take the time to learn how to do nursing and be socialized into nursing as a profession. As a student, you are given time to work through the things you are learning. You have time to stop and ponder and sit and talk with a patient. Your learning time is different from the time during which you will work as an LPN. The principles of behavior are the same, however. As

a student, you should learn all you can and practice the skills taught you until you can do them perfectly. That is true of all skills, including the skills of communication.

When you communicate in the clinical area, you should use the information presented earlier in this chapter. You need to apply listening, questioning, and friendly conversation skills. The great challenge of applying what you've already learned is that the clinical setting is more complex than the school setting. There are physicians, nurse practitioners, nursing assistants, families, and patients. Add to that list the housekeeper, the dietary aide, the physical therapist, and the pharmacist, to name a few others. You have a major responsibility as a future LPN to communicate effectively with all people necessary to provide the highest level of care. How do you do that?

To communicate effectively in the clinical setting, use the following communication principles:

1. Follow the communication concepts previously discussed in this chapter.
2. Think before you speak. Always consider what you are sharing and with whom it is appropriate to share. Working in the hospital or nursing home is not the same as having lunch with your friends at school. At lunch, you may feel free to say whatever you want. That is not acceptable behavior in the clinical setting.
3. Be quiet and gentle in your communication. Patients are sick, families are grieving, and staff members generally are stressed. If you are sensitive to the environment and learn to speak quietly and gently, you will not add to the stress or distress of others. The contradiction to this concept is when there is an emergency or reason for alarm. If there is an emergency, communicate it to others in a loud, firm voice so that you will get their attention. Do not scream or run because it could cause panic among the patients and families.
4. Ask only appropriate questions. You are encouraged to ask all pertinent questions about the patient for whom you are giving care, but do not ask questions about other patients. Review the section of confidentiality if necessary. If you are not giving care to the person about whom you are making inquiry, it is inappropriate and unprofessional for you to ask questions about that person.
5. Do not talk about patients or their families in inappropriate places; this includes the elevator,

lunchroom, or hallways of the facility. Maintaining patient confidentiality is a professional obligation.

6. Be respectful in your communication with others. Treat physicians and nursing assistants with equal respect. Treating patients and their families with respect is essential and should come automatically to you.

7. Do not hesitate to find out what you don't know. This may be information about a drug you are asked to give or what laboratory results might mean. Don't "pretend" you know things and through this behavior possibly harm a patient. One of the principles of being a professional is being a lifelong learner. Generally, this means you should find out what you don't know or collect information about which you are unsure. This could be summarized as "get to the truth!"

The importance of what you do in the clinical area cannot be overemphasized. A critical part of that work is based on accurate and meaningful communication. Take the time you have now as a student to practice and ask for feedback on your communication skills in the clinical area. Your objective is to be a wonderful LPN, and practicing is one of the ways to achieve that goal. The skills necessary to be truly therapeutic with patients are crucial to being a meaningful nurse. Generally, nurses spend 85% of their time communicating with others, including patients, their families and friends, the interdisciplinary and nursing staff, and physicians. The list grows when you add people such as volunteers, human resource personnel, and education department personnel. Your job as a nurse is to communicate with multiple and diverse people successfully.

There are several effective tools commonly used to communicate important information about patients to physicians or from one caregiver to the next. These tools are also useful when communicating patient needs to other health-care providers, such as a respiratory therapist or a physical therapist.

- The SBAR tool (Table 11-1) can be used during shift changes or at any time there is an unexpected change in the patient's condition.
- CUS is a tool that can be used any time there is a concern for patient or employee safety and you feel you are not being heard during the communication process. CUS stands for I am

TABLE 11.1 SBAR COMMUNICATION

Situation	LPN identifies what is going on with the patient.
Background	LPN provides the clinical facts surrounding the problem.
Assessment	LPN offers a suggestion about what may be wrong with the patient.
Recommendation	LPN makes a request or suggests a specific action.

Concerned. I am **Uncomfortable**. This is a **Safety** concern.

- The Two-Challenge Rule is a tool that can be used if you think your initial communication approach has not been effective. You will state your concern twice and make sure the individual with whom you are communicating acknowledges your concern. The goal of this strategy is to assure that what you are trying to communicate is being heard and acknowledged by the other person.

Although these tools are generally used to communicate information regarding patients, these strategies can also be used by nurse managers to promote effective communication among staff.

REFLECTIVE THINKING

How can the SBAR tool be used in your personal life to improve your communication with those around you? Record your thoughts in your class notebook.

Successful communication is an art form that is based on the concept of caring for the other person and ensuring that the communication is successfully received and acknowledged. As a manager, you have the responsibility of accomplishing work through others. A major part of how you make that happen is through successful communication. Work does not get done if people do not know how important it is, how to do it, or what to do if there is a problem in achieving the objectives. It is your job to communicate with other employees in a way that allows this information to be shared. Clear and accurate communication in the clinical setting can enhance employee performance and ensure patient safety.

All communication has a goal. If you are telling a joke, the goal is to get the other person to laugh. If you are frustrated, the goal may be to share your frustration with the person involved and clarify what has happened. If you are giving a report, your goal is to give only accurate and pertinent data about the patients to the oncoming nurse. Even casual or "silly" communication has a purpose. The receiver also has goals. For the nurse taking your report, the goal is to receive and record accurate and pertinent data about the patients. For the listener to the joke, it is to have a good laugh. For the person who is involved in your feelings of frustration, it is to clarify the problem and continue with the work at hand.

Edwin Markham, quoted at the beginning of this chapter, conveys the basic premise of caring communication. He refers to the Golden Rule and simply asks that humans live it rather than just quote it. This requires a commitment from you.

FAILED COMMUNICATION

Most nurses have experienced what I refer to as failed communication. Failed communication is an interaction in which the communication that was planned or anticipated did not occur. Often the communication that does take place involves frustration, anger, crying, "storming away," and other nonproductive and noncaring behaviors. You recognize from these interactions that the intent of the conversation was not achieved and that something negative occurred even though you are not sure how it happened.

Generally, failed communication happens when people's feelings are "hurt" or when people are so frustrated that they raise their voices and make negative and unpleasant utterances. (That is a polite way of saying they lose their temper!) It also can happen when people refuse to share their genuine feelings about a situation and nod their head and say, "Yes," or, "Of course," without other input or clarification.

Your work as an LPN is critical to the people in your care. As a nurse manager, your realm of

interaction increases, as does the complexity of what you need to communicate. The impact of a failed communication on your part and its consequences may fall on more people in your role as a nurse manager than it would as an LPN. The ability to recognize where your failures occur and the type of person with whom they most commonly occur is important to preventing them.

A failed communication often is one that is unconsciously put on a "tape" in your head and is played repeatedly. A failed communication just doesn't feel right, so your mind takes it and keeps playing it in an effort to understand what happened or to justify what you did. I am sure everyone reading this text has had the experience where an interaction has been uncomfortable or negative and it keeps replaying in your mind. You have thoughts like, "I should have said this," or "Why didn't I think of this example to use?" You can be enjoying a few minutes of relaxation and suddenly that failed communication tape starts playing in your head again. It is symptomatic of something being wrong and generally takes a great deal of energy and time from your daily life to resolve. The most effective solution is to avoid the same type of failed communication by improving your skills with others.

As you read about failed communication tapes, did one come to your mind? It may be something that has happened recently or an old event that took a great deal of time and energy when it occurred. Generally, it is a communication with someone who either got angry or caused you to get angry, or it is with someone who told you what to do without clarifying the reason or giving you an opportunity to express your feelings about what was said. This person expects immediate and unquestioning obedience to all demands, often causing a tape to be made and replayed. As you think about your failed communication tapes, consider what type of person is usually in them. Often it is one or two personality types that "costar" with you in such tapes. It is important for you to identify who those people are and develop skills for working with them.

Feedback

Feedback is a step in the communication process that assists in preventing or correcting failed communications. It is a simple idea; however, it requires skill and self-confidence to implement. When you think that a communication is on the verge of failing, you need to stop the communication process from continuing in the "failed" direction and get the conversation moving in another direction away from the failure. This skill is most effective when you can see that the communication is not working because of the responses you are receiving from the other person. When that happens, it is crucial to the success of the interaction for you to use feedback.

Feedback should be part of every communication to verify that the message you wanted to give was received by the listener. Feedback requires acknowledgment of what has been said. You may say, "Please share with me what you understand from what I have just told you." The listener is now able to state what has been heard. A direct approach such as this gives you the opportunity to listen to the feedback and verify that it is correct, clarify the parts of the feedback that are not accurate, and reinforce the aspects that were correct. The concept of asking someone to restate the message you have attempted to deliver (remember that it is not "delivered" unless it is properly understood) should not sound like a psychiatric communication approach. Do not use the phrase, "I hear you telling me . . ." with other professionals; this can doom a communication quite forcefully. Your response needs to sound like you want to know that the person has understood your message and the details of what you had to say. It is important to observe the nonverbal communication of the person and respond to any messages from that source that you receive. If an assignment seems to be understood, but the person does not express any excitement over doing it, you should address that nonverbal response. You could explain to the person the importance of what has been asked and, if it is appropriate, reinforce the significance of the role you have given the person. Clarifying combined verbal and nonverbal messages is an important aspect of feedback.

Do you understand why I said that it takes skill and self-confidence to use feedback? A manager needs to have the ability to be comfortable using feedback without it making the listener uncomfortable or feel devalued. This is done easily if a caring approach is used. Your questions regarding understanding the message should be asked in a nonthreatening manner and with a focus on the goal of communication—that the message is received. You need to have the time to participate effectively in the communication process. The concept of feedback requires time and effort. The effort that goes into the effective use of feedback is worth your time because it is more likely to bring about results. The message has been received and understood, and the instructions contained within the communication are acted on properly and effectively.

Communication Blocks

Inadequate or absent feedback mechanisms are one block to effective communication. The absence of feedback is not the only block to good communication. Other examples that you should know about and be prepared to deal with in your role as a manager follow.

A communication block occurs if either the sender or the receiver has a preconceived opinion of what is going to be discussed during a communication and the preconceived opinion is wrong. An example is an employee expectation of a good evaluation that results in a salary increase. If an employee comes to you for an evaluation with that idea in mind, and the evaluation that you give is focused on skill deficits that need to be mastered, the communication becomes blocked. You talk about skills and ways to improve them that the employee does not recognize as being a problem; this may result in a defensive and angry communication that does not allow your intended message to be received. The solution for this block is to listen so that you understand what the employee is thinking and expecting. If you do not know what is going on in the other person's mind, there is little hope for an effective communication.

Physical disabilities can be a communication block if you are not aware of the disability or do not know how to communicate successfully with the disabled person. Students generally learn about disabilities in their nursing classes and develop skills in working with people who have them during clinical experiences. Physical disabilities that affect communication include blindness and deafness. Each block deserves a specific intervention for the communication to occur in a meaningful way.

Personal physical health and emotional health also are potential blocks to communication. Such a block could come from you or from the person with whom you need to communicate. Because you are a nurse, you can readily understand the block that would come from a migraine headache, a miserable cold, or emotional strain, such as the

FOCUSED LEARNING CHART
Communication Blocks

Effective managers do all they can to recognize and avoid communication blocks.

COMMUNICATION BLOCK	EXAMPLE
Expectations not met	Expecting praise, but receiving criticism
Lack of physical or emotional well-being	Physical pain such as a migraine, depression, or stress
Inadequate communication skills	Frustration from failed communications
Lack of appropriate feedback	Misunderstandings
Physical disabilities	Communication with someone who is blind or deaf

death of a loved one. These and other illnesses and experiences can cause a person to be less effective not only in their communication skills but also in many areas of life. One way to resolve this block is to ask people not to work when they are physically ill or emotionally distressed. Most organizations recognize the need for people to stay home when they don't feel well and provide sick leave. Often, individuals need the support and approval of their manager to stay home without feeling guilty.

Language and cultural differences can also provide communication blocks. Employees and patients are more diverse in health-care organizations today, which can create issues when trying to communicate. For more information on cultural concerns, refer to Chapter 12.

There are other blocks to communication that may be particular to you or the place where you work. Recognize these blocks and develop strategies for successfully managing them. That is one of the hallmarks of a good manager—a person who is prepared.

TYPES OF COMMUNICATION

There are four styles of communication that are commonly used: assertive, aggressive, nonassertive, and passive-aggressive. Assertive communication is the most positive type of communication and for most of us does not come naturally but can be developed with some practice. Aggressive communication promotes only the needs and desires of the communicator during the communication process. This is a very noncaring style of communication. Nonassertive communication occurs when the communicator does not express her thoughts and feelings

and leaves the interaction feeling as though her needs are not being met. When using passive-aggressive communication, the communicator appears passive during the communication process and then acts out negatively in an indirect manner at a later time. People who use this style of communication usually feel powerless and unable to deal with other individuals in a direct manner. Determining the style you most commonly use when communicating with family and colleagues is important if you want to develop good communication skills.

Assertive Communication

Assertive communication is a skill crucial for the nurse manager to develop and use effectively, especially if it is not already present in one's communication repertoire. A focus on assertive communication can improve you personally and professionally and can enhance the entire profession of nursing.

Assertive communication is the ability to express yourself and protect your rights without violating the rights of another person. This is a communication style that is often contrasted with aggressive, nonassertive (passive), and passive-aggressive communication. A classic example is someone speaking to you in an angry, yelling manner. First, that is a violation of your rights as a person; most aggressive behavior is. If you yell back, you also have been aggressive. If you turn and walk away or say something like, "You're right, I should have done it your way," you have been passive and have allowed the other person to violate your rights by being aggressive toward you. If you say something placating and walk to the break room where you yell at the person in front of others, you are being passive-aggressive. This is a violation of the rights of the aggressive person.

The professional and caring way to communicate is to use assertiveness techniques because they do not violate anyone's rights and they protect your rights as a person. You may be wondering just what your rights are. Everyone lives what they have been taught their rights are, but at this point in your professional work, you, as the LPN, need to identify and understand those rights for yourself.

Melodie Chenevert (2007), a nurse who has spent a great deal of her career assisting nurses to understand the critical concept of assertiveness, has compiled 10 basic rights of health professionals:

1. You have the right to be treated with respect.
2. You have the right to a reasonable workload.
3. You have the right to an equitable wage.
4. You have the right to determine your own priorities.
5. You have the right to ask for what you want.
6. You have the right to refuse without making excuses or feeling guilty.
7. You have the right to make mistakes and to be responsible for them.
8. You have the right to give and to receive information as a professional.
9. You have the right to act in the best interest of the patient.
10. You have the right to be human.

Chenevert states that these basic rights belong to each nurse, but the individual person is responsible for acquiring the rights for himself or herself; no one is responsible for providing them. The use of assertiveness is necessary for you to achieve and maintain these rights.

Nurse managers who are assertive are more effective in their jobs than nurse managers who are not. They are able to express themselves honestly, openly, and responsibly. The communication style you choose comes with a payoff for you and consequences for the person with whom you are communicating. Your objective should be to make the "consequences" positive ones. The classic example of aggressive communication is anger. If you are venting angry feelings to someone, usually you feel better when you are through because getting rid of the angry feelings felt good, and the power that accompanies aggression generally makes the person using it feel superior. These are payoffs. You feel better, and you feel superior. The person against whom you aggressed may comply with your request because of fear of your aggression; however, that person may seek revenge or hold a grudge against you because of the manner in which you treated him or her.

The consequence for the passive person is the feeling of never getting what you want. The other person in the communication never learns what it is that the passive person wants or needs. When the need is that for a patient, the most severe tragedy of this type of communication can emerge.

Assertive communication often is not a communication style that "comes naturally"; it must be learned. What was the most difficult skill you learned in the nursing laboratory while you were in school? Was it to insert a nasogastric tube or a bladder catheter? Perhaps it was doing sterile dressings. If you are not already assertive, developing this skill can be as or more difficult than the skill that initially troubled you in the nursing laboratory. Assertive communication requires practice, requests for feedback from others, and support from colleagues who recognize what you are trying to master; it is work: focused, concentrated, good old hard work! After you have mastered assertive communication and incorporated it as a natural reaction in communication, you may notice a profound difference at work and in your personal life. Some people may not understand how to respond to the new you; take the time to teach them what you are doing. Others may be offended because they do not understand the reason for your change; perhaps they learned to depend on your passive nature. They also need to be taught. As a nurse manager, you cannot be successful unless you communicate assertively.

Generally, aggressive communication does not take this extreme form, but it can. Remember, it always infringes on the rights of others.

With that serious comment in mind, consider the following basic format for assertive skills (it is simple to remember but a challenge to apply and use consistently). When someone has transgressed on your rights as a person (i.e., raising their voice at you), this is an effective format to use as a response.

1. "I feel . . ." (describe the feeling you have because of the behavior, such as feeling devalued as a manager).
2. "When you . . ." (share the specific behavior that is bothering you, such as talking about you when you aren't there).
3. "We should . . ." (describe your thoughts regarding a solution to the problem, such as needing to meet privately to discuss the problem).

Using this approach doesn't seem natural to most nurses. Take a moment and practice the format, filling in the appropriate words for something that has recently happened in your life. Remember that you do not want to violate someone else's rights or to have your rights violated. This direct and objective information does exactly that for the people involved in the communication. You are honest, you share the problem, and you do it without hurting the other person.

One of the rules in making assertiveness work is the use of "I" messages. Generally, people are socialized to blame others for the mistakes that occur. I don't know how this blaming became a socially acceptable method for sharing a problem, but somewhere, somehow, it did. It is part of the defensive nature that seems natural to humans. It is the desire to protect oneself while blaming others. I hope you can see immediately why this type of communication is absolutely unacceptable for a licensed nurse of any level. The blaming and defensive nature indicates an inability to assume responsibility for what has been done or what is being felt. Nurses have to assume absolute responsibility for the work they do, and the words they say to people. An LPN doesn't look at the family members of a patient who received a dangerous dose of medication and point a finger at the RN or the physician and scream, "They made me do it!" You quickly recognize that as unprofessional behavior. Nurses must assume responsibility for all their actions; that is part of the professional code. The same is true with communications. The nurse needs to assume responsibility for all personal feelings. These feelings are shared by using "I" messages.

The use of "I" messages, such as "I feel devalued when you . . ." or "I feel frustrated when you . . ." allows the nurse to take responsibility for personal feelings and share them honestly with the appropriate other person. This approach prevents the other person from being blamed by you and from becoming automatically defensive toward you. Have you ever done something (probably as a child) and expected to get screamed at about it? It is such a surprise when the possible "screamer" comes to talk to you instead and shares personal feelings, a description of the problem, and a suggestion for a solution. Assertive communication preserves the integrity of both people in the communication circle.

Another aspect of assertive communication is based on the right to say no. Many nurses are socialized to say yes to even impossible tasks. Examples of this are being called at 6:00 a.m. every day that you have a day off to see whether you can come into work, being asked to work a double shift, or being requested to take an extra patient load or work without pay because there has been too much overtime used in the last pay period. Every person has the right to say "no." The assertive format for doing so follows:

1. Start your reply with a simple "no."
2. Give a brief explanation using an "I" message; for example, "I am not able to come into work today to help cover the day shift because I have family commitments."
3. Honor prior commitments. This means that whether you have family or any other commitments, you have the right to honor them without feeling guilty or defensive.
4. Suggest alternatives. This depends on the situation and your knowledge base as to what else can help solve the problem.

Assertive communication also is characterized by apologizing. If an apology is warranted and sincere, it is acceptable to apologize once. Any additional statements of apology—overapologizing—are a passive behavior and do not enhance your efforts to be a nurse manager. Have you had interactions with people who apologize and then do it again and again about the same issue? It is uncomfortable and meaningless after the first apology. The additional apologies indicate a lack of self-confidence and a passive nature.

Aggressive Communication

Aggressive communication violates the rights of people and is not based in caring theory in any way. Aggressive communication does not enhance the lives of individuals giving or receiving it. Instead, it is oppressive communication that keeps people from meeting their needs and making progress on Maslow's human needs pyramid. It achieves short-term results, but the consequences in terms of the reactions of others are difficult to manage over the long-term.

Nonassertive Communication

Nonassertive (passive) communication is similar to becoming a victim to someone else's communication, wishes, and desires. A nonassertive communicator ignores his own feelings and needs and avoids voicing his opinions to placate another person. It causes negative feelings that often are ignored until they are too overwhelming, and then the passive person becomes aggressive. It is a way to keep temporary peace, but it does not resolve problems and is ineffective in the long term. Passive communication definitely is not based in caring theory and does not allow either the aggressor or the passive person to move up Maslow's pyramid. It is stifling and limited in promoting individual worth. People who are victims of spousal abuse are often passive individuals living with aggressive people; this is perhaps the most graphic description I can share with you.

Passive-Aggressive Communication

Passive-aggressive communication is a common form of communication. It occurs when an individual seems agreeable during the communication process but responds negatively afterward. To avoid participating in passive-aggressive communication, you must have knowledge of it and consciously not allow it to happen.

REFLECTIVE THINKING

Being able to apply the assertiveness format for effective communication takes practice. Follow the format listed here and complete three brief scenarios with situations from your life. Record these in your class notebook and be prepared to discuss them in class. You may want to take a situation that has recently been incorporated into one of your mental tapes. There may be a frequently occurring communication problem that you recognize as something that violates your rights, or you may want to look around you and take a situation that "might" happen, and because it might occur, you can begin practicing for it. Use the following format and make detailed notes in your class notebook:

"I feel . . ."

"When you . . ."

"We should . . ."

How is passive-aggressive behavior manifested? It is complaining to the wrong person, talking about people when they are not there, and being unkind and uncaring. I often see passive-aggressive communication in the halls of the university where I teach when the students are upset with a faculty person. Instead of taking the problem to the person, they stand around and complain. Sometimes they go to the dean to complain without ever sharing their feelings with the faculty person. In hospitals and nursing homes, I notice this during reporting or in the break room, where people air all their frustrations about another person. The communication often is mean-spirited, devaluing, and uncaring. It is not helpful information, but instead a negative venting. The tragedy is that the problem only escalates because of the way it is handled. There is seldom a constructive resolution.

People who use passive-aggressive communication are not professional. They are not focused on resolving problems and helping others to understand, learn, or change. Generally, they are not interested in learning and changing themselves. This type of communication does not belong in any professional arenas, and it is time for it to be stopped in nursing.

OTHER FORMS OF COMMUNICATION

As a nurse manager, you may find as part of your job that it is necessary to write e-mails and letters and to complete evaluation forms (Box 11.1). It is important that you have developed the ability to use written English properly to perform these responsibilities well. Take advantage of opportunities for writing while you are in school. Value written feedback and corrections that come to you

Box 11.1 Writing an Appropriate E-Mail

1. Do not put anything in an e-mail that you would not want to see on the front page of a newspaper.
2. Do not include any confidential information about patients or employees.
3. Make sure you have addressed the message to the appropriate person.
4. Be sure to check who is "included" in the message's recipient list.
5. Provide brief information in the message, no more than one or two paragraphs.
6. Bullet the information for easier reading.
7. Be sure to proofread your message.
8. Take the time to determine whether an e-mail is the best method to communicate your message.

from faculty members. Read professional journals to see how other people write proficiently, and seek help if this is a weak area for you.

All written work you do as a nurse manager should be assertive in its approach. Do not be passive or aggressive. Write your ideas in a clear manner with "I" messages, and if there is a problem, make suggestions for correcting it. People and the work they do are the most critical aspects of delivering excellent nursing care. The use of caring approaches that value the other person is important.

Communication in meetings is another concern for some managers. If you are conducting the meeting, be sure to prepare an agenda ahead of time. It is important not to waste your time or that of others, so be sure the meeting is necessary and worth the time spent by the people attending it. Set beginning and ending times for the meeting, and do not alter them. If the entire agenda has not been covered when it is time to close the meeting, assure people that the remaining items will be dealt with at the next meeting or in an e-mail. Allow all interested people to share their ideas. Decide ahead of time on which items the group can make decisions and about which ones you simply want more information so you can make the decision. This should be clear to the people attending the meeting.

If you have been asked to attend a meeting, be hopeful that the manager has an agenda and has sent it out early so that you can be prepared. If there is a topic scheduled for the meeting that you think may be yours to present, but that information is unclear on the agenda, simply ask what is expected of you. Always go to a meeting prepared to share your best information and willing to give your best effort in working with the committee members. Act interested, get involved, and support the worthy ideas of others. If there is a point of confusion or conflict, use your high-level assertive communication techniques to resolve the problem. Communicating effectively is one of the highest level performances of the human mind.

For an individual to manage multiple words and thoughts and to place them into sentences and ideas in milliseconds is a phenomenal feat. This is something you have been doing for most of your life. The purpose of this chapter is to assist you in enhancing the skills that you already have to manage the business of nursing on a higher and more meaningful level. Remember that it is better to commit the Golden Rule to life instead of to memory only; that is how caring managers work.

REAL-WORLD CASE STUDY

■ You are one of two evening team leaders on a medical floor of a busy metropolitan hospital. The unit has recently returned to team leading as a staffing pattern because several RNs have been laid off throughout the hospital. You are new in the role but think you are well prepared because of your experience and your clinical background. The problem is that the other employees, physicians, and patients do not understand the role in which you have been placed. You do have strong support from the unit nurse manager and the RN with whom you work. Tonight you are working with an RN, the charge nurse, who is new to the unit and the role of LPNs as team leaders. The unit is full, with 40 acutely ill people. The rest of the staff are regular staff members who know the unit and the patients and have worked with you in the past. By all indications, it will be a difficult shift. You have a patient who has terminal cancer and is on frequent pain medications. The charge nurse is unwilling to give you the second set of narcotic keys because you are "only" an LPN. This is a major inconvenience and the first time you need to get medication for the patient, it takes an extra 15 minutes to locate the RN and get the keys. This results in wasted time for you and a longer time of discomfort for the patient.

You have decided to talk to the RN about the problem.

1. What communication approach do you plan to use?
2. What other skills do you need to implement for the conversation to go well?

Key Points

- Communication occurs only after the sender and the receiver have understood the meaning of the message. A good communicator asks appropriate questions and uses effective listening skills. Anxiety, stress, fatigue, and interruptions are barriers to effective listening. Being a good communicator takes practice.
- When communicating in an academic setting, you should use active listening skills, ask appropriate questions of student peers and instructors, learn to read nonverbal communication, and engage in friendly conversation. Using these skills will enhance your learning experience in the classroom.
- When communicating in a clinical setting as a student, remember to use these communication principles: Think before you speak, be quiet and gentle in your communication with patients and family, ask appropriate questions, maintain patient confidentiality, be respectful in your communication with others, and do not hesitate to find out what you don't know.
- Failed communication is an interaction in which the communication that was planned or anticipated does not occur. Failed communication usually occurs when people are frustrated, so they raise their voices and make negative or unpleasant statements. The ability to recognize when communication failure occurs and the type of person

with whom they are most common is important in preventing future communication failure.

- Leaning to be an assertive communicator is important for a nurse to be successful in the professions. SBAR, CUS, and the Two-Challenge Rule are three effective communication tools to use when communicating with other healthcare professionals. Nurse managers can also use these tools to communicate with staff during difficult situations.
- There are four common communication styles: assertive, aggressive, nonassertive, and passive-aggressive. Assertive communication is the most positive type and keeps the rights of others in mind. Aggressive communication tends to be one-sided and violates the rights of others. Nonassertive communication does not allow for the expression of thoughts or feelings by an individual, leaving their needs unmet. Passive-aggressive communication is used by an individual who feels powerless and unable to deal with others in a direct manner.
- Other forms of communication used by nurse managers include e-mail, letters, and other written reports. It is important that you learn to use written English properly to perform these functions well. Take advantage of opportunities to write while you are in school and learn to value feedback from you instructors on your written work.

ANSWERS TO REAL-WORLD CASE STUDY

It is a busy shift, and it may seem easier to endure the behavior of the RN than to deal with the situation. At least, this is your first reaction. After thinking about it for a few minutes, however, you realize that would be passive behavior and is not the type of communication that you want to participate in even for one shift. You want to scream at the RN, "Look at the unnecessary pain you made the patient experience!" Of course, you recognize that as aggressive behavior and equally unacceptable as a communication style. You take a deep breath and plan how you can communicate with the RN in an assertive way.

This is not an easy problem to solve. Because the shift is so busy and because you are still new at being a team leader, it requires a great deal of energy from you to do the job. You recognize that you may have to work with this RN again. She has also violated your right as an LPN to feel valued in your work and to have a work environment that allows you to give the best possible care to the patients, that is, keys to the narcotic room. Resolving the problem effectively is important.

You think about the recommended sequence for communicating with someone in an assertive manner. As a reminder it is:
"I feel . . ."
"When you . . ."
"We should . . ."

1. Now you need to fill in the blanks with the problem that you are encountering. It could be something like:
   - "I feel devalued as a team leader and licensed nurse when you do not allow me to carry a set of narcotic keys that are needed by me every 2 to 3 hours for Mrs. F. . . ."
   - "We should identify a solution to this problem quickly so that Mrs. F. can get the best care possible during the remainder of this shift."

2. It is impossible to predict accurately how the charge nurse may respond to your comments. Your hope is that she understands what you are saying and the reason for your comments and gives you the narcotic keys. If that does not happen, you may need to use the skills of active listening and caring theory; if there is not a resolution between the two of you, you may have to explain the problem to your nurse manager and discuss the issue with him or her.

REVIEW QUESTIONS

1. The process of active listening requires the listener to do which of the following? Select all that apply.
   1. Observe nonverbal cues provided by speaker.
   2. Allow the person to finish speaking before you respond.
   3. Think about what you want to say so you are ready to respond.
   4. Focus on what the person is saying.

2. The LPN has a difficult time communicating with a coworker. Which statement best describes what she might do to improve the communication process?
   1. Ask for suggestions from other coworkers.
   2. Pay more attention to the nonverbal cues used by the coworker.
   3. Avoid having conversations with the coworker.
   4. Tell the coworker that she needs to learn how to communicate better.

3. Feedback should be part of every communication to verify that the message you wanted to give was received by the listener.
   1. True
   2. False

4. The nurse manager is discussing an important situation with an employee and is not sure the employee understands the importance of what is being said. Which communication tool would be the best tool for the nurse manager to use?
   1. Two-Challenge Rule
   2. SBAR
   3. CUS
   4. All of the above

5. When communicating with employees, the nurse manager uses an approach that clearly states what the employee needs to know but uses a caring approach. This is an example of
   1. Passive-aggressive communication.
   2. Assertive communication.
   3. Nonassertive communication.
   4. Aggressive communication.

References

Chenevert, M. (2010). *Mosby's tour guide to nursing school: A student's road survival kit* (6th ed.). Philadelphia: Elsevier.

Clochesy, J. M., Dolanskym, M. A., Hickman, R. L., & Gittner, L. S. (2015). Enhancing communication between patients and healthcare providers: SBAR3. *Journal of Health & Human Services Administration, 38*(2), 237–252.

Web Resources

Developing Communication Skills www.mindtools.com/page8.html

12

Considering Culture

CAROLYN ANITA JONES
AND CORY MOSS

KEY TERMS

Cultural blindness
Cultural competence
Cultural imposition
Culturally competent health care
Culture
Culture shock
Diversity
Ethnicity
Ethnocentrism
Inclusion
Prejudice
Race
Stereotyping

CHAPTER CONCEPTS

Culture
Leadership and Management

LEARNING OUTCOMES

1. Define culture.
2. Identify one's own personal cultural framework.
3. Explain the value of respect for and sensitivity to the patient's cultural beliefs, values, and practices.
4. List the eight descriptors used to define cultural competence.
5. Explain the eight barriers to cultural competency development.
6. Perform a cultural assessment.
7. Describe the relationship between diversity and inclusion.

All things are connected. Whatever befalls the earth, befalls the children of the earth.

—Chief Seattle of the Suquamish & Duwamish

I remember as a young nurse I was assigned to the daily care of a young monk who had been admitted from a nearby Catholic monastery. Because of the vow of silence this Frenchman had taken, he had not learned English. I was assigned to him throughout his hospital stay because I spoke conversational French. What I thought of as an opportunity to "brush up" on my French became a profound cultural experience.

The monk had major abdominal surgery and refused to take the intramuscular narcotic analgesic ordered for him by the surgeon. It is crucial for a postoperative patient to take pain medication so that he does not suffer pain unnecessarily and can move and ambulate with less pain, which aides in preventing pneumonia and blood clots, and in stimulating circulation, to carry oxygen and nutrition to the tissues thereby promoting healing. I immediately discovered I had a problem that exceeded the language barrier.

I knew enough French to talk to the patient more about his view of the illness experience he was having and about his pain management. I learned that he was offering the pain to God as a symbol of his willingness to do all that he could to serve Him. Although I am not Catholic, I could understand his decision because I was educated in a Catholic school of nursing. It was clear to me that his religious desire (his cultural basis) was not compatible with an optimal postoperative recovery. What was I to do? I would like to clarify that this problem would not occur in today's health-care world because of preoperative teaching. Such teaching was not done when I was a young nurse.

There were two concepts in the treatment of the monk that I could not ignore as a professional nurse: (1) The Patient Care Partnership gives every person the right to refuse treatment, and (2) as a nurse, I have a responsibility to provide culturally and linguistically competent care. What did I do to meet the cultural and linguistic needs of the young monk, avoid misinterpretation or misunderstanding due to the language barrier, and still give him excellent nursing care? The solution was challenging. See whether what I did relates to your solution.

Once I understood the problem, I immediately notified my nurse manager. I recognized at an early point in my career that experienced nurses knew many things I had yet to learn. After the nurse manager and I discussed the situation, I returned to the monk prepared with some paradigm-shifting ideas. They were requests for him to consider: (1) taking the medication 1 hour later than it was ordered (i.e., his medication was ordered every 3 to 4 hours as needed; would he consider taking it every 5 hours?); (2) taking the medication orally (slower to reach the bloodstream and take effect) every 3 to 4 hours; or (3) taking medication 20 minutes before each time he was to ambulate (provided the previous time administered was at least the minimum time period). Some of these options may have needed approval from the patient's physician.

Before I could share the options with the monk, I had to teach him about the healing aspects of pain management—in French no less! Once he understood the pain management concepts, I talked to him about the three options I had described, and we worked to find one that was acceptable. He chose the oral medication because it did not relieve all of the pain. It was a solution that assisted him in the healing process and in meeting his cultural needs. I could not have managed the situation well without the leadership of my nurse manager. Our objective was to give culturally competent care as an integral part of quality nursing care.

REFLECTIVE THINKING

Consider the options you could use to promote a more positive postoperative recovery for the Catholic monk described here. Take the viewpoint that you are an atheist and an experienced postoperative nurse who knows the importance of pain medication as it relates to healing. Put your best thinking in your class notebook so your ideas can be shared in class. Feel free to ask more experienced nurses their opinion and consider whether their ideas are good solutions for you.

WHAT IS CULTURE?

Culture is a way of life that involves unique characteristics of human beings, wherein they share a pattern of learned behaviors such as customs and moral conduct. The Frenchman in my story at the beginning of this chapter belonged to the religious culture of Catholic monks who had taken a vow of silence and offered their very lives to God. A family is another type of cultural group wherein unique characteristics are shared between the members of the family.

My grandparents were immigrants to the United States. Their nationality is Danish and English. This is my cultural heritage. Right now, my personal culture is that of rural Utah, higher education, and nursing. I retain aspects of my grandparents' European culture because they passed it down to me as they lived their lives.

Culture also encompasses the interpretation of the behavior of others and goes beyond a person's nationality, ethnicity, or race, although as our population grows increasingly more diverse, ethnicity and race are often used interchangeably. The term *ethnic* is defined as concerning a group of people within a cultural system who desire or are given a distinct classification based on traits such as religion, culture, language, or appearance (Venes, 2016). *Race* refers to a set of distinct characteristics such as skin color that are genetically and biologically transmitted (Andrews & Boyle, 2016).

For example, genetic predisposition for sickle cell anemia affects people of African and Mediterranean decent; predisposition for Tay-Sachs disease affects Ashkenazi Jews; Native Americans and Hispanics have a high prevalence of diabetes mellitus. Other cultural health problems are related to social behavior, such as intravenous drug use and HIV.

Just as you have your own culture, so do families and communities. People with a similar cultural background tend to live near each other. An example is the presence of a Chinatown in many big cities, such as New York and San Francisco. There often are similar sections of the city where whites, Latinos, and blacks live in separate cultural groups. Harlem in New York City has a long and dynamic history of African American culture.

The concept of culture also includes the group values, customs or traditions, rituals, communication styles, language, behavior, and social practices. The visible aspects of culture that assist in defining it to others are obvious factors, such as how the group dresses and their food, art, and buildings. The smell of Chinese cooking and the beauty of the unique buildings in most Chinatown sections of a city are distinctive.

The less visible aspects of culture include values, norms, worldviews, and expectations of the members of the cultural group. An example is the coming-of-age rites that exist for teenagers, such as a Jewish boy's bar mitzvah at age 12 or a teen getting a driver's license at age 16. Another example, although a less positive one, is the initiation rites for gangs. These rites vary from group to group, but are a significant factor for each gang; they represent the gang's culture.

Health care has its own culture. A subgroup of that culture is nursing. Overall, the culture provides care for others. Nurses are expected to be a culture of caring people who are clean and efficient. They also are expected to be intelligent, quick thinking, and willing to serve others. They have to be flexible to cover health-care needs 7 days a week ("24/7") and on holidays. One aspect of the nursing culture that I really appreciate is the general ability to solve problems.

POPULATION MOSAIC OF THE UNITED STATES

Dealing effectively with cultural diversity is an essential aspect of effective nursing care. When comparing the U.S. census of 2000 with the census of 2010, there are some interesting trends that will have an impact on the diversity of people to whom you will give nursing care. You need to be aware who your current and future patients are to be an effective manager.

The Population Is Growing

The population of the United States is growing. The U.S. Census Bureau reported a population increase from 309.76 million on the 2010 census to an estimated 324.33 million in June 2016. The predictions are that the number of citizens in the United States will continue to grow to 400 million by 2051 (U.S. Census Bureau, 2014). So when you feel like your units are "just too full" and that there are heavy assignments to make, you need to realize that there simply are more people who need health care. How does that affect you as a manager specifically in terms of a nursing shortage?

If your management position requires you to work with "hiring and firing" and other critical staffing issues, you need to plan for a continuing growth in patient population.

The Emerging Majority of People of Color

The population of the United States is becoming more diverse. The increased diversity adds to the richness of the mosaic of people you will encounter as a nurse. White Anglo-Americans are currently the dominant culture in North America. Historically and socially, Latinos have been considered part of the white population. More recently, the census has gathered information on Latinos as a separate category because of their growing numbers. The ratio of minority group members to the non-Latino white population is increasing every year. In the next half century, the United States is projected to grow increasingly diverse, with racial and ethnic minorities increasing from 32% of the population in 2010 to more than 50% by 2044, thereby becoming a plurality nation in which the Caucasian population remains the largest single group and no group is in the majority. Also, by 2060, nearly one in five individuals within the United States will have been born in a foreign country (Colby & Ortman, 2015).

What does this shift in population mean to you as a nurse manager? The significance is that you need to be prepared to meet the needs of an increasingly more diverse population of people. Many nurses find that learning Spanish is a helpful tool. If you are not interested in learning a new language, you need to be sure there are interpreters available where you work. The interpreters could be placed on a call list and should include the languages common to your community. Box 12.1 provides suggestions for identifying an interpreter. With awareness of the increasing diversity of the population, you need to plan accordingly. Remember the significance of my meager French while working with the monk? How could his needs have been met without some awareness of what he was trying to say? Understanding, through language, is essential to quality care.

Care of diverse populations requires more sensitivity to and awareness of their cultural needs. Do you understand the different religious and social needs of the diverse persons to whom you give care? Entire books are written and multiple Internet sources are available that list the differences in religions and worldviews of different cultures. That is not the purpose of this chapter. Instead, the idea is to build your awareness of the significance

Box 12.1 Using Interpreters

1. Offer communication and language assistance to the patient with limited English proficiency.
2. Inform the patient that language assistance is available free of charge.
3. It is best to use a certified interpreter who is trained in the health-care field, such as a bilingual employee. Do not use family members as interpreters.
4. If the interpreter is not trained in the health-care field, be sure the interpreter is familiar with medical terminology and understands the health issue to be discussed.
5. Be sure the interpreter is fluent in the language of the patient as well as the nurse.
6. Ensure the interpreter is acceptable to the patient.
7. Facilitate the success of a triad interaction, which is an interaction among three people—in this case, the patient, the interpreter, and the nurse—by conferencing with the interpreter before and after the interaction with the patient.
8. Speak in short sentences, allowing interpretation at the end of each sentence.
9. During the interaction, seat the patient, interpreter, and nurse/health-care provider in triangular positioning (triad) so that the interpreter hears and interprets all statements and never answers for the patient.
10. Some facilities require the use of an interpreting service, which may be provided in person, via the Internet, or via telephone (speaker phone), for all three parties to hear. One company that provides interpreting services is Language Line (http://languageline.com).
11. Provide easy-to-understand translated materials (signage, such as consent forms, instructions, and health education materials).

Source: Adapted from Hill, S. S., & Howlett, H. S. (2013). *Success in practical/vocational nursing* (7th ed.). Philadelphia: Saunders.

of cultural diversity and how to look at and care for all individuals through a culturally aware lens.

The Population Is Aging

The population of older people in the United States is increasing. Currently, 14% of Americans are aged 65 or older. Projections of the population of this segment in the next census in 2020 indicate a 10.6% increase from the 2010 census. The percentage is expected to increase to about 21% by 2040 (U.S. Department of Health and Human Services, 2016a). The number of people in this age category has grown consistently since taking the census began. The increased elderly population is attributed to advances in preventive health care, immunizations, improved nutrition, and advancements in pharmaceutical science that allow people to live with multiple chronic diseases.

Most elderly people are placed on busy medical and surgical units where their uniqueness (the culture of aging) is not addressed. I often hear nurses complain about older adults being too slow, too fragile, and hard to communicate with because of hearing or visual losses. When I hear such comments, I wonder what these nurses expect. The elderly, after all, are *old*! It should be expected that they move more slowly, hear less clearly, and have visual problems.

If you are the nurse manager for a gerontological unit, recognize that aging has its own culture and staff accordingly. Nursing personnel need to be given permission to move at the pace of the elderly person. It takes time and requires skills that are not needed with other patients. The manager needs to assure the staff that they will have an assignment that will give them the time necessary to

The growing number of older adults in the health-care system requires more specialized care from nursing staff.

care for the elderly properly, with sensitivity to the culture of growing old.

Poverty as Another Aspect of Culture

There are many definitions of poverty. According to the national guidelines for poverty, a person is poor if he or she has an income of $11,880 a year or less. For a family of four, the guideline is $24,300. The number of people currently below the poverty level in the United States has decreased since 2012 (U.S. Department of Health and Human Services, 2016b).

The culture of poverty has a direct impact on the health of people before they present to you for nursing care. It also affects the quality of care based on insurance and other financial considerations. Higher income is related directly to overall health for the following reasons (Spector, 2017):

- It increases access to health (insurance and mobility).
- It allows people to live in neighborhoods that are safer.
- It makes better housing possible.
- It enables people to avoid living in environmentally hazardous areas, such as waste sites or places with industrial pollution.
- It provides more opportunity to engage in health promotion.
- It generally ensures work-based health insurance.

People who lived at or below the federal definition of poverty often did not have health insurance. In 2010, the percentage of people without health insurance was 16.3%; this equated to almost 50 million Americas. Of that number, 23.1 million were non-Hispanic whites, 15 million were Hispanics, 12 million were blacks, and 9 million were Asians. There were also 7.3 million uninsured children.

On March 23, 2010, the Affordable Care Act (ACA) was signed into law by President Barack Obama. This legislation was responsible for the most sweeping health-care system reforms since the 1965 passage of Medicaid and Medicare. The ACA, which provides Americans with better health security by putting in place comprehensive health insurance reforms, actually includes to two pieces of federal legislation: (1) the Patient Protection and Affordable Care Act and (2) the Health Care and Education Reconciliation Act, Children in low-income families may qualify for insurance through the federally funded Children's Health Insurance Program (CHIP).

Poverty, along with the other issues mentioned in this section, has its own culture. It is challenging to be poor. Consider, for example, having to decide between getting a prescription filled or buying food for one's family. Poverty limits transportation to get to clinic appointments or to visit a loved one who is in the hospital. What happens to the children while a parent is ill and there are no funds to pay for child care?

In general, poverty breeds a sense of helplessness and hopelessness. When individuals are raised in poverty, they generally do not have the opportunity to seek skilled job training or higher education. The lack of additional education leads to employment in lower-paying jobs. Without adequate access to health care, health problems go untreated, creating more barriers to education and employment opportunities.

What can you do to help these individuals? People who live in poverty need more time to examine their health practices with you, your staff, or a social worker. They need to be recognized as people who are valued. Often basic information is missing from a poor person's knowledge base regarding health. An assessment to determine what should be taught to them is crucial. A caring staff (you are the role model and teacher for caring) and time to meet the needs of this social culture are required.

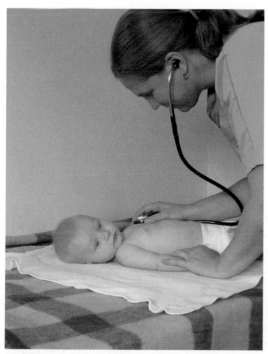

A child accessing health care using CHIP.

Once I worked with a service organization to take health care and other services to the Indians in the mountains of Guatemala. I will discuss cultural shock later, but I did experience genuine cultural shock. One mother of five died because of a tooth abscess. No one in the village knew what to do about it, and there were no dentists or antibiotics available in the high mountains where she lived. Preventive health care practices, such as tooth brushing and flossing, had never been done in their village, which made dental teaching a priority. The same tragedy could occur in poor and crowded environments in the United States. A mother who is exhausted from child care and her job and a father who is absent or working two minimum wage jobs may not realize that tooth brushing is not happening. Do the children get new toothbrushes every 6 months as recommended? Are there biannual visits to the dentist? Is everyone taught and supervised in tooth flossing? Tired parents who feel either helpless or hopeless may not attend to these basic needs. In such a situation, an effective nursing assessment and intervention can have a great impact.

Gender Roles and Human Sexuality

During the 20th century in the United States, the role of women changed dramatically. The role of women has expanded from childbearing and child care to include active participation and leadership in the workplace. The feminist movement has championed this change in roles and has increased awareness of the multiple roles and opportunities available for women.

In addition to the increased opportunities for women, there have been increased rights for the lesbian/gay/bisexual/transgender (LGBT) population and recent laws supporting same-sex marriages. The culture of the United States and the laws, in some states, have increased awareness of LGBT persons. The advances in the women's movement and the sexual orientation movement have changed the culture of the United States.

As a nurse and a nurse manager, it is essential that you role model and promote acceptance of these cultural changes. The expanded roles of women and recognition of homosexual and other sexually oriented lifestyles and rights have heightened consciousness about full opportunities consistent with the American values of individualism, equality, and political freedom.

Some women are criticized for working outside of their home; gay and lesbian people are beaten and even murdered because of their sexual orientation. These behaviors are an example of radical reactions to cultural change. Objective approaches are critical to support all people within their cultural framework of thinking and to provide culturally competent care.

PERSONAL CULTURAL COMPENTENCY

Cultural competence is one of the expectations of nursing similar to skills in using sterile technique. A simple definition of *cultural competence* is awareness and acceptance of cultural differences. As we encounter a significantly increasing diversity among patients and coworkers, it is essential to be culturally competent (Box 12.2). It is my premise that you cannot understand, be sensitive to, and respect the cultural differences of others until you have developed your own cultural awareness.

Think back to the story of the monk. I tried something different to accommodate his religious culture. In addition, the nurse manager was trying to meet his cultural needs by assigning me to work with him because we shared a common language. It was easier for me to understand his culture because I graduated from a Catholic school of nursing and studied French. My educational culture allowed me to meet this patient's needs more effectively.

Having the ability to adapt the nursing care you provide to the culture of others is an important part of patient-centered care.

The initial step in developing cultural competence skills is to spend time focusing on your personal cultural background. You need to understand yourself before you can understand others. Consider the cultural groups to which you belong. You have a family group, fellow student nurses, a circle of friends, the people with whom you work, and perhaps a religious group. Beyond that, you may belong to a soccer team or reading club, a volunteer organization, or an online support group. Each of these separate aspects of your life has its own cultural nuances. The complexity comes as you weave them together into your personal culture. The way to identify your own culture is to examine all aspects of yourself and see how they have intertwined.

When you understand your personal cultural characteristics, you can relate better to the cultural needs of others. As the nurse manager, you need to assist the staff to realize that culture is much more than skin color or country of ancestry or personal origin. Culture is the accumulation of one's life and makes people who they are.

REFLECTIVE THINKING

Spend time thinking about your personal culture. What formulates your standards and dreams? How do you communicate (e.g., quietly, assertively, aggressively, kindly, and in what language[s]) and why? Do you live an active or sedentary lifestyle? How do you experience illness? How do you treat it? Which do you value more, art or sports? Were you raised in a city or a rural area? Are there other nurses in your family and other people who have gone to college as you are doing? Do you know the stories of your ancestors?

Talk to people who are in your cultural world. Ask them questions and spend time considering aspects of their lives that contribute to who you are. Then make a list of your cultural characteristics. Record this list in your class notebook, and be prepared to discuss it in class.

Box 12.2 Developing Personal Cultural Competence

Developing personal cultural competence involves:

- Valuing diversity
- Conducting self-assessments
- Developing self-awareness
- Being sensitive to the needs of others
- Having cultural knowledge and an understanding of other cultures
- Having a nonjudgmental, open-minded, and objective attitude
- Having sensitivity and empathy and avoiding the use of stereotypes

Thoughts on Cultural Competence

A crucial aspect of being culturally sensitive is to recognize that one member of an ethnic group is not always the same as the next. There are several ethnic groups among Asian Americans/Pacific Islanders. As a child, I remember thinking that Tahitian dancers were Hawaiian. Both types of dancers had dark skin and long black hair, and they danced beautifully. When I was older, I recognized that the music and type of dancing were different, as were the language and the geographic origins of the dancers. Knowing the difference between these two types of dancing may not seem important to you in your role as a nurse. Imagine you are in an emergency department, however, when a dark-skinned, dark-haired young man in a Polynesian dancing costume is admitted for burns. To give culturally competent care, it would be important for you to ask the patient and his family whether there are any cultural issues that need to be addressed to give this young man good care. You may find out about the pride Samoan fire dancers have in what they do and the shame they feel when they sustain serious burns.

There are more than 500 recognized tribes of American Indians in the United States. To be culturally competent, it is important to recognize that each American Indian tribe has distinctive cultural concepts. If you had a Navajo family unexpectedly lose their child on the pediatric unit where you worked, you would be able to understand their sorrow at such a tragic loss. I am sure you would extend yourself to them by being available

This photo shows four generations of women from a Japanese family. What do you know about Japanese culture that will tell you who, in this picture, will make the health-care decisions?

to discuss the loss of their child. How would you feel if every time you brought up the child's death, the family rebuffed you? In this scenario, the parents complete the arrangements necessary and leave the hospital without seeing the social worker you had arranged to talk to them. Perhaps you would go home that evening feeling like you let the family down during such a catastrophic experience.

What you don't know is that traditional Navajos do not discuss death. Many believe discussing future or untoward events will lead to their occurrence. By not talking about the deceased person, the bereaved family members do not delay the transcendence of the spirit by listening to the grief of loved ones. Other American Indian tribes do not have the same culture surrounding death.

If you work at understanding yourself and your personal culture, you will be better able to recognize and meet the cultural needs of others. That is culturally competent care, your goal for this chapter. Remember that developing cultural competence is a process and your cultural competence will develop over time.

HOW TO DEVELOP CULTURALLY COMPETENT CARE

Culturally competent care is care given that meets the cultural beliefs of an individual. Eight descriptors are used to define cultural competence, as follows:

- *Integration* of your nursing knowledge with the cultural needs of the patient results in the patient being better informed and, it is hoped, more cooperative with the health-care regimen.
- *Understanding* that meeting cultural needs assists in improving health and health-related outcomes is important for every nurse.
- *Respect* for another person's cultural needs inspires the trust two people can have for each other and fosters cooperation.
- *Communication,* based on cultural understanding, provides a strong bridge to identifying the overall needs of a patient.
- *Sensitivity* to another's cultural needs provides a mechanism for health-related needs to be met more successfully.
- *Dignity* is a crucial aspect of holistic care and does not exist without an understanding of culture.

- *Knowledge* about culture comes only with effort. A benefit to having that knowledge is the opportunity to meet the overall needs of the patient.
- *Acceptance* of the beliefs and characteristics of another person is essential for culturally competent care to be given.

Do these characteristics seem like aspects of yourself you would like to develop? It sounds like caring, holistic nursing to me. Go back over the eight characteristics. You may not see a reason for doing so, but please trust me and do it. This time read them carefully and slowly. Think about each one as though you were the patient. Do you want people to be sensitive to your cultural needs and accept them? Which aspects of your personal culture are the most important to you in a health-care situation? Is it important to you to be treated with dignity? How knowledgeable do you want your caregiver to be? By rereading the characteristics of cultural competence and personalizing them, I am hopeful that you will begin weaving them into your personality as a nurse.

In your work in nursing, the health-care institution or organization that employs you has a responsibility to provide cultural competence training to prepare you and your coworkers for the diverse populations you will serve. You may also decide to take continuing education training online or in person. The Office of Minority Health of the U.S. Department of Health and Human Services provides quality literature, links, and free online continuing education coursework and credit for health-care providers, including nurses. On this same Web site, they provide Standards for Culturally and Linguistically Appropriate Services (CLAS). CLAS services are respectful of and responsive to individual cultural health beliefs and practices, preferred languages, and communication needs of patients in multiple health-care settings.

Now that you understand the behaviors necessary for cultural competence, you need to know how to develop it for yourself. There are five steps in the process. Because you are in a nursing program, I am going to assume that you find people interesting. That is the foundation for step one, cultural desire.

Cultural Desire

Because you find people interesting, you probably have developed a desire to understand what makes people different. That is the desire to understand

culture. Pretend you are a new nurse assigned to two teenagers on the oncology unit. Their situations are very emotional because both girls are terminal, yet the teens and their families are handling things differently. You are interested and pay attention to the activities and communication dynamics of each family. You have the desire to know what is causing the differences in behavior.

Cultural Awareness

As you give your care, you recognize that the two patients and their families share many similarities. Each of your patients is from two-parent families with three children. The most significant similarity is that both families are very concerned about their critically ill teenager and appear to love them deeply. Despite the similarities, their behavior is different.

Tina's mother always looks harried and often sleeps while she is with her. The dad is worried and pensive and never seems to relax. He carries a short strand of beads in his hands and constantly moves his fingers from bead to bead while he is repeating words you don't understand. The little brother and sister are often with the parents. They appear bored and restless and frequently cry. You wonder why.

Sarah's mother is with her constantly, and she seems to be crying whenever you go into the room. The father comes in the evening and only stays a few minutes. There often are many visitors for Sarah. You wonder whether it is too many. While the visitors are there, they stand in a circle and appear to be praying. The room is always crowded and noisy because of these small prayer groups. Sarah has multiple copper and silver bracelets on her thin, weak arms. She gets a new one almost every day. The bracelets are noisy and inconvenient. You wonder whether they could be put in a drawer at bedtime.

As you process the holistic needs of these teenagers, you need to come with respect for the beliefs and values of each person and appreciation for their cultural differences to meet their holistic needs.

Cultural Knowledge

You are assigned to give care to the terminally ill teenagers for 5 consecutive days, and you want to give excellent holistic care to them and their families. You recognize that you know how to give personal care and to manage the medications and other therapies required for them. You do not know how to meet their cultural needs. You are seeking knowledge, so you review records of previous admissions and literature on the cultures of terminally ill patients. You also seek insight from individuals who share the patients' cultural backgrounds and an experienced nurse.

During your "knowledge-seeking" you learn several helpful traits and cultural values. The experienced nurse knows both families because they have been bringing their children to the hospital during the course of the disease. Some of the things your colleague shares with you include the following:

Tina's family

- Father is unable to work because of a disability from his previous job as a construction worker. He is concerned about the hospital bill and asks the price of everything that is used for Tina's care.
- Mother works part-time nights as a waitress and cannot afford child-care services.
- The family is Muslim and has strong spiritual beliefs.
- They are a close family without extended family support because of their conversion to Islam.

Sarah's family

- Siblings are older than Tina's and are a strong support to their parents at this stressful time.
- Father is an executive in a large corporation.
- Mother does not work outside of the home.
- The family has strong Christian spiritual beliefs.
- They are a close family with strong extended family support.
- The family has many friends from their religious group.

From this information, you recognize that despite the similarities in the families, they have different cultural backgrounds. As you leave work that evening, you go to the hospital's library and check out a book suggested to you by the experienced nurse. The topic of the book is the impact of social issues on the dying experience. You read as much of the book as you can that evening.

Cultural Skill

Now that you have gained some useful knowledge, it is time to apply it. You know theoretical concepts from the book and learn personal information from the individuals who share the patients' cultural backgrounds and also from the experienced nurse. How will you put that together to develop skills in delivering culturally competent care? If you were in the classroom or a nursing laboratory, you would practice with feedback from the faculty person. You now are in a situation, however, where you have 4 more days to give care to these girls and their families. It is not an ideal situation, but a real one. The way to avoid "practicing" skills while actually being expected to deliver them is to pay attention to information such as that provided in this chapter and practice while still a student.

In this situation, you need to be honest with the persons involved. Let them know what your desire is, which is excellence in care. Then ask them to share with you the needs they have that you can fulfill. Inquire about their beliefs, practices, and values relating to illness. Obtain cultural information along with the health history. Make some suggestions from what you learned the previous day. Keep the communication focused on meeting the needs of everyone involved, with the patients as the priority.

Cultural Encounter

The cultural encounter is the time you actually deliver culturally competent care. Have you thought of some things you could do to assist these teens and their families to manage their situations? What are the problems, and how can you meet them?

Perhaps Tina's parents need to talk to a social worker about making payments for the hospital bill and resources for child care so that they will be less worried about the bill and can spend more time with Tina without the unhappy younger children present. The mother is working evenings as a waitress and needs her rest during the daytime. If she won't stay at home and sleep, can you arrange for a comfortable bed for her to be brought to the room? What do you need to know about the Muslim religion and death rituals that will help the staff and the family prepare for Tina's death?

Because Sarah's mother isn't working, is she spending too much time at the hospital? Should she be encouraged to get more sleep or to do other things to take care of herself? Are the rooms big enough to accommodate the siblings? Is there a place where Sarah's extended family and friends could be while waiting to see her? This would keep the confusion in her room at a lower level and might provide Sarah with more restful time.

Or is the confusion (your perspective) and the continuous prayers a solace to Sarah? You need to find out.

Both are religious families. Identify what church or mosque they attend and obtain the name and phone number of their religious leader. Seek the assistance of your hospital pastoral care services. Ask the patients and their parents what you can do to assist them in their religious practices.

What is the meaning of the copper and silver bracelets that Sarah keeps receiving? Are they necessary? You want to discuss this because the bracelets are heavy and noisy. Do they bother Sarah? Is there an alternative cultural item that can be given to Sarah that isn't noisy? After making inquiries, you discover that in Sarah's community, the bracelets are given to young women to ensure them health and joy. This assists you in understanding why Sarah insists on wearing them.

These are just a few ideas that reflect culturally competent care. Excellent nursing care is not simply doing the technical tasks. Excellence comes when caring, individualized, holistic care is given as well. Cultural competence is a prerequisite to that type of care.

 ## BARRIERS TO CULTURAL COMPETENCY

For some people, it is challenging to admit the need for cultural awareness. They may think they know enough about other cultures or simply are not willing to learn. Some Americans today have the perception that new immigrants to the United States, such as Arabs, Asians, Indians, and Mexicans (both legal and illegal), are taking away American jobs and priorities. This discriminatory perception fosters prejudice that is only further compounded by the ignorance of cultures of the new people entering the country. After all, who is not of immigrant descent, except Native Americans?

As a professional person, it is your responsibility to recognize any personal barriers to cultural competency and deal with them. A lack of cultural accommodation denotes a lack of quality nursing care and may lead to accidental or deliberate prejudicial acts. If you identify any of the following barriers to cultural competency as obstacles within yourself, seek the guidance and support of someone who can assist you to gain insight and resolve the problem.

The greatest barrier to cultural competency is *ethnocentrism.* This is a concept that indicates that one person's culture is "the best." The most devastating examples of ethnocentricity are the "ethnic cleansings" that occurred in Germany during the Holocaust and, more recently, in Bosnia, the former Yugoslavia, and Darfur. The horrific acts performed on the victims and the large number killed, simply because of their race, is overwhelming and horrific ethnocetrism.

A minor example of ethnocentricity could have occurred while you were reading this chapter. Remember the information about traditional Navajo Indians and their reaction to death? It is such a strong reaction that they abandon their homes when a death occurs there. Did you think that was strange? Unacceptable? Stupid? Curious? Interesting? Amazing? Evaluate your response, and determine whether it had any undertones of ethnocentric thinking. Many people have ethnocentric attitudes without realizing they do. How does this happen? Generally, it is because the person lives in a homogeneous society where there is not much cultural diversity.

The concept of *cultural imposition* is similar to ethnocentrism. It occurs when one person imposes the rules of his or her culture on another person. How does that look in a health-care setting? If you have a devout Muslim in the hospital, you should deal with the need of the person to face east and pray several times a day. If you choose to impose the culture of the hospital on the person, you would interrupt his prayers to give medication or give him his bath during prayer time simply because it is more convenient for you. The idea motivating cultural imposition is that you impose your cultural or personal needs on to the person. The term *cultural blindness* also could be used here. It occurs when a person refuses to recognize the cultural needs of another person. Both of these concepts stem from ethnocentrism and are unacceptable for you or the staff you manage. *Stereotyping, prejudice,* and *racism* have similar unpleasant characteristics, and all of them interfere with excellent nursing care and quality relationships among people. Have you ever been the victim of stereotyping, prejudice, or racism? Consider these possible situations. If you had a young Mexican man as a patient, would you stereotype him as a gang member when, in reality, he was the son of a minister? It is possible. Suppose you had an 81-year-old woman in for postoperative care.

FOCUSED LEARNING CHART
Barriers to Cultural Competency

The following definitions will assist you in understanding barriers to cultural competency:

ETHNOCENTRISM

A belief that one's own way of viewing and experiencing the world is superior to other perspectives (Venes, 2016)

CULTURAL IMPOSITION

Imposing one's culture on another person's culture

CULTURAL BLINDNESS

Refusal to recognize the cultural needs of another person

STEREOTYPING

Assuming that all people of one culture or race have the same personal characteristics

PREJUDICE

Strong negative feelings for persons of a specific culture

RACISM

Racial prejudice

CULTURAL CONFLICT

Conflict that is based on ethnocentric thinking

CULTURAL SHOCK

Emotional shock experienced by being immersed in a different culture.

Would you assume she would be boring, repetitive, and confused because of her age? If so, that is *ageism,* which is similar to racism and sexism. None of the "isms" belong in professional nursing. As you give care to the woman, you discover that she has a PhD in history and has traveled the world. Her stories are articulate and interesting. She also is a "dynamo" who wants to get better and is wearing you out with all of the walking she is doing.

Prejudice is an uncomfortable concept. Racial prejudice is common and historically has been directed toward people of color. If you had a certified nursing assistant with whom you worked frequently who admitted to hating black men because she had been raped by a black man, what would you do? The young woman is prejudiced after having such a horrible experience. You have empathy for her feelings, yet she needs to seek counseling so that she does not stereotype and consider all black male patients to be rapists. I suggest you talk to her, encourage her to seek counseling for her trauma, and teach her the concepts shared in this chapter. Then give her as much support as you can to work through the

problem. Prejudice never is a successful approach to human care.

The final two barriers to cultural competency are cultural conflict and cultural shock. They are not the same, but they both fit on this list as potential hostile encounters. *Cultural conflict* occurs when you enter a power struggle with another person (the patient). Let me remind you what happens in a power struggle: *No one wins.* If you look at our war-torn world, you will see that power struggles are a continuous aspect of our global society. Wars are continuous acts of society that make the point; no one is the winner in a power struggle.

REFLECTIVE THINKING

Take some time and determine whether you ever have been the victim of stereotyping, prejudice, or racism. These behaviors could have occurred because of your cultural background, where you live, hair color, style of dress, weight, language, gender, age, education, or any one of a number of other factors. Record in your class notebook the experience you had and your feelings about it. Were you hurt, frustrated, or angry? Record in your notebook your behavior during the experience. How did you handle the situation? What was the outcome? This may be personal and painful, but it is important to recognize how such behavior generally makes a person feel. What, if anything, would you change about your response were you to experience this situation again? Carefully record your experience and feelings, but share in class only the things you feel comfortable telling others.

What if you refused to let the Muslim pray at the specified times? Refused to allow a young, "almost" mother continue with her desire for a natural birth because of the pain you sensed she was experiencing? Restrained the wise old woman with the PhD? Refused to release the body to the Navajos until they spoke with the social worker? All of these behaviors demonstrate cultural conflict. Can you recognize that the conflicts are based on ethnocentric thinking? It is the foundation of all cultural competence barriers.

Cultural shock occurs when you are immersed into a culture and are literally emotionally shocked by it. Remember the shock I felt when I saw the mother of five die of an abscessed tooth in Guatemala? Cultural shock happens to some new graduates who discover the real world of nursing is caring for 8 to 10 patients rather than the 1 or 2 patients that were assigned during student clinical rotations. For a short time, I taught in an Arab college of nursing in the West Bank of Israel. I was in cultural shock. Everyone spoke English, but there were modern Arab women and others who wore traditional clothing including face covers. These women couldn't imagine a woman giving care to a man. I quickly recovered, but while I was in shock, I was not optimally effective. If you find yourself in that situation, get help to understand the culture. You won't be effective while you are in culture shock.

COMMON ETHNIC GROUPS IN THE UNITED STATES

Although I have made the case that ethnicity is not culture and that all persons of a similar group are not the same culturally, I do not know a way to share general information about different groups

of people without discussing their ethnicity. There are five predominant ethnic groups of people living in North America. As you give nursing care to these people, remember them as individuals. Take the time to get to know them as people rather than as members of a group of people. Yet, you still need to know some basic information about each ethnic group.

European Americans

The 1600s and 1700s saw large numbers of Europeans immigrate to the United States. These predominantly white people left environments of oppression or poverty or both to discover a better life for themselves and their families. The descendants of the European immigrants constituted approximately 77% of the people in the United States. This number is slowly decreasing (U.S. Census Bureau, 2015c).

The Europeans brought with them a strong individualism, work ethic, and the ability to conquer nature because many were farmers. These ethnic groups focus on strong family units but tend to maintain individual freedom as their strength.

Native Americans and Alaska Natives

The indigenous peoples of North America make up 0.2% of the total population and live across the United States and Alaska (U.S. Census Bureau, 2015a).

Many Native Americans moved to more urban areas, although many continue to live on rural reservations. It is common for traditional Native Americans to adhere to folk medicine, and many may consult a tribal medicine person or religious leader before going to a health clinic.

Common health problems include diabetes, obesity, infectious diseases, alcohol abuse, tuberculosis, and suicide. Years of racism, oppression, and dehumanization have left many Native Americans distrustful of the white health-care system.

African Americans

African Americans represent a strongly heterogeneous population that constitutes almost 14% of the U.S. population (U.S. Census Bureau, 2015b). Many African Americans are descendants of African slaves who were brought unwillingly to the United States. Others are recent immigrants from Africa and the Caribbean Islands.

Common health problems include cancer, stroke, diabetes, heart disease, and homicide. High morbidity and mortality rates are directly proportional to socioeconomic factors such as lifestyle behaviors, social environment, and lack of access to preventive health care. African Americans are becoming more health conscious and seeking health screenings and treatment. Health literacy tends to vary by generation.

Asian and Pacific Islander Americans

Asian Americans constitute approximately 6% of the U.S. population (U.S. Census Bureau, 2016a). Most Asian Americans live in California and Hawaii; more than half of Hawaii's population is Asian American (U.S. Census Bureau, 2016a). The people in this category come from a wide variety of countries, including China, Japan, and Korea, with Chinese people representing the largest group of Asian Americans. There also are numerous immigrants from countries, such as those of the Pacific Islands, Vietnam, Cambodia, Thailand, Laos, and India. The culture of each country varies and challenges the nurse to understand each cultural group and individual.

This population is one of the healthiest in the United States, although cancer, heart disease, and stroke are the leading causes of death (Centers for Disease Control and Prevention, 2016). The health-care practices of Asians vary according to their country of origin or ethnic heritage. Individuals may practice home treatments, acupuncture, the balance of hot and cold according to the cause of disease and how disease should be treated, or health practices associated with their religious preference (AARP, 2015).

Hispanic Americans

The Hispanic American population makes up 17.6% of the U.S. population, making this group the largest ethnic minority in the United States (U.S. Census Bureau, 2016b).

This population includes emigrants from Mexico, Spain, Puerto Rico, Cuba, Dominican Republic, and Central and South America. The predominant religions are Catholicism and Pentecostalism. The family and extended family are important, and the family unit generally is patriarchal.

Many members of this cultural group hold traditional health beliefs, with folk healers being used in some situations. Hot and cold remedies are used for many maladies. Spiritual elements, such as worship of saints and the use of talismans, also are common. Common health problems in some Hispanic groups include cancer, diabetes, heart disease, and unintentional injuries.

 CULTURAL ASSESSMENT

To obtain the information you need to give culturally competent care, do a cultural assessment. The cultural assessment will yield data for the nurse to develop a care plan that includes cultural needs and interventions. If you spend time thinking through how to ask cultural questions along with the general health questions already required of you, this will not take much time and will not be yet "another piece of paper" to complete. When the questions about the patient's culture are integrated into the full assessment (physical, psychological, spiritual, and cultural), you ease the patient's responses to any one part of the assessment. To gain insight into a patient's beliefs about his or her health, you need to ask only three questions:

1. What makes you sick?
2. What do you do when you are sick?
3. What makes you better?

The answers to these questions will give you a great deal of insight into the impact personal culture has on the process of illness and wellness.

Now think logically. What else do you need to know as basic cultural information?

- The primary language is crucial because you may need an interpreter.
- Are there special foods the person feels are necessary for healing? Traditional Latinos believe the "hotness" of the food (e.g., chili peppers for heat) affects healing.
- What is the family situation, and what role does the family play in the person's health beliefs? Does the husband or oldest son need to make the decisions because of the culture of the family?
- What are the person's spiritual beliefs as they relate to illness, wellness, and death? On the nursing unit it may be necessary to accommodate last rites for Catholics; priesthood blessings for Mormons; or the presence of a Voodoo doctor, shaman, or other spiritually guided healer.

The questions listed in Box 12.3 can give you the basic information you need to give culturally competent care. When you know the answers to

Box 12.3 Basic Cultural Assessment

1. What language do you speak?
2. What makes you sick?
3. What do you think made you sick this time?
4. What do you think made it start?
5. Are there any particular concerns or fears you have about it?
6. What has this sickness changed about your daily living?
7. What do you do when you are sick?
8. What usually makes you better?
9. What have you done about it this time?
10. Are there special foods you need to assist you in getting better?
11. Tell me about your family and how they can help you to feel better.
12. What are your spiritual beliefs as they relate to your illness?
13. What treatment do you expect to receive?
14. What do you expect to be the result of this treatment?

these questions, you will be able to make further inquiries based on those answers.

This is a simple assessment and includes information you need from every patient admitted to your facility. The point is to ask the questions with a broader understanding of the cultural information you need in order to give excellent care. I suggest you take these questions and interview at least seven people. You may find the answers interesting. Use your own family members, roommates, and other friends for your practice interviews. By using people you know, you should be more comfortable during the interview. That is the objective of practicing—to be comfortable using the questions in your clinical practice.

HIRING AND MANAGING A DIVERSE WORKFORCE

Many health-care organizations believe the strategic management of diversity and culture is necessary for success. Diversity among nurses may be based on ethnicity, race, socioeconomic status, gender, language, religion, and other demographics. The concept of creating a culturally competent organization is not new to health care. In 1965, the Equal Opportunity Commission established important elements for workplace diversity. Since that time, health-care organizations have implemented various ideas and perspectives to improve the workplace surroundings of employees (Nolen, 2016). A couple of the main factors in U.S. health care that drive the need to become a more diverse workforce are the surrounding communities of health-care providers and the populations they serve. Most health-care organizations are part of and centered in their respective communities and cities. According to national census statistics, our communities are growing larger and more diverse each day. Yet research shows that health-care organizations have not done enough to increase employee diversity and mirror the patient communities they serve (Yeldell, 2015).

To meet the needs of diverse patient populations, organizational values and management policies should include diversity as a goal. Nurses and nurse managers need to be involved in developing these policies. Employing a more diverse staff should be initiated at the recruiting and hiring stages, and should be adequately managed and maintained throughout the employee's time with the organization. Over the past few years, the concept of inclusion has been added to diversity policies among health-care organizations. Inclusion, which is defined as specific employee behaviors and how you manage them, and employee diversity, which is defined as the demographic characteristics or mix of a group, must be part of a strategic plan if organizations desire to provide culturally competent care to their patients. Inclusion considers the different personnel; their own behaviors, personalities, and skills; and how these differences can positively impact patient outcomes. A health-care organization's diversity generally increases when it hires applicants with diverse social characteristics and implements inclusion practices to take advantage of varied employee experiences (Guajardo, 2015).

Inclusion begins with recruiting and hiring for gender and ethnic diversity. Hiring efforts may be adjusted to recruit from different geographic locales. Once employees are hired, inclusion practices should allow for staff ideas, suggestions, brainstorming, and discussions of problems and potential resolutions. These processes will foster inclusion, build team unity, and create a diverse team environment. It is important to note that human resources staff should have proper policies in place to assure that the activities and responsibilities of management and hiring personnel allow for diverse applicants and encourage inclusion at all levels.

Hiring activities could focus on recruiting applicants with varied clinical experiences. This process of hiring is the responsibility of both nurse managers and the human resources department. Nursing departments often get in a hiring rut of recruiting nurses with similar backgrounds or experiences, but that does not need to be the case. Human resources can consider qualified applicants from differing clinical backgrounds and provide a robust training and orientation program, which will ensure diversity and inclusion.

Managing staff is more than overseeing employee performance related to policies and procedures; it is about managing personnel and their behaviors and skills. Staff members often come from varied backgrounds and differing cultural beliefs, with a need to be included in a team environment. Management of diversity and inclusion centers on individual employee values, varying personal beliefs, and performance outcomes (Farr & Cressey, 2015). By working closely with staff, nurse managers get to know the individual strengths and characteristics of each employee and can use what they've learned about each employee's personal beliefs and values to help each nurse provide the best possible patient care. During this process, differences among the nurses are valued and respected, creating an environment of trust. The successful management of and respect for the differences among nurses allow for safe cultural expression within employee settings (Vogel, 2015). Nurse managers should consider the differences among their nurses, their prior clinical experiences, their credentials, and their individual personalities and characteristics, and then think about how best to create working teams to ensure nurses achieve the best patient outcomes. This is diversity management. This approach allows for staff inclusion and creates the best opportunities for success of all employees. When managers create diversity among staff, it ensures a better working environment for nurses, a happier and more successful team of nurses, and excellent patient care.

REFLECTIVE THINKING

Spend time thinking about your workplace surroundings in a current or prior job. Do you work within a diverse group? What are some of your coworkers' similarities and differences? Does your workplace practice inclusion? Give an example.

Maintaining Diversity

Organizations should first assess their current situation and determine what positive changes can be made to ensure diversity (Nolen, 2015). An organization's assessment of its commitment to and practices related to diversity can include both individual and organizational assessments, which could help the nursing team unify in efforts to become more diverse. With regard to diversity, be aware that when individuals self-evaluate, they tend to rate themselves higher than they may really be, which creates a false belief about their attitudes and behaviors related to diversity. This false assessment may have a negative impact on an organization's diversity goal.

A specific plan to maintain diversity and inclusion should include several of the following points:

- Each nurse manager plays a key role in sustaining diversity and, although individual commitment is necessary, a team approach to diversity and inclusion will help ensure this as a sustainable policy within the organization.
- Diversity strategies are most successful when they are implemented both at the organizational and departmental levels.
- The focus on process and outcomes is best managed in smaller settings such as individual units in which hands-on managers can have an immediate impact.
- Efforts to maintain and monitor the commitment to diversity should be discussed and evaluated frequently (Villarruel, Washington, Lecher, & Carver, 2015).
- Organizations may utilize minority programs such as affirmative action or minority scholarship resources to increase diversity among nurses and to develop a foundation for inclusion. Diversity must be embraced thoroughly by management and should be practiced by both clinical and administrative staff.

Diversity and Quality Care

As patient populations continue to grow and become more diverse, so does the need for corresponding diversity in nurses and other health-care providers. There must be a clear effort on behalf of health-care providers to establish diverse organizations. A positive climate of diversity and inclusion improves employee morale, increases employee retention, and increases the quality of care. This increased commitment to diversity by employees is positively reported on in patient satisfaction surveys and is evidenced by improved patient outcomes. The acceptance of diversity policies by organizational leadership and nurses enhances employee engagement and is proved to increase nurses' overall performance. Individual employee standards may not always align with health-care organizations' standards, but nurses who are led and motivated by patients' diverse values and concerns are more patient centered and provide more personalized care.

NURSE MANAGERS AND CULTURE

As a future nurse manager, you need to understand the significance of culture on two levels: (1) patient care and (2) personnel management. The concepts of culturally competent patient care and hiring a diverse workforce have been discussed in this chapter. How can you apply what you have learned to the responsibility of personnel management?

When you are interviewing someone for a position on the unit you manage, it would be wise to share the unit's cultural beliefs. This statement will sound like the nursing philosophy of the unit and could read something like the following: *To give excellent, culturally competent care to all patients.*

It is important to observe whether the potential employee can support that philosophy as well as to ask about the candidate's knowledge and understanding of her or his personal culture. Another matter of significance is to provide education to all new employees about culturally competent care. An effective manager cannot assume that all employees will know what that phrase means. The nurse manager needs to ensure a method for sharing culturally specific information about patients and families with all staff members as an integral part of the assessment and records. Is that in report, on the care plan, or both? You may have other ideas; it does no good to have information about a person if it is not shared with everyone giving care to that person.

There are other considerations for you as a manager. If you have a Hispanic nurse on your unit, will you always assign her to the Hispanic patients? Would you do the same with an African American nurse and patients? If you do, you are practicing stereotyping in your management style. It is not true that Hispanic patients want only Hispanic nurses or that African American patients only want African American nurses. Embrace the diversity of your staff as well as the patients.

A Final Story

Mr. Ibaka, an elderly man from Laos, immigrated to the United States to live with his son and daughter-in-law. Mr. Ibaka was ill and eventually was diagnosed as having Hansen's disease, more commonly known as leprosy. He was referred to the public health system for treatment with medication that would cure the disease.

The public health nurse took a young woman who spoke Laotian with her to visit Mr. Ibaka and serve as interpreter. The interpreter followed the instructions of the nurse exactly. She explained the disease to Mr. Ibaka, showed him the medication, and taught him and his daughter-in-law how to take it. Then she made the final explanation to him. It was simply that if he did not take the medication, he would be deported because the disease was contagious.

The nurse and the same interpreter went to visit Mr. Ibaka 1 month later. His condition had worsened slightly, and he had not taken the medication except for four or five pills. The same information was given to him that had been given to him on the previous visit. There was special emphasis on deporting him if he did not take the medication.

The third visit was 1 month later. The nurse was unable to obtain the services of her usual interpreter and asked a colleague who also was Laotian to go with her to visit Mr. Ibaka. Her colleague agreed. When they arrived at the house, the Laotian colleague took off his shoes and bowed as he greeted the old man. This had not been done previously. He sat near Mr. Ibaka and talked of life and the coming springtime. After several minutes of general discussion, the interpreter asked Mr. Ibaka how he was feeling. He responded, "Not well." He went on to explain that the pills made him sick, so he didn't like to take them. After some time had passed, he also confessed to the younger man that he had committed a horrible crime during the war and he felt the leprosy was his punishment.

The interpreter worked with the nurse to get a doctor's order for a lower dose of the medication with the hope that the side effects would be lessened. Then the nurse and the interpreter made a home visit one day with the medication and wood, hammer, nails, and paint. With his supplies, the interpreter and Mr. Ibaka together built a shrine in the backyard where Mr. Ibaka could pray for forgiveness of his crimes. Mr. Ibaka also took the medication because the side effects were diminished. This is a true story and is a classic example of why cultural competence is integral to quality health care in an increasingly diverse population.

REAL-WORLD CASE STUDY

Mal de Ojo (The Evil Eye)

■ Mary Dixon, a licensed practical nursing (LPN) student, was assigned to work with Ms. Alder, a registered nurse, in the hospital's postpartum clinic. Mary was excited to be able to work with Ms. Alder because of her reputation for providing valuable learning experiences for students assigned to her clinic. Ms. Alder had worked in the postpartum clinic for 7 years and understood what experiences would be helpful for Mary's learning needs.

Mary came early to the clinic so she could orient herself to the surroundings and meet Ms. Alder. Ms. Alder was friendly and introduced Mary to other clinic personnel. Mary was taken on a tour while Ms. Alder explained to Mary what her assignments would be. Mary was delighted that she was going to have experiences in using the information from her maternal/child class. Mary had done well in understanding the LPN's responsibilities in caring for mothers and children and was excited and nervous at the same time. She wanted to help her patients and did not want to do anything that could be harmful.

The first few hours went well. Mary was able to complete all of her assignments and enjoyed what she was doing. Ms. Alder was complimentary of the care Mary was giving to each of her patients. Mary felt this was the place she wanted to work when she finished her LPN program and was licensed.

Mary expected to see new mothers and their babies and was surprised at the number of immigrants and refugees who came to the clinic. Mary found it exciting to be working with women from other cultures and wanted to help them to feel comfortable and welcomed in the clinic.

Ms. Alder asked Mary to care for Mrs. Martinez's 3-year-old daughter, Maria, while the nurse practitioner examined Mrs. Martinez and her new baby. Mary was delighted. Maria was a beautiful child, and Mrs. Martinez had dressed Maria in a blue-and-white jumper and had put blue butterfly clips in her ponytails. Mary told Mrs. Martinez that Maria was a beautiful child. She complimented Mrs. Martinez for the way Maria was dressed for the visit to the clinic as she touched Maria's shoulder. Without saying a word Mrs. Martinez grabbed Maria and her baby and left the clinic. Mary could tell Mrs. Martinez was very upset.

Mary was upset and asked Ms. Alder what had happened, as she did not understand what had gone wrong. Mary's comments were meant to be complimentary and positive. Ms. Alder took Mary into the conference room and invited her to sit down at the table. Ms. Alder went to the kitchen, got Mary a drink of juice, and then asked what happened.

Mary explained how she had admired the beautiful little girl, Maria. Mary thought she was giving Mrs. Martinez a compliment and did not mean to say anything offensive. Ms. Alder softly explained to Mary that in some cultures you can put a spell, or a hex, on children by admiring them without touching them at the same time. This is called the evil eye, or *mal de ojo*. It was all right for Mary to admire Maria, but Mary needed to be touching the child as she talked with Mrs. Martinez.

Mary wanted to know what Mrs. Martinez would need to do to remove the spell from Maria. Ms. Alder said a *curandero*, a healing person, would use a cultural practice to remove the spell, and Maria would be fine. Ms. Alder said she would call Mrs. Martinez the next day to check on Maria and make another appointment to complete the postpartum examination.

Assignment

Write a cultural scenario following the format of the *mal de ojo* story. Describe the setting, persons involved, and a cultural experience related to health-care practices and beliefs. Write about something you know and make it interesting. This assignment should not be longer than one page. Use your best writing skills and be prepared to submit your scenario in class. Sharing scenarios with your classmates and reading theirs will assist each of you in being better informed.

Key Points

- *Culture* is a way of life that involves unique characteristics of human beings, wherein they share a pattern of learned behaviors such as customs and moral conduct. It also involves shared attitudes, beliefs, and language.
- The population of the United States is increasing and becoming more diverse. Care of diverse populations requires more sensitivity to and awareness of their cultural needs. To meet the needs of diverse patient populations, organizational values and management policies should include diversity as a goal. Nurses and nurse managers need to be involved in developing these policies.
- *Cultural competence* is awareness and acceptance of cultural differences. As we encounter a significantly increasing diversity among patients and coworkers, it is essential to be culturally competent. It is an important nursing skill that must be developed by all nurses in order to meet the varied needs of patients. In order to manage a diverse workforce, nurse managers must also understand the importance of cultural competency when developing their management style.
- Eight descriptors are used to define cultural competence: *integration* of your nursing knowledge with the cultural needs of the patient; *understanding* that meeting cultural needs assists in improving health outcomes; *respect* for another person's culture; *communication* based on cultural understanding; *sensitivity* to cultural needs; *dignity,* which is crucial to providing holistic care; *knowledge* about culture, which comes only with effort; and *acceptance* of the beliefs and characteristics of another person.
- You, as a nurse, cannot understand and respect the cultural differences of others until you have developed your own cultural awareness. It requires open-mindedness and tolerance to be able to adapt to the culture of others. Take the time to focus on your own personal cultural background by considering the groups to which you belong. When you understand your personal cultural characteristics, you can better relate to the cultural needs of others.
- As a professional, it is your responsibility to recognize any personal barriers to cultural competency that might hinder your ability to provide safe care to patients or as a nurse manager to appropriately manage employees. Barriers to cultural competency include ethnocentrism, cultural imposition, cultural blindness, stereotyping, prejudice, racism, cultural conflict, and cultural shock. The greatest barrier to cultural competency is ethnocentrism.
- There are a number of common ethnic groups in the United States, including European Americans, Native Americans and Alaska Natives, African Americans, Asian and Pacific Islander Americans, and Hispanic Americans. The Hispanic population has had the highest increase over the past several years. Nurses need to learn about the cultural needs of the various ethnic groups in an effort to provide culturally sensitive care. Providing culturally sensitive care improves patient outcomes.
- A cultural assessment is used to obtain culturally specific information needed to provide individualized care for diverse patients. A cultural assessment consists of questions designed to identify how a patient perceives his or her health needs based on cultural nuances. As part of their skill set, nurses need to learn how to competently perform a cultural assessment.
- *Inclusion* refers to specific employee behaviors and how they are managed. Nurse managers should participate in the development of inclusion policies for their organizations, which should include recruiting and hiring for gender and ethnic diversity. *Diversity* is defined as the demographic characteristics or mix of a group. Health-care organizations should assess their organizations to determine what positive changes can be made to ensure diversity in the workforce.
- It is important for every nurse to understand that meeting cultural needs of diverse patients assists in improving health and health-related outcomes. Respect for another person's cultural needs inspires trust between the patient and the nurse and fosters better cooperation.

ANSWERS TO REAL-WORLD CASE STUDY

You can base your scenario on a real-life experience or write a scenario based on information you have gathered about a particular culture. Whatever approach you take, have fun with the writing process. As part of the scenario, you want to include the setting where the interaction occurred. Was it in a clinical, workplace, or social setting? Who were the individuals involved?

Also include health-care practices and beliefs related to the individuals involved in the scenario. You might want to refer to the cultural assessment information in Box 12.3 for suggestions about information you can include in the scenario. Be sure to address how cultural concerns in your scenario could be addressed.

REVIEW QUESTIONS

1. The nurse manager has made it a point to get to know her employees and use any differences in their personalities and behaviors to benefit patient care. Which term best describes this concept?
   1. Diversity
   2. Inclusion
   3. Cultural competence
   4. Cultural blindness

2. Mrs. Behar is about to have lunch and discovers a pork chop on her tray. She is upset because she is Jewish. What would your culturally competent response be?
   1. Here is the menu; just take a look and I will be happy to order what you prefer. I will take this plate back.
   2. You didn't state your race or a diet preference on your admission form.
   3. The nurse who admitted you must have thought you were white.
   4. Here is the menu; just call the dietitian and tell them you do not eat pork so they won't send it to you again.

3. Mr. Obanta, a 72-year-old Nigerian, is noncompliant with his tuberculosis (TB) medication orders. You and the staff interpreter go together to his home to reassess him and develop a plan to resolve the problem. Mr. Obanta says he feels the illness is punishment for his sins and the medication causes his stomach to be upset. Which of the following nursing interventions would you and the interpreter choose to implement?
   1. Speak with your supervisor regarding discharging Mr. Obanta for non-compliance.
   2. Speak with the physician regarding a smaller dose and take tools to build a prayer stand for Mr. Obanta to pray for forgiveness of his sins.
   3. Get an antacid for Mr. Obanta to take before his TB medication and pray with him through his daughter as the interpreter.
   4. Talk with Mr. Obanta's daughter and suggest she give the medication to her father with milk.

Continued

4. Mrs. Kihega, a 40-year-old Kiowa Native American, is coming in to the clinic for an annual checkup. During your assessment, which of the following questions is culturally oriented and appropriate to include?
   1. Do you know how to give a shot?
   2. Can you afford to pay for this office visit?
   3. How have you treated illness in the past?
   4. What is your occupation?

5. The nurse assigned to Mr. Jones is aware of her personal fear of African American men and utilizes her self-awareness to maintain her cultural competence. Without this knowledge and skill, she would not be aware that judging Mr. Jones based on preconceived ideas is considered:
   1. Ethnocentrism.
   2. Cultural shock.
   3. Cultural imposition.
   4. Inclusion.

References

AARP. (2015). The health and healthcare of Asian Americans and Pacific Islanders age 50+. http://www.aarp.org/content/dam/aarp/home-and-family/asian-community/2015-01/AARP-Report-Health-and-Healthcare-AAPIs-50-Jan2015.pdf

Andrews, M. M., & Boyle, J. S. (2016). *Transcultural concepts in nursing care* (7th ed.). Philadelphia: Wolters Kluwer.

Centers for Disease Control and Prevention. (2016). Health of Asian or Pacific Islander population. http://www.cdc.gov/nchs/fastats/asian-health.htm

Colby, S., & Ortman, J. (2015). Projections of the size and composition of the U. S. population: 2014 to 2060: Population estimates and projections, current population reports. Retrieved from https://www.census.gov/content/dam/Census/library/publications/2015/demo/p25-1143.pdf

Collini, S. A., Guidroz, A. M., & Perez, L. M. (2015). Turnover in health care: The mediating effects of employee engagement. *Journal of Nursing Management, 23*(2), 169–178.

Farr, M., & Cressey, P. (2015). Understanding staff perspectives of quality in practice in healthcare. *BMC Health Services Research, 15*(1), 123.

Guajardo, S. A. (2015). Assessing organizational efficiency and workforce diversity: An application of data envelopment analysis to New York City agencies. *Public Personnel Management, 44*(2). doi:10.1177/0091026015575179

Hill, S. S., & Howlett, H. S. (2013). *Success in practical/vocational nursing* (7th ed.). Philadelphia: Saunders.

Nolen, L. (2016). Recruiting a diverse workforce. Retrieved from http://www.advanceweb.com/jobs/healthcare-news/hr-employee-recruitment-articles/recruiting-a-diverse-workforce.html

Spector, R. E. (2017). *Cultural diversity in health and illness* (9th ed.). New York: Pearson Education.

U.S. Census Bureau. (2014). 2014 national population projections. Retrieved from http://www.census.gov/content/dam/Census/library/publications/2015/demo/p25-1143.pdf

U.S. Census Bureau. (2015a). Facts for Features: American Indian and Alaska Native Heritage Month: November 2015. Retrieved from https://www.census.gov/newsroom/facts-for-features/2015/cb15-ff22.html

U.S. Census Bureau. (2015b). Facts for Features: Black (African-American) History Month: February 2015. Retrieved from http://www.census.gov/newsroom/facts-for-features/2015/cb15-ff01.html

U.S. Census Bureau. (2015c). Quick Facts: United States. Retrieved from http://www.census.gov/quickfacts/table/PST045215/00

U.S. Census Bureau. (2016a). Facts for Features: Asian/Pacific American Heritage Month: May 2016. Retrieved from https://www.census.gov/newsroom/facts-for-features/2016/cb16-ff07.html

U.S. Census Bureau. (2016b). Facts for Features: Hispanic Heritage Month 2016. Retrieved from http://www.census.gov/newsroom/facts-for-features/2016/cb16-ff16.html

U.S. Department of Health and Human Services. (2016a). Administration on Aging. Aging statistics. Retrieved from http://www.aoa.acl.gov/Aging_Statistics/index.aspx

U.S. Department of Health and Human Services. (2016b). Poverty guidelines. Retrieved from https://aspe.hhs.gov/poverty-guidelines

Venes, D. (Ed.). (2016). *Taber's cyclopedic medical dictionary* (23rd ed.). Philadelphia: F. A. Davis.

Villarruel, A., Washington, D., Lecher, W. T., & Carver, N. A. (2015). A more diverse nursing workforce. *AJN: The American Journal of Nursing, 115*(5), 57–62.

Vogel, L. (2015). Is your hospital culturally safe? *CMAJ: Canadian Medical Association Journal, 187*(1), E13.

Yeldell, C. (2015). Healthcare report card reveals lack of supplier diversity. *Crisis, 122*(2), 40–41.

Web Resources

Culturally Competent Nursing Care www.thinkcultural-health.hhs.gov

National Standards for Culturally and Linguistically Appropriate Services (CLAS) in Health and Health Care www.pcpcc.org/resource/national-standards-culturally-and-linguistically-appropriate-services-clas-health-and

Transcultural Nursing Society www.tcns.org/

U.S. Department of Health and Human Services, Office of Minority Health https://minorityhealth.hhs.gov

United States Census 2010 www.census.gov/2010census

13

Understanding Benefits of Change

SALLY CANTWELL

KEY TERMS

Change
Change agent
Change by drift
Evidence-based practice
Planned change
Transition

CHAPTER CONCEPTS

Collaboration
Communication
Evidence-Based Practice
Spirituality
Stress

LEARNING OUTCOMES

1. Discuss the value of planned change in the nursing profession.
2. Identify the importance of decision making as it is outlined in the process of driving and restraining forces.
3. List and describe the three stages of Kurt Lewin's change theory.
4. Write a paragraph on the role of the LPN as a change agent.
5. List three of the five common mistakes that are made when using change theory.
6. Describe the use of evidence-based practice as a tool for improving patient care.

Great ideas are often opposed by violent reactions of mediocre minds.

—Albert Einstein

The concept of change often makes people uneasy and causes them to feel less secure than they did before the suggestion or enactment of a change. Why does that happen? What concepts underlie the philosophy of change? Most important for the nurse manager, how can those "violent," negative, or resistant reactions be overcome so that effective changes can be made in the health-care system?

I know you are experiencing changes in your professional life as you read and study the information in this book. In Chapter 11, you were presented with the information necessary to become an assertive nurse. How difficult has it been for you to implement those concepts? Once you became comfortable with the techniques and began using them regularly, how did people react to the changed you? Generally, there is a reaction from people who were accustomed to your behavior who then try to understand why you have become assertive. People who are unaccustomed to assertive communication skills may think that you are being aggressive because it is such a change from your previous, perhaps passive, behavior. It is interesting to participate in a change such as communication style and observe the impact it has on other people.

Change is important; without it, health care still would have nurses sharpening needles before sterilizing them for reuse. Without change, there still would be polio wards or units in every hospital with iron lungs. Without change, the role of the licensed practical nurse (LPN) would be nonexistent, and nurses still would be educated in hospitals where they provided much of the nursing labor free as part of their learning experiences. Without change, people and organizations become stagnant, no progress occurs, and the status quo becomes acceptable to everyone.

As an experienced nurse, I invite you to embrace change, analyze it as it comes, and make well-thought-out decisions regarding changes proposed to you. Make changes yourself! The skills for accomplishing this task are given to you in this chapter. You have the ability to process problems, define possible solutions, and propose better ideas or solutions as others consider change on the management team. If people have been uncomfortable with the change in your communication style, continue to be consistent, provide clarity, and challenge others to rise to understand the benefits of well-designed changes. You should not be the same nurse after you study and process this information. This is something for you to look forward to happening.

WHAT IS CHANGE?

Change involves altering the flow of events in any situation, such as in your life, the lives of patients, or an organization. Some people mutter, "Why would I want to change? There is no advantage in it for me!"

I want you to take the time to ponder two questions and write your responses (see the Reflective Thinking feature). To respond to these questions effectively, you must have self-awareness and the ability to use your imagination. You need to envision, to see the potential, and to create with your own mind what does not exist but could exist in your life. Change is not easy, but it can be valuable.

To paraphrase the late Stephen R. Covey (2013), effective people make changes. Effective people are not problem oriented; they are opportunity oriented. Are there opportunities in your personal life or your career that you have been ignoring? What opportunities do you need to recognize, understand, and pursue? You or, where appropriate, a team of colleagues are the people who can and should identify existing opportunities and implement the changes necessary to capitalize on them.

Most changes involve a reaction from someone or somewhere in the organization. This is the concept Einstein was trying to share in his quote at the beginning of the chapter. Change evokes reactions from people who are unwilling to learn or focus on understanding the opportunity that change can bring. You need to accept negative reactions as inevitable. If you work in an organization that does not produce such a reaction, you are fortunate. The same is true in your personal life. If you suggest change—based on opportunity and creative thinking—to your family or significant others, and no negative reaction occurs, again you are fortunate. Even the decision to go to school for your LPN license caused changes in your personal life, and some people responded to those changes. You are home less often, your free time is spent studying, and you are more tired than you were before you went to school. Others have to adjust to the impact of all of these changes not only on your life but also on theirs. A healthy adjustment to the change is a healthy life transition. There are critical transitions you need to make when moving from being a student nurse to being an LPN. The transitional concepts in this chapter will add to what you already know and will assist you with the change process throughout your career.

REFLECTIVE THINKING

Thoughtfully answer the following questions from Stephen Covey's book *The 7 Habits of Highly Effective People* (2013):

1. What one thing could you do regularly (something you are not doing right now) that would make a meaningful, positive difference in your personal life?
2. What one thing in your professional life would bring similar results?

Because of the history of nursing, the oppression of the profession, and the socialization of women, nurses often have not been taught or had role models for the process of taking advantage of opportunities and making changes. This is your opportunity to make meaningful changes personally and professionally.

EFFECTIVE DECISION MAKING DURING CHANGE PROCESS

There are two common ways change occurs. One is planned change, and the other is change by drift, or accidental change. Planned change needs someone like you to eventually serve as the change agent. This usually is someone with experience and skill in the change process. You may not feel qualified for that role right now, but you should keep it on your list of things to learn to do. There may be a time in your future when being a major change agent is critical to the work you are trying to accomplish. This role requires the ability to work well with others, to teach and explain, and to implement change through the use of change-making skills.

Planned change often comes from a committee or an administrative group. Much of the more recent change in health care that has resulted in management jobs for LPNs has come from administrative groups who have tried to avoid the financial crises

that threaten U.S. health-care systems. Planned change is a well-thought-out and deliberate effort to make a change. The usual way an LPN is involved in a planned change is through receiving the instructions of the change and being asked to implement them at the bedside of patients. The LPN is the person the change maker is trying to teach and work through to implement the change. It would be worthwhile to think back to planned changes in which you have been involved. If you have not had that experience, keep it in mind for the future because change is inevitable.

Change by drift, or accidental change, is unplanned change that occurs because of an imbalance in the system. Because people have not been taught about the forthcoming change and have not had an opportunity to be involved in it, change by drift is generally met with resistance, even hostility. Current nursing leaders agree that much of the change in the nursing profession has been unplanned or forced on the profession by other groups, such as physicians or administrators. Consequently, changes have not had a strong nursing

When implementing planned change, an educational program is helpful. It ensures that everyone has the same information about the suggested change.

FOCUSED LEARNING CHART
Choose Your Change Process

CHANGE BY DRIFT

Problematic

Unplanned change

Outcome unsure

PLANNED CHANGE

Most desirable

Well-organized plan

Identify driving and restraining forces

Unfreeze

Move

Refreeze

basis. Nursing should be defining its own needs for change and designing plans for implementing those needs.

Decisions regarding change need to be concrete and made according to a plan for change to be successful. Short-term and long-term decisions are necessary to invite change to occur. For example, you and the other nurses on your unit may think there is a strong need for shift report to be done with more efficiency and more information. This change demands short-term and long-term plans that require decisions to be made before the implementation of the change.

Similar to the nursing process, you need to determine what the problem is. Perhaps you and others are merely feeling frustration after report is given and have never discussed what is causing those feelings. The first decision may be to plan a meeting in which the process of report could be discussed freely (perhaps the supervising nurse should not be present so that people can be more comfortable sharing their feelings). Meeting together as a group is not an easy process; it involves people admitting that report is not perfect; it is often difficult for people to admit that problems like this exist.

It is wise to select an informal leader among the nurses and to discuss your feelings with that person before suggesting a meeting be organized. Is the feeling of frustration something specific to you alone, or do others feel it? You need to recruit people who understand what you want to discuss or

change. As awareness grows, so does the desire to have a meeting to discuss the problem. It is wise to keep your supervisor involved in every aspect of what you are thinking and doing.

After the meeting occurs, accurate, validated information can be used to design the necessary changes. This information can be used to set goals and determine the methods for achieving the goals. The process allows everyone to be involved, a crucial aspect of making change. The decisions that are made by the group or an assigned individual are crucial to the success of the desirable changes.

Change by drift is undesirable because of the distress it brings to people who are either asked or required to make change without knowing why or being involved in the change process. It also resembles the idea of "putting out fires" instead of planning and making decisions that prevent the fires. Good change theory requires solid and reliable information on which effective decisions can be made. Change by drift does not allow that to happen.

KURT LEWIN'S CHANGE THEORY

Many change theories are available for learning or review. Kurt Lewin's (1951) theory is the grandfather of change theory. It is not complicated, it makes sense, and it is user-friendly. If you choose to continue your education, you may encounter additional change theories. It would be interesting for you to compare them with Lewin's theory because most change theorists admit that they used his as the basis for developing theirs. Lewin addresses three phases of change—unfreezing, moving, and refreezing—which are based on two concepts identified as *driving* and *restraining forces.*

Driving and Restraining Forces

One of my mottos for trying to understand people instead of judging them is "There is a reason for every behavior." Accepting this statement is important in understanding the two concepts of driving and restraining forces. There is a reason for everything you do. Somewhere in your conscious or subconscious mind, you have made the decision to adopt certain behaviors at work, at home, or in social situations. Some people dress flamboyantly and others dress conservatively. Some people are conscientious about getting to work on time and others are always just a few minutes late. Our minds are so incredible that we, as people, often do not realize the work the mind goes through to determine, from the millions of possible behaviors that are available, which ones we choose to exhibit. This process is done through identifying the driving and restraining forces for exhibiting behaviors.

REFLECTIVE THINKING

Briefly describe two "change by drift" changes you have experienced. How were you affected by the change? Who else was involved, and how were they affected? Record your thinking.

Let me provide you with a very practical application of driving and restraining forces. For most North American teens, decisions are based on promoting acceptance in one's peer group. Consider the following example: You are 15 years old and have been invited to Sara Martinez's birthday party. Sara is the most popular girl at school, and boys will be at the party. You are extremely excited and can hardly wait until the night of the party arrives. Your parents are conservative and do not want you going to boy-girl parties or dating until you are 16 years old. You have been well taught throughout your upbringing to obey your parents and respect their decisions. You also have a keen conscience that says lying, especially to your parents, is wrong.

The decision you have to make is whether to go to the party. To do so, you have to lie directly or by omission to your parents and risk being caught in the lie. You love your parents and do not want to disobey or disrespect them. These are the restraining forces: the realities that tell you not to participate in the behavior you are considering. The driving forces, or the things that urge or motivate you to participate in the behavior, include your desire to have fun and be accepted by your peers and to experience the excitement of your first boy-girl party. They are powerful driving forces.

If the person making the decision is familiar with change theory, these issues are considered carefully and a decision is made. You plan either to lie to your parents or to tell your friends that you are unable to attend the party. Both of these behaviors are a change from your normal behavior. Theoretically, this decision is made with careful consideration. In actuality, young people generally do not go through such a detailed cognitive process to make social decisions. Often their decisions are made more intuitively without going through the formal decision-making process. This response is individualized in people of all ages.

The identification of the concepts of driving and restraining forces in making a decision about change is crucial for professionals who assume the tremendous responsibility of being an LPN. This is a key factor in implementing planned changes that are made by the institution, by your work team, or by you personally. If you are considering a change in any of these arenas, you should make a two-column list with driving forces in one column and restraining forces in the other. Perhaps you are trying to decide which job to take when you graduate from school. You should prepare a sheet of paper for each position you are considering, carefully listing the driving forces and the restraining forces. After you have these two lists clearly identified, information should be available for you to make the decision to stay where you are currently working or change to a new job. Not attending to this critical first step in all planned changes often results in many changes being made by drift instead of being thoroughly scrutinized.

Planned change is the most desirable form of change, and it depends on making meaningful decisions. A conscious effort to list driving and restraining forces as they relate to the change being considered provides a solid foundation for incorporating change theory.

Unfreezing

After thinking about the planned change and after the decision has been made to make a change, the first phase of change according to Lewin's change theory (1951) is unfreezing the people who are to be affected by the change. The concept of unfreezing allows people to know what is going on and what is being considered. In contrast, when people do not know what is happening and the reason for it, they strongly resist the change. Changes that are not understood or are seen as unnecessary at best "rock the boat" and at worst threaten one's sense of stability and ability to cope with the environment. Managers should not be surprised when people resist change. It is a natural response to trying to maintain the current environment. Many people think that even the unpleasant known is better than the unknown. These tendencies explain why unfreezing is the critical first phase in the actual change. An effective unfreezing assumes that driving and restraining forces have been considered, and good decisions have been made regarding the proposed change. This concept of change theory assures everyone involved that the change is being made for a good purpose.

The act of unfreezing individuals or an organization is the ability to get them to recognize that a change is needed for progress. There are two practical rules to be used in this process:

1. Do not try to implement the change until unfreezing has taken place.
2. Provide psychological safety for people involved in the change.

Rule Number One

Rule number one addresses the most common mistake made in introducing change. Perhaps the decision making, based on driving and restraining forces, has been done well. The people trying to implement the change have a clear knowledge base about the change and its many ramifications. Because they have done such a good job of research and are convinced of the merits of the change, they often forget that others who will be affected by the process do not have the same knowledge. Unfreezing means that knowledge is shared and, most important, understood. The act of unfreezing means that the people involved in the change understand the reason for the change and its process and that they accept the information and the decision to make the change as the best possible decision.

Rule Number Two

When considering the need to provide psychological safety for the people asked to make the change, it is crucial to give them enough time to understand and adapt to the change. The managers planning the change need to allot enough time for everyone to come to an understanding. To push the change without that time factor would cause psychological stress to the people involved. This stress does not help the process. Psychological safety also calls for involvement of the people who have to make the change in the decisions and planning of the process. This involvement is crucial to planning change effectively.

The problem with planned change is that it requires an undetermined period of time; it is seldom a brief period. Administrators pressure managers, managers pressure staff, and the time-consuming process of making effective change becomes a quick fix that ends up being a change by drift. Change takes time, and people need to be involved and feel psychologically safe with the process and the change itself.

Moving

After people have been unfrozen concerning the proposed change, they are ready for the second phase of change proposed by Lewin (1951)— moving. If, as a manager, you try to implement the change and you meet resistance, you need to admit that you are not through with the unfreezing process. Unfreezing is essential before implementing the change, and it may take a great deal of time.

You can tell people are ready to make the change (are unfrozen) when they appear eager to start the process, or they begin the change without you formally implementing it. Unfrozen people are eager to move, which is the actual implementation of the change. The unfreezing process leaves people feeling unbalanced or ready for something else. This unbalanced feeling is referred to by some as *hyperenergy.* This energy indicates that the person or team is ready to move ahead. This is a critical time for the manager and an opportunity that should not be missed. If the manager misses the cues of hyperenergy and does not provide the leadership necessary for the change to happen, people use the energy in other ways that often are not constructive. When the people involved in the change are ready, the manager needs to have the plan in place to accommodate their needs.

To implement the moving process, a strong sense of support is needed for the change efforts being made. Problems may occur, and mistakes may be made. The manager needs to support people in these real reactions to something new. Mistakes should not be criticized but instead used as positive learning experiences. The manager generally needs to spend more time with staff to teach and reinforce the process with which they are engaged. This is one reason for a good manager not to introduce many changes at the same time. The manager and the employees need to focus on and become good at the current change.

Other management considerations during this phase of the process include providing opportunities for success in the change for individual employees or teams of employees. Allow people to talk about their feelings so that they can vent frustration and possibly anger. Listen to these comments without reacting negatively. Express appreciation to people for the feedback and process with them the possible solutions for the problem that has been expressed. Make sure you, as the manager, are trustworthy; this keeps communication lines open and allows you to hear all the feedback about the change.

Another suggestion is to take care of yourself so that you can be an energizer for the change. You need to exhibit enthusiasm for the change and have energy to continue processing it. You can see why change is a challenge, and the skills of the manager must be well developed and focused.

Refreezing

The third and final phase of Lewin's change theory (1951) is that of *refreezing*. This is a great time in the change process because the actual change has happened. What is needed in this phase is the

During the moving stage of Kurt Lewin's change theory, it is important to give people time to examine the change and to talk about it with each other.

ability to stabilize and integrate the change so that it becomes a part of the regular work of the unit, team, hospital, or agency.

This formalization of the change requires support systems, such as policies and procedures that allow the change to be firmly embedded in the organization. It also needs teaching and clarification of the change to new employees and possible new members of the management or administrative team. The change should be evaluated periodically for effectiveness and efforts required to maintain it. These responsibilities fall to the manager of the change, or the change agent.

ROLE OF THE LICENSED PRACTICAL NURSE AS CHANGE AGENT

What is a change agent? A change agent is an individual who acts as a catalyst for change through a methodical process that includes identifying needs, planning and implementing the change, and evaluating the effectiveness of the change. You may be feeling uncomfortable with the idea that you have to assume responsibility as a change agent in your job as a nurse manager. This is the same feeling that your employees have when change is introduced to them without enough information to make their roles clear. It is a good idea for you to acknowledge the feelings you are having right now so that you can recognize them when they are expressed by the people you manage.

Most major changes come from the administration or the formal nurse manager. That person may be an LPN. Many LPNs are directors of nursing for nursing homes, the nurse manager for a unit, or a shift manager. As a new graduate, you generally are not asked to assume a major role in identifying needed changes and implementing them. Your role initially is to participate in change as introduced to you by your manager. Take that challenge and place it within the framework of the information provided here. This information gives you a method to understand the process and observe how others play out their roles and responsibilities in the process of change. It also provides you with the opportunity to learn more about the change process and its implementation. Get involved and observe, then process what you experience with your mentor or another trusted colleague. This type of active participation gives you experience in making change successfully.

As you move from a novice nurse to one with more experience, you may find changes on your unit or shift that you would like others to consider. If you are the shift manager, it is your responsibility to take your ideas and observations to your manager and to process them. If your manager agrees with what you have identified as a needed change, enlist that person's help in planning a strategy for implementing it. Ask your manager to be closely involved and perhaps mentor you through your first management adventure in the change process. By working closely with a manager, you can initiate the change you want and develop more awareness and skills during the process.

Eventually, you may be in a position in which you make the decisions regarding change for an organization larger than a unit or shift. When this happens, you can appreciate and use all the experiences you have had in making changes. You can look back at what you have done and identify the successes, the mistakes, and possibly some failures—otherwise known as learning and skill development. If you go about mastering the ability to be a change agent with a strong mentor or support person, none of the mistakes or failures should involve compromising colleagues or patients. Instead, you have the background to identify changes that need to be made and design plans for effective change. The process of making needed changes is crucial to the nursing profession.

Following are the most common mistakes made during the change process that are important for you to recognize and to avoid:

• Not using planned change process
• Not identifying clearly the driving and restraining forces
• Not allowing enough time for effective unfreezing to take place
• Not providing psychological safety for people going through the change process
• Not solidifying the change with procedural change and support

Well-planned change is crucial to the continued growth and success of the nursing profession (Box 13.1). It is important for the LPN to be a part of planned change as it occurs. The change process and its common pitfalls are pointed out to you so that knowledge and skills in change theory can be learned over time. Awareness of the

---

Box 13.1 Things to Remember When Planning a Change

1. Change takes time.
2. It is natural to resist change.
3. Consider restraining and driving forces.
4. Make sure everyone understands the reason for the change and its process.
5. Give individuals time to adapt to the change.
6. Involve individuals in the decision making and planning.
7. Support individuals going through change.
8. As manager, exhibit enthusiasm for the change.
9. Develop new policies and procedures to support the change.
10. Evaluate the change periodically.

---

process of change and its implications on self and others is crucial to caring theory practice. It also is important in placing people on a higher level of Maslow's hierarchy of needs pyramid. If people are threatened by the change, and the implementation of the change is poorly done, then people regress in their placement on the pyramid and do not contribute as much to society in general or nursing in particular. Sometimes people regress to the violent reactions referred to by Einstein. This reaction occurs because someone has not planned the change well, which is a tragedy when considering the multiple and demanding changes that face the nursing profession on a regular basis.

Evidence-Based Practice

A planned change you will be experiencing in your practice relates to the use of current evidence in patient care. *Evidence-based practice* (EBP) is a term that has become more common in nursing and assists nurses in providing the best care possible for patients. So, what is evidence-based practice? Quality and Safety Education for Nurses (QSEN) has defined EBP as integrating "best current evidence with clinical expertise and patient/family preferences and values for delivery of optimal health care" (QSEN Institute, 2014).

Much of the work we do as nurses has been developed from evidence collected and then shared. Florence Nightingale was one of the first nurse researchers. She documented information regarding conditions at the hospital in Crimea. She was able to show an improvement in patient outcomes by improving the environment. This observation led to an emphasis on the patient environment in patient care. Changes in health care have continued based on current information available. This information comes from many sources including written records, statistics, and research. These sources allow comparisons of health outcomes and lead to changes in care. Did you know that nurses no longer wear the white caps designating a registered nurse because research found the caps carried microorganisms that contributed to increased infection rates? Insulin administration is another example of evidence that changed practice. When insulin was first discovered, it was not known how much needed to be administered to those with diabetes. Patients would inject an amount that looked adequate; if they became light-headed or weak, they were given extra food. If they were urinating frequently, more insulin was injected. It was through research that dosage was standardized, checking for blood sugar levels was incorporated, and the use of multiple daily dosing was implemented. These changes have improved the lives of patients living with diabetes.

It is important as a nurse to be aware of research that could affect the patients under our care. As a manager, you will want to keep current on research and examine evidence relating to your field of employment. It is valuable to know what is dependable and valuable evidence. Certain Web sites, such as www.cdc.gov, www.nih.gov, and www.cochrane.org, are peer-reviewed, monitored, and kept up to date by governmental and professional agencies. As you review current evidence and research, it is important to examine the information critically to determine whether the information is reliable. This critical examination would involve looking at a study for its ability to be applied to other people or areas in health care, any strengths and weaknesses it may have, and its statistical or clinical significance. This examination will help you determine whether the new information would be useful in your practice area. By performing this critical examination, you will be able

to determine whether the implementation of a new policy or practice would lead to improved patient care. The new practice could also increase patient safety or the safety of the employees. It could decrease cost to the facility or improve employee satisfaction. These are benefits that would warrant a change. If a decision is made to implement a change, it would be good to review the change process at the beginning of the chapter. Remember, not everyone gets excited about change!

TRANSITIONS

Understanding transitions is an important aspect of understanding change theory. Transitions are a significant process of change that revolve around human experience and that can be developmental, situational, or organizational. Because transitions are interconnected with the evolution of the human being and the world, understanding transitions has rich significance for your personal and professional life and for nursing as a science of human caring.

A Story

A young girl watched curiously as the butterfly thrashed and jostled itself within its cocoon, desperately trying to escape its stiff confinement. The girl was moved with compassion because she sensed the exhaustion and desperation that the butterfly was experiencing. So to help the butterfly, she gently opened the cocoon, releasing the insect from its entrapment and suffering. To the little girl's dismay, the butterfly teetered on the ground and soon died. Moved to tears, the child told her mother about what had happened and asked for some explanation. "My dear," the mother said, "it is only through struggling out of the cocoon that the butterfly becomes strong enough to fly" (QualifeQuest, 1998).

Understanding Transitions

Whatever your age, you have experienced a lifetime of transitions. High school graduation, loss of a job, marriage, significant illness, death of a loved one, divorce, pregnancy, and relocation to a new state are some of the life events that you might have experienced. These events were marked by endings and beginnings and new phases of life change known as "transitions." Some of these transition events were marked with joy and celebration, and others were marked with a deep sense of loss and sadness. Whether pleasant, painful, anticipated, unexpected, temporary, or permanent, by their nature, all transitions evoke some degree of stress.

Transitions also can lead to personal renewal, growth, mastery, transformation, and a positive change in self-concept, self-esteem, and role performance. You should work toward these outcomes as you move through your LPN program.

Transition is a fundamental concept in developmental, change, stress, and adaptation theories that you will learn in your nursing program. Tyhurst has been credited with introducing the dictionary definition of *transition* into the mental health literature in 1957. He traced the term from the Latin verb *transire,* meaning "to go across," and defined *transition* as a passage or change from one place, state, or set of circumstances to another. Tyhurst studied three major life transitions: retirement, migration, and disaster. Although these are vastly different human experiences, he noted the following four features common to the transition events he studied:

1. A phase of turmoil
2. Disturbances in bodily function
3. Mood and cognition changes
4. An altered time perspective

Have you experienced these features of transition? If so, take a moment and think about them. Did you have all four features or just one or two? What was the transition that stimulated feeling these symptoms of transition? Now think about your patients. Do you recognize any of these features in the behavior you see in them? Can you think of one particular person and identify what the transition was that caused these symptoms to be exhibited? This is a good topic to discuss with your nursing and non-nursing friends or your family because everyone experiences transitions.

Transitions are processes of change that are lasting in their effects, force one to give up how one views the world and his or her place in it, and necessitate the development of new thinking and skills. It is important for you to recognize and manage the transitions in your own life because of the dramatic changes they require from you.

Transitions can be developmental (aging, adolescence), situational (divorce, illness), or organizational (downsizing or corporate restructuring).

Health-illness transitions are changes in health status, role relations, expectations, and abilities. Multiple transitions occurring simultaneously are particularly challenging and common. A health-illness transition precipitated by a severe stroke can require a person to relocate to a hospital, followed by a second or even third relocation to a nursing home. At the same time, the individual can experience a significant role transition caused by job loss and loss of a prized family role, such as "breadwinner." A basic principle you need to understand is to consider all transitions within the framework of change, then personalize them to the person who is ill.

The time span of a transition extends from the first anticipation of transition until a sense of stability in the new situation has been achieved. That can take weeks, months, or, in unsupported transitions, years. A transition is evaluated in terms of its significance or meaning to the individual's well-being. When a favorable outcome is anticipated, the situation is viewed as positive.

Because transitions necessitate new thinking and skills, they often are perceived as challenging. For example, a young man or woman thrust into parenthood often begins to view himself or herself differently from the carefree teenager of earlier times. The world of parenthood is much more complex with its many demands and responsibilities. New skills—parenting skills—have to be developed to meet the challenges effectively.

Transitions are characterized by a sense of uncertainty, disconnectedness, loss, incongruity between past expectations and present perceptions, and a lack of familiar reference points and guidelines. I am sure you experienced some of those emotions when you started school. Responses to a transition include disorientation, distress, irritability, anxiety, depression, and changes in self-esteem. Some of the characteristics of a transition that vary among individuals include duration (temporary or permanent), scope and magnitude (minor or major disruption), effects, and the extent to which the transition is anticipated and voluntary.

Observation of transitions has revealed the following questions that influence the outcomes:

1. How involved is the individual in the transition process (i.e., something like unfreezing)?
2. How extensive is the change?

3. Is the person prepared for the change?
4. What are the personal characteristics (i.e., strengths and weaknesses) of the individual experiencing the change?
5. How does the individual perceive the change (e.g., threatening, unnecessary, positive)?
6. What is the strength of the support systems for the change (e.g., family, environment, professional assistance)?

SUNSHINE ACRES LIVING CENTER

by Marilyn Krysl, RN

The first thing you see up ahead is Mr. Polanski,
    wedged in the arched doorway, like he means
    absolutely to stay there; he who shouldn't be
    there in the first place, put in here by mistake,
    courtesy of that grandson who thinks he's a
    hotshot, and too busy raking in the dough to
    take time for an old man.
If he had any place to go, you know he'd be out
    instantly, if he had any money.
So he intends to stay in that doorway, not missing
    a thing,
and waiting for trouble.
Which of course will come.
And it could be you—you're handy, you look
    likely,
you have the authority.
And you're new here, another young whipper-
    snapper, doesn't know ankle from elbow,
but has been given the keys.
Well he's ready, Polanski. So you go right to him.
Mr. Polanski, good morning—you say it in Polish,
which you learned a little of when you were little,
and your grandmother taught you a little song
    about lambs,
frisking in a pen, and you danced a silly little
    dance with your
grandmother while the two of you sang.
So you sing it for him, here in the dim, institutional
light of the hallway, light which even you find
insupportable, because at that moment it reminds
    you of the light in the hallway in the rest home
    where, when your grandmother died, you
    weren't there.
So that you're also singing to console yourself.
And at the moment you pay her this silly little tribute.
Mr. Polanski steps out of the doorway.
He who had set himself to resist you,
he who made himself a first,

Mr. Polanski, contentious often combative and al-
    ways inconsolable hears that you know the song.
And he steps out from the fortress of the doorway,
begins to shuffle and sing along. (Krysl, 1994)

This poem captures many aspects of human relationships and struggles. If you have time, discuss your insights about the poem's message with colleagues. As an LPN, you will have many opportunities to meet the Mr. Polanskis of the health-care world, to engage in a healing relationship with older adults for whom transition brings a deep sense of loneliness, powerlessness, and loss of control. You will be the healing environment for others, and they for you.

Transition Into a Licensed Practical Nurse Program

There is little question that acceptance into an LPN program brought you happiness and a deep sense of pride. It affirmed that others thought you would be successful in a challenging profession and in a rigorous nursing curriculum. At the same time you were accepted into the program, it is fairly safe to say that you experienced, to some degree, flashes of self-doubt and fear about academic performance and standards, school-related costs, fitting in with faculty and peers, disruption to your household, and changes in family roles. One change, such as entry into an LPN program, sets up a whole chain of other related changes—nothing insurmountable, but definitely changes that make your life more "complex." Forget the simple life; it is largely a myth anyway. Embrace the complexity of every day. Learn to appreciate and love it, for it is woven into the intricate fabric of your experiences.

What was the start of your transition? A gradual awakening, a deepening awareness or insight about yourself and your values, a crisis, or something else that made you realize you needed to change? These common transition beginnings led you to where you are now—in the thick of studenthood and a new phase in your life.

Transition as an In-Between Place

The short essay by Parry (1991), "Parable of the Trapeze," captures the idea of transition as an in-between place poignantly. I have shared this essay with numerous student groups who are entering and exiting a nursing program, and it metaphorically describes their experiences.

PARABLE OF THE TRAPEZE: TURNING THE FEAR OF TRANSFORMATION INTO THE TRANSFORMATION OF FEAR

Sometimes I feel that my life is a series of trapeze swings. I'm either hanging on to a trapeze bar swinging along, or for a few moments in my life I'm hurtling across space in between trapeze bars.

Most of the time, I spend my life hanging on for dear life to my trapeze-bar-of-the-moment. It carries me along at a certain steady rate of swing, and I have the feeling that I'm in control of my life. I know most of the right questions and even some of the answers.

But, every once in a while as I'm merrily (or even not so merrily) swinging along, I look out ahead of me into the distance and what do I see? I see another trapeze bar swinging toward me. It's empty and I know in that place in me that knows that this new trapeze bar has my name on it. It is my next step, my growth, my aliveness coming to get me. In my heart-of-hearts I know that, for me to grow, I must release my grip on this present, well-known bar and move to the new one.

Each time I am filled with terror. It does not matter that in all my previous hurtles across the void of unknowing I have always made it, I am each time afraid that I will miss, that I will be crushed on unseen rocks in the bottomless chasm between bars. I do it anyway. Perhaps this is the essence of what the mystics call the faith experience. No guarantees, no net, no insurance policy, but you do it anyway because somehow to keep hanging on to that old bar is no longer on the list of alternatives. So, for an eternity that can last a microsecond or a thousand lifetimes, I soar across the dark void of "the past is gone, the future is not yet here." It's called transition. I have come to believe that this transition is the only place where real change occurs. I mean real change, not the pseudo-change that only lasts until the next time my old buttons get punched.

I have noticed that in our culture this transition zone is looked upon as a "no-thing," a no-place between places. Sure, the old trapeze bar was real, and that new one coming towards me, I hope that's real too. But, the void in between? Is that just a scary, confusing, disorienting nowhere that must be gotten through as fast and as unconsciously as possible? NO! What a wasted opportunity that would be. I have a sneaking suspicion that the transition zone is the only real thing and the bars are the illusions we dream up to avoid where the real change, the real growth occurs for us. Whether or not my hunch is true, it remains that the transition zones in our lives are incredibly rich places. They should be honored, even savored. Yes, with all the pain and fear and feelings of being out of control that can (but not necessarily) accompany transitions, they're still the most alive, most growth-filled, expansive moments of our lives.

So, transformation of fear may have nothing to do with making fear go away, but rather with giving ourselves permission to "hang-on" in the transition between trapezes. Transforming our need to grab that new bar, any bar, is allowing ourselves to dwell in the only place where change really happens. It can be terrifying. It also can be enlightening in the true sense of the word. Hurtling through the void, we just may learn how to fly. (Parry, 1991)

Do you remember your first days in class and clinical areas or anticipating your first examination? Although no single examination should ever define a person's competence, the first LPN examination seems like it surely will. Students often feel threatened because of the fear that the results of early examinations will affect how an instructor views them during the rest of the program. Feeling anxious, undereating or overeating, nausea, diarrhea, disrupted sleep, and obsessing about all the possible outcomes are possible reactions. Feeling insecure is common when you leave the world of the familiar and comfortable to embrace the new and uncomfortably strange. It also is common for a person in transition to feel psychic stress, lose track of time, and feel a bit disoriented. Think for a minute about an older person entering a hospital or nursing home or having to leave a familiar home to move into a new city. Have you observed the discomfort and disorientation that accompanies those changes? If you haven't, be alert to this phenomenon in your future practice. Remember what coming into a new program and a new place felt like to you.

Facilitating Transitions

Researchers and authors offer strategies for you to give yourself the greatest advantage in experiencing helpful and healthful, satisfying transitions. These strategies are introduced here.

Let Go

Making endings during transitions often clears the way for new beginnings. Creating a new reality entails relinquishing the previous one and admitting that the old way is gone. This may mean letting go of a relationship with someone, an object, a lifestyle, experience, or what one believes to be the "self."

For students entering a nursing program, letting go of past behaviors, relationships, and attitudes is often accompanied by serious bouts of ambivalence and confusion. For example, if you are a wife, a mother, employed outside the home, an active community member, and now a new LPN student as well, major issues involving letting go are likely, especially letting go of roles. "Let go of what?" you ask. "Everything I do is important." If you cannot let go of some degree of child care and housework while you are going to school, you likely will feel debilitating fatigue, and your energy for excellent work will be depleted. It is not reasonable to think of giving up your children, your spouse, or your home responsibilities to go to school. (It is perfectly normal to entertain those thoughts for a few brief minutes, however!) It is reasonable and necessary to decide whether financial aid could help you cut down on extra employment stressors and enable you to devote more time to family or curriculum demands.

You are a nursing student entering an important profession. Maintaining a passion for nursing most likely will compete with other things you like to do. Clear decisions about priorities will not make guilt or ambivalence go away totally, but they will make the goals more realistic and achievable.

Understand Your Own Characteristic Style of Coping With Endings

In an effort to understand how you cope with ending, you may find value in "touring your life history," noting all the endings along the way. What you bring with you, to any transitional situation, is the style you have developed for dealing with endings. Endings are the first phase of transition. It is not unusual for students who begin a program of formal study to have to leave jobs, relocate to a new community, separate from family and friends, and relinquish lifestyles incompatible with serious study. Some endings are easier to make than others.

Develop New Skills

The nature of any transition is that the person experiencing it frequently feels less than totally prepared or adequate to meet its demands. The popular quip that is filled with practical wisdom simply states, "Get over it." Most of us in and out of transition realize that life always gives endless opportunities to learn new things about ourselves and whatever we're trying to do at the time. Most of us learn when we need to learn. We can learn anything if we are forced or motivated to do it. A colleague recently said to me, "Learning is hard. Knowing is fun." Give yourself time and space to try new skills, to feel less than brilliant in the learning process. You will feel better and have more fun after you know what you are doing, and that takes time and experience.

What new skills do LPN students most often need to transition successfully through the program? The following skills are mostly relational but are not as easy as they seem because of the prevalent individualistic "bootstrap" mentality that keeps us believing that we have to do it all—independently. The short list of skills includes the following:

1. *Seek out appropriate people for help,* such as financial aid directors, faculty, and family members.
2. *Use free or low-cost resources* that can change the quality of your life in school (tutoring, writing and term-paper workshops, study skills classes, reading improvement sessions, computer classes, and practice laboratories).
3. *Talk to people who know you* and whose feedback about your strengths and weaknesses, thinking, and performance is trustworthy and objective. This includes, but is not limited to, professional counselors, friends, family, and faculty.
4. *Make friends with your local or school librarians,* and visit the library often. It is not unusual for students who have been out of school for a while to feel anxious in libraries and avoid using them. With so many resources available online, the library is a great place orient yourself to the proper use of these changes. Newer library technology need not intimidate you.
5. *Plan your time.* Time management more likely will result in adequate sleep and a better balance of recreation and social activities with

study time. Try keeping a log of how you spend your day for 1 week. It could give you useful insight into where and how you spend that precious gift called time.

Develop Your Spiritual Self

Spirituality is a powerful force that propels us into a search for meaning and purpose in life. It is a different concept from that of religion. Research has shown that nurturing the spirit is a major reconciling force during transitions. For some, the nurturing aspects might include prayer, meditation, reading, yoga, discussion groups, or music. Persons who are uncomfortable with these approaches will find their own path in their spiritual journey, but all will likely find spiritual nurturance in loving relationships with others—God, a Higher Being, friends, and those who bring hope, peace, and meaning to their life. Spiritual nurturance leads to greater self-acceptance, courage, and self-appreciation. The spiritual dimensions of our lives connect us with our deepest human struggles and pain. Take time to visit yourself.

Appreciate and Create Rituals

Rituals are traditional ways every society uses to mark life transitions with their characteristic endings and beginnings. There are many rituals and ceremonies surrounding birth, death, marriage, graduation, confirmation, illness, and developmental age-related milestones, such as "sweet 16" parties and "over-the-hill" birthday parties. Some rituals are embedded in religious tradition, but all are embedded in broadly defined culture.

Rituals are rich ways of reaffirming values and one's unique cultural heritage, celebrating events of special meaning, and connecting the past and present with the future. In most nursing programs, there are unique ways that faculty and older

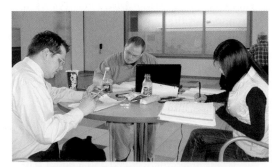

Transitions make it necessary to ask for help from others, such as a study group in mathematics.

students initiate newcomers into the program and celebrate certain program milestones. Many nursing ceremonies are rich in history, symbols, song, and readings. Be alert to the importance of ritual in your life and transitions. Help create meaningful rituals for yourself, your family, and your friends.

Whether public or private, rituals often help us cope with endings and beginnings. They are important markers in life. As an LPN student, you will learn the importance of creating healing environments in caring for patients of all ages and the role of ritual in that process. Your awareness of rituals in your own life will help you better appreciate its significance in others' lives. Talk with other students and faculty about rituals in your nursing program. It is important to create and incorporate rituals and ceremonies in various phases of your journey through the program. Using symbols, such as candles, lamps, books, joining hands, flowers, bestowing pins, and other meaningful things, is often more powerful than words in conveying meaning and significance.

Summary

The skills needed for successful transition are primarily relational: relationship building, communication, and self-awareness. Critical thinking skills involved in planning and effective problem-solving are important in your efforts to decide on what resources you need to succeed in making transitions. It takes some level of resolve and commitment to reach out for these resources.

Whether or not you are always aware of it, every decision you make has one or more values associated with it. If you truly value yourself, you will not engage in negative self-talk, abuse your mind and body with unhealthy substances, or allow yourself to get so run down that you cannot function effectively. If you value the LPN program goals and your opportunity to become a successful nurse, you will find ways to give your studies and positive relationship building high priority. Value people over things.

▊ FINAL THOUGHTS

You will likely find that exiting your program is as challenging as entering it. The LPN students in my courses talk openly about their fear of graduating; taking the National Council Licensure Examination for Practical Nurses (NCLEX®-PN); finding employment; going back to the same institution with a different credential; and, most of all, wondering whether they have the "stuff" to do the job, to handle competently and confidently the problems that arise in nursing practice. Even though the program you are in is solid and has equipped you well for practice, these fears are common. Commit yourself to lifelong learning. Avoid worrying about arriving because, in reality, you are always in process. Look for first-employment settings that have good transition programs for new employees. Health-care settings that have good transition programs frequently are committed to mentoring, supporting, and teaching new employees over weeks and months. You also need to develop relationships intentionally with more experienced nurses. Most of all, when you start your first position as an LPN, remember what you know about transitions and be patient with yourself. Practice liking who you are, with all of your vulnerabilities, strengths, and limitations. It is wise to accept the reality of change.

A question I have heard prospective students ask is, "What if I begin nursing school and find I really dislike it?" That question is relatively simple to answer: Do something else where you will find pleasure. I believe one's major should be selected on the "pleasure principle." Pick what you believe will give you the most enjoyment. What you most enjoy studying will draw your mind in the liveliest way to being educated. I hope that each of you will find true enjoyment studying nursing and in preparing yourself to be an LPN. Never be afraid to change your mind. Whatever your goal, be optimistic about your ability to change, to succeed, and to grow in new ways.

REAL-WORLD CASE STUDY

■ As a student, you probably have not had many opportunities to work with the process of planned change in nursing. After you graduate, those opportunities may be presented to you at irregular

intervals and with differing roles for responsibility. You can work on change strategies right now to assist you in developing this critical management skill. Take the answers you wrote to the two questions by Stephen Covey at the beginning of the chapter through the planned change process (Reflective Thinking, page 197).

1. How would you go about implementing the changes you wrote that would make a positive difference in your life?
   a. *The first question:* What one thing would you do regularly (something you are not doing now) that would make a meaningful, positive difference in your personal life?
   b. *The second question:* What one thing in your professional life would bring similar results?
2. Now design a plan of change for each of the preceding two questions. Each plan should include the following components:
   - Assessing the reality of the change you desire
   - Identifying a mentor
   - Listing the driving and restraining forces
   - Deciding which strategies to use to unfreeze others who may be involved or affected by the change
   - Describing how you expect the people involved in this change to behave when they are ready to move into the change
   - Determining how you can refreeze the change so that it endures
   - Deciding which strategies to use so that you can avoid the common mistakes made when implementing change

For each of the two questions, plan the implementation of the change within the framework described. You may add other ideas or material to the change process. This exercise should be thorough and meaningful to you. It is going to be time-consuming, which is the watchword of making change.

Key Points

- Change is an opportunity and an absolute in your personal and professional life. Understanding the need for change and the role it plays in our lives provides a strong foundation for success in personal and professional circumstances.

- Decisions regarding change need to be concrete and made according to a plan for change to provide success. The reason for the proposed change should be determined and decisions regarding the final outcome of the change should be made before the implementation of the change.

- Change is more effective when it is planned rather than occurring by accident. Poorly planned change often results in others being unhappy and the outcome being ineffective.

- Driving and restraining forces are concepts that influence how and why individuals make decisions the way they do. Identifying these forces in making a decision about change, whether to the institution, your work team, or personally, is crucial for professionals who assume the responsibility of being an LPN.

- Unfreezing, moving, and refreezing are the three phases of change from Kurt Lewin's change theory. Applying the phases independently of one another will not bring about positive implementation. It is important to understand that the three phases of this change theory are a process that requires time and attention to the environment within which the change is occurring.

- Being a successful change agent is the result of experiences that influence our learning and skills development.

- When considering change, such as by implementing a new policy or procedure, knowing and evaluating quality resources for evidence-based practice is paramount to your success as a nurse manager. As you review current evidence and research, it is important to examine the information critically to determine whether the information is reliable and safe for practice and patient care.

- Transition traditionally has four common features: a phase of turmoil, disturbances in bodily function, mood and cognition changes, and an altered time perspective. Transitioning into the role of a student in an LPN program is challenging. Understand up front that this is a complex time in your life. Set priorities and organize all aspects of your life to be better prepared for this new phase in your life.

- Balancing multiple roles as an LPN is a complex process, often contributing to our stress levels and challenging our coping mechanisms. Know and continue to develop coping mechanisms that work for you, including knowing and developing your spiritual self.

- Understand and create rituals that bring value to your journey through change. All individuals focus on different rituals that bring them the organization and peace they are seeking. Give yourself time to discover what yours are and you will have more joy in your journey.

ANSWERS TO REAL-WORLD CASE STUDY

The following is an example of what these answers might include, but the response to this case study will most likely be different for everyone.

1a. In my personal life, I would like to make a significant change of eating healthier on a regular basis. To go about making the daily change of eating healthy, I would make a list of healthy recipes, make a grocery list, then make a meal plan (including a calendar) to increase the chance of my being successful.

1b. In my professional life, I would like to be a more effective listener. To begin, I know I must talk less and listen more. Taking this mind-set with me into meetings will be the foundation for this change.

2a. I am extremely busy, so I know that the reality of this change is possible, but will not come easily. I will need my husband to be on board so he won't be bringing home junk food and will sit in on meal planning, so the whole family is happy with the meals. This increases the likelihood of sustaining the eating healthy vision. I need the help of my friends/family who have been successful with meal planning and eating healthy foods, so I am choosing my sister to be my mentor. I believe everyone in the family must be ready; the meals need to be planned and the shopping done prior to starting. I think it is unwise to assume we will be sugar-free, fat-free, etc., so increasing healthy foods is a good place to start. This will also help to make these a life change and not a fad diet change.

2b. Professionally, I want to improve in my leadership, and effective listening is a strong skill to have. I know it is absolutely possible. I have already spoken with my boss and a peer to give me feedback following meetings. This will allow me to immediately see areas where I could have listened instead of spoken. Specifically, I need to allow others to find their own answers and solutions to problems. In order to decrease frustration and to endure this change, I will not get frustrated with feedback or my slow progress in achieving this goal. I will remind myself that this is a process, not an immediate change. I do not feel this is an outward plan to share with others, except for those I am seeking feedback from. Knowing this is a marathon and not a sprint will keep me focused on the end goal, which is improved communication through utilizing effective listening.

REVIEW QUESTIONS

1. A nurse manager would like to employ Kurt Lewin's change theory. She knows she needs to create a plan that utilizes Lewin's theory in the correct order. Which of the following reflects Lewin's phases of change applied in the correct order?
   1. Unfreezing, moving, refreezing
   2. Unfreezing, driving, restraining forces
   3. Moving, unfreezing, refreezing
   4. Driving, restraining forces, unfreezing

2. An LPN working on the floor comes across two other employees who are complaining about their recent schedules. In order to be an effective change agent, the LPN's best response would be which of the following?
   1. When speaking with the employees she states, "Just call in sick for the shifts you don't want to work."
   2. Joining in the conversations, she states, "My schedule has a lot of problems with it too."
   3. Rather than speaking with the employees, she goes to the nurse manager and says, "Jody and Marsha are always complaining about the schedule."
   4. As she approaches the employees, she engages them in a conversation and states, "If you had the opportunity to make changes to the schedule, what would they be?"

3. The LPN is concerned about his facility's current policy on wound-dressing changes. Which of the following are appropriate resources to verify workplace policies are congruent with evidence-based practice guidelines? Select all that apply.
   1. www.cdc.gov
   2. www.nih.gov
   3. www.Wikipedia.com
   4. www.WebMD.com
   5. www.Cochrane.org

4. The LPN student is struggling with balancing his personal life with the demands of nursing school. Which of the following skills will be least likely to help him through this transition process?
   1. Plan your time.
   2. Seek out appropriate supportive resources.
   3. Just get over it and keep pushing forward.
   4. Seek out a faculty mentor.

5. The reason change can be distressing to individuals is that they function more often in the change-by-drift process than in planning for change.
   1. True
   2. False

References

Covey, S. (2013). *The 7 habits of highly effective people: Powerful lessons in personal change.* New York: Simon & Schuster.

Krysl, M. (1994). Sunshine acres living center. Dreamcatcher's Workshop. Denver, CO: University of Colorado Health Sciences Center.

Lewin, K. (1951). *Field theory in social science.* New York: Harper & Row.

Parry, D. (1991). Parable of the trapeze. In *Warriors of the heart*. Bainbridge Island, WA: Earthstewards Network.

QSEN Institute. (2014). Knowledge, skills, and attitudes (KSAs): Evidence-based practice. (Current definition) Retrieved from http://qsen.org/competencies/pre-licensure-ksas/

QualifeQuest. (1998). Denver, CO: QuaLife.

Tyhurst, J. S. (1957). The role of transition states-including disasters-in mental illness. In R. Keith Cannon (Chair), *Symposium on Preventive and Social Psychiatry.* Symposium conducted at the meeting of Walter Reed Army Institute of Research. (pp. 149–172). Retrieved from https://books.google.com/books?hl=en&lr=&id=YFArAAAAYAAJ&oi=fnd&pg=PA149&dq=The+Role+of+Transition+States+-+Including+Disasters+-+in+Mental+Illness&ots=pDSFtX7iM7&sig=zcUASoG85Z1XsoMTqqfvqzRKoy0#v=onepage&q=The%20Role%20of%20Transition%20States%20-%20Including%20Disasters%20-%20in%20Mental%20Illness&f=false

Web Resources

Nursing Theories: Lewin's Change Theory www.nursing-theory.org/theories-and-models/Lewin-Change-Theory.php

Transition www.wmbridges.com

14

Setting Meaningful Priorities

KEY TERMS

Decision making
Decision-making process
Personal mission statement
Personal value statement
Prioritization

CHAPTER CONCEPT

Critical Thinking

LEARNING OUTCOMES

1. Discuss the process of setting personal priorities.
2. Demonstrate how to write a personal values statement and a personal mission statement.
3. Discuss the importance of using Maslow's hierarchy and Watson's theory for sctting priorities.
4. Demonstrate the use of a decision-making process.

Priority setting is not for the weak or timid.

—Author Unknown

Can you imagine the leader of this country setting a political priority as "ice cream in every home" as opposed to the protection of U.S. borders? Or a teacher setting the priority for her class as "two-thirds of the members will receive an 'F' grade" instead of working toward achieving maximum learning for each student? I am certain these priorities are of concern to you! The purpose of this chapter is to assist you in being able to set meaningful priorities in both your personal and professional lives. When several serious concerns are being thrust at you to sort out and prioritize, you need to be able to make decisions quickly to be an effective nursing leader.

It has been said that you can take a horse to water but you can't make it drink. That is true for people who need to set priorities but are hesitant to do so. As a manager, you need to coach and teach the people you manage the importance of priority setting.

SETTING PERSONAL PRIORITIES

Let us take some time to examine setting personal priorities. This is something you do every day. Setting priorities, also known as *prioritization,* is the process of designating something more important or determining the order in which to deal with a task. Do you remember the two types of change discussed in Chapter 13? They were "planned change" and "change by drift." Change by drift, the less desirable of the two types of changes, occurs when you are unclear about your priorities. I am assuming that your current priority is to complete school successfully. That is a planned change. It is clear what your priority is because you have planned it. You work hard to achieve this priority, and you sacrifice much.

You may have set other priorities as well—to improve your health, develop more patience, learn to tango, or run a marathon. Will any of these things happen "by drift"? It is doubtful. Each concept suggested is challenging and requires focus and effort to achieve. Yes, it must be a priority!

How do you set your priorities? First, you use your personal value system to determine what is of value to you. Personal values are determined by your cultural, social, and philosophical background. Then you plan activities that fulfill your personal values. You also might have a "type" of mission statement that runs through your family. For me, it was a strong work ethic. This mission statement developed because of my hard-working

Danish ancestors. They passed on the concept of "hard work reaps its own reward" to their children and descendants because hard work is what kept them fed and together.

When you consciously put your personal values and your mission statement together, you have a clear road map to follow in terms of setting your priorities. So what are they? Can you identify what has meaning for you? What is worthy of being a priority for you?

REFLECTIVE THINKING

If you have not written your personal values statement, now is a good time to do it. It is important for you to be clear about what is of value to you. Your values statement could be a sentence, a paragraph, or longer. If you spend time pondering it and actually take the time to write it, you will be further ahead in life than many other people. Persons without clear values become confused when major decisions need to be made quickly. They flounder in their lives and do not achieve their most pressing desires.

Write your personal values statement and share it with someone important to you. Such personal statements are often not to be shared with the general public. However, if you feel that you can share yours, come to class prepared to do so. It may be helpful to someone who is struggling to write his or her own.

My personal values statement comes from what I was taught by my parents. Your values statement might be based on your religious or cultural beliefs. Mine is: "I believe in being honest, true, benevolent, and doing good to all people." With this values statement, I am clear about where I set my personal priorities. There is no confusion, no wondering what to do, no stress.

My mission statement is simple. It is influenced by my hard-working ancestors, but what it says is my own purpose in life. It is: "I will be a loving mother and wife, an effective teacher, and a benevolent person throughout my life."

REFLECTIVE THINKING

All health-care facilities and academic institutions have mission statements. Do you know the mission statement for your school? It would be interesting to see what it is. More important, however, is for you to identify your own personal mission statement. What are you about? What is it you want your life to mean? Now take the time necessary to identify your personal mission statement. What do you really want to achieve in life? What are your foundational concepts for living? Ponder this assignment and record it. Again, this may be too personal to share in class, but you should share it with someone. That makes it more real.

With this statement clearly stated early, I have been able to achieve all three "missions." Whenever I had a hard decision to make, these are the three things that influenced what I did. I am hopeful you will seriously consider writing your mission statement for life (realize it may change as you progress through life) and use it whenever you need help in focusing your personal energy.

If you have sincerely completed both Reflective Thinking assignments, you are ready to move forward with the information in this chapter on setting priorities. It is important that you identify your own priorities before you take on the priorities of the clinical world.

APPLICATION OF MASLOW'S AND WATSON'S THEORIES

At this point in the book, you know a great deal about the theories of Maslow and Watson. They are respected examples of a framework for setting

meaningful priorities. What do I mean when I say that? It is simply to think of every situation according to Maslow's hierarchy of needs. Who is involved in the priority setting, and where are they on the hierarchy? Then stop and consider whether you are making a decision that is based on the caring framework of Watson. If you learn to allow these two ways of thinking to guide your priority setting, you will be successful at setting meaningful priorities.

There is a priority in nursing that should never be ignored: The most ill person gets the most immediate treatment, in other words, that person is the priority. This is the thinking for triage in an emergency situation. People are assessed and tagged and then receive treatment according to the criticality of their needs. Treating the most critical person first is a sovereign rule in nursing. This may seem clear and easy to understand; however, because nurses are human, things can become confusing. Another way to determine priorities is by considering the urgency of the priority. Is the activity urgent and important or important but not urgent? See Table 14.1.

Here is a possible scenario:

You are one of two team leaders on the evening shift of a small surgical unit. The other team leader is a registered nurse (RN) with years of experience. You have worked on the unit for 3 months. You have a new postoperative patient who is complaining of severe pain and whose color is pale. You have checked his dressing, which is dry. His vital signs are normal except for a slightly elevated pulse (92 bpm). He is diaphoretic, and he has not responded to the pain medication you gave him 30 minutes ago (intramuscular [IM] injection).

You go to find the RN so she can assist you in assessing the problem. She left the floor for her evening meal and will not be back for 30 minutes. Because it is evening, the unit is full of visitors and patients walking in the halls or sitting and talking. As you are processing what to do for the patient, a physician comes on the unit and demands your help. He has a list of equipment he wants "now" and then demands assistance in doing a procedure on his patient. His patient is 3 days postoperative and will be discharged the next day. You are the only licensed nurse on the floor and have to decide what to do.

His demands for equipment and assistance are usually done by preordering the equipment and doing the procedure on the day shift when there are more licensed personnel on the unit. In addition, you realize his patient cannot be discharged as planned without the procedure being completed. How do you prioritize what to do next?

You are weighing a potentially critical patient against a patient ready to be discharged. The decision should be easy. However, it isn't, is it? According to Maslow's hierarchy, you would like to maintain your dignity by not having a conflict with the physician, particularly in front of the audience of patients and family members. You realize the physician may become angry with you for not meeting his needs immediately. For some people, that would be reason enough to do as he demands and leave your new postoperative patient for another 20 to 30 minutes. How would you choose your priority? What is urgent and important? What is important but not urgent? Neither the physician nor his patient is in danger; therefore, your responsibility is to the new postoperative patient. This is basic Maslow's hierarchy thinking and something you should be able to do without hesitation. Now that the decision is made, how will you manage meeting that priority within Watson's framework of caring? There are several things you can do, but any or all of them should be done quickly so you can focus on your most ill patient.

TABLE 14.1 EXAMPLES OF URGENT AND IMPORTANT TASKS

Urgent and Important	Important But Not Urgent
• Patient with changing vital signs	• Staff training on a new piece of equipment
• Teaching a patient how to administer insulin	• Teaching a patient about preventive care
• Not enough staff for the next shift	• Preparing a budget report that is not due for 6 weeks
• Project with an immediate deadline	

REFLECTIVE THINKING

Make a list in your class notebook of a minimum of five things you could do to manage this priority-setting situation. Come prepared to bring them to class to discuss with your classmates. I think you will be interested in how each person would resolve this problem.

The following is a list of what I would do:

1. Contact two certified nursing assistants (CNAs). Send one to the cafeteria to ask the RN to return to the floor and meet you in your patient's room. The second CNA should go to clean holding and get the equipment the physician wants.
2. Explain to the physician that you have a potentially critical patient, and you need to contact his physician immediately. Whatever his reaction (anger or concern), you need to let him know you have done all you can do for him at the moment. You may want to use the Two-Challenge Rule mentioned in Chapter 11.
3. Call the new postoperative patient's physician and using the SBAR technique (situation, background assessment, recommendation) explain your assessment and concerns. Be factual; do not let the stress of the physician with the procedure deflect your attention from what you need to share with your patient's physician.
4. Go to the ill patient's room and do whatever the physician asked you to do or stay with the patient and be reassuring until the RN returns from dinner.
5. When the RN returns, give her report in a "succinct manner and ask her to assume responsibility for the ill patient (that is appropriate because of her years of experience and licensure).
6. Go assist the other physician. You can easily do that because the equipment is now in the room.
7. Be careful to speak to everyone involved in this scenario with respect and caring.
8. When the situations are resolved, sit down with the RN and determine how to handle this type of priority setting in the future. Ask her questions and clarify anything that was difficult for you.

Whew! That took effort, skill, and knowledge application, didn't it? With the new roles being given to licensed practical nurses (LPNs), it is essential that you develop the ability to set priorities and meet them, whatever the challenge.

Let us consider something that is not so complicated. You are the team leader in a long-term care facility. It is lunchtime, and you have a heavy noon medication pass. You know that legally and ethically medications need to be administered to residents within 30 minutes of the time they are scheduled. Your cart is ready and you are moving down the hall toward the lunchroom when someone taps you on the shoulder. It is the daughter of one of the residents who is terminal. She is crying and asks to talk to you. Previously you have been very supportive of her and have assisted her with the grieving process. What is the priority? Do you pass the medications or talk to the grieving daughter?

Passing the medications is both ethically and legally correct. It also meets the physiological needs of the residents according to Maslow's theory. This definitely is a priority. The grieving daughter is in need of attention that is caring (Watson) because emotionally she cannot move up Maslow's pyramid until she works through her grief. Her needs are a priority as well. What decision do you make and how do you make it? Ponder this dilemma and make some notes regarding what you will do. My first question is, Did you learn from the last case study? In that situation the LPN used others to get the help she needed for the patients. She asked the two CNAs to get the RN and the equipment for the physician; she asked the RN to manage the care of the ill patient while she assisted the physician. What you need to learn from this is that others should be used for the good of the residents in this and most cases. You do not have to do everything alone. Health care should be the best example of teamwork there is because of the impact it makes on the lives of others.

PRIORITY SETTING IN THE CLINICAL ARENA REQUIRES TEAMWORK

You can often set your personal priorities by yourself. You may intermittently need the assistance of others, but, as an adult, you can set and meet many of your priorities independently. That generally is not true when dealing with other human beings.

Here is what I would do to manage the last case study, but remember to value your own thinking if your solution is not the same as mine. Consider the solutions of your classmates and take the best from others' thinking to add to your own.

1. I would secure the medication cart and take the daughter to a private place to talk to her briefly. I would listen to her immediate concerns and then . . .
2. I would ask her whether the social worker or charge nurse or whoever is appropriate in your setting (most nursing homes have a social worker on duty) could talk to her about her concerns and feelings. Then . . .
3. I would pass the medications. I hope I started early to pass them (say, 11:30 a.m.) so this interruption wouldn't put me off more than 15 minutes, and I would have until 12:30 p.m. to finish the medication pass.
4. I also would remember the rule of delegation. Once I am sure the person I am delegating to has the skill level to handle the problem, I would let him handle it. Let the social worker do her job in assisting the daughter. This does not mean you do not take an interest or demonstrate caring behavior, but you do not take back what you have delegated to someone else.

Here is another priority-setting problem for you to consider. Once, when I involved students in gathering data for a research project, an interesting priority-setting dilemma occurred. The students were shadowing licensed nurses on the intensive care unit (ICU). The nurses did not know why the students were there. The responsibility of the students was to observe when and how often the nurses performed hand hygiene and whether the hand hygiene was appropriate. I was shocked to learn that some nurses did *not* perform hand hygiene as was appropriate. One wore the same pair of gloves all morning and did not change them until lunchtime. She washed her gloves while they were on her hands throughout the morning, but not between each patient contact, and she never changed gloves! Another person simply did not take the time to wash her hands unless she got something messy on them (that happens frequently in an ICU); she never wore gloves. There were other infractions of the hand hygiene rules we readily accept as nurses, but these were the two worst.

Herein lies the dilemma. The students shadowing these two nurses worked in the same hospital. They did not want to report what they observed for fear of being a "tattletale" about it. The students discussed with each other the possibility of altering the data. That would have been a very serious infraction of research ethics. They decided to give me the correct data but talked to me about their concerns.

Here is the second aspect of the dilemma. When doing research, the participants (in this case, the nurses who were inappropriate in performing hand hygiene) sign an informed consent form. In this form, both information and assurances are given to the research participant. One of the assurances is the statement that the results of the research will not be identified by individuals but instead as a group. It also says that the participant's behavior will not be reported to his or her supervisor.

In summary, there were two nurses who were very inappropriate in their hand hygiene technique. They were endangering their patients and possibly each other (I am sure they were spreading bacteria). The students met their priority of being ethical when they submitted to me the correct research data. Now, what was I to do? I could not report the individuals to their nurse manager without breaking the dictates of the informed consent form, a legal document. But how could I live within the framework of my mission statement, or Watson's theory of caring (protecting the patients), or recognizing that there is a "reason for every behavior" and try to understand the behavior of the nurses according to Maslow's hierarchy of needs theory?

What would you do? Let the potentially lethal situation go unattended or intervene in it? The answer to the dilemma did not come to me easily. I had the priority of protecting all patients from anything that may endanger them. I also had as a priority to conduct ethical research, which meant not breaking the statements in the informed consent form. What did I do? I met both of my priorities by meeting individually with each nurse. I carefully explained that the students did what was ethical by honestly reporting the data. I also clarified that I would be keeping the contract made in the informed consent form; however, I wanted to discuss their behavior with them. One nurse became very angry with me and told me that it was none of my business how she delivered nursing care and left my office upset. The second nurse was apologetic and said she had no excuse except that it always is so busy on the ICU. We often see each other, and I have never mentioned it again.

My approach to the two nurses was kind and professional. I did not make accusations but simply told them what had been reported through the research data. I was not judgmental or critical, simply honest. In that way, I was trying to establish my solution on both Watson's and Maslow's theories and make it clear that the patient's safety was my priority. Do you think it worked? What could I have done that would have been more effective? Talk about this with your colleagues and fellow students in order to have the advantage of other people's thinking. It should be interesting.

NEED FOR PRIORITY SETTING

If you know the mission statement and values of your place of employment, you are better able to fulfill successfully the requirements of your job. The ability of a nurse to set priorities is of monumental importance in health-care facilities. YOU are the patient advocate; YOU are the 24-hour caregiver; YOU are the one to make decisions that determine life or death, permanent damage, or prevention of permanent damage. YOU are the linchpin that ties the entire picture of health care together.

The one constant in today's health-care system is that tomorrow it will change. Tim Porter-O'-Grady, a nursing futurist (someone who makes his living as a predictor of what will happen in the future for nurses), challenges nursing leaders and managers to be prepared for the changes that will come. This means working with the changing priorities of your organization and being able to change your own priorities if you can personally accept them. For example, I could not work in a long-term care facility that pursued active euthanasia. It does not fit in with my personal values, and I would have to seek another job immediately.

You, as a leader, will have to be a lifelong learner and share your new knowledge and skills with your staff. You need to continue to use "best evidence-based practice," as mentioned in Chapter 13. You need to keep your personal values system and mission statement representative of the new things you learn. Then your big responsibility is to role model them to your staff and provide an environment for healing that is best for sick patients. There are problems in health-care delivery, and you are the most qualified person to intervene clinically. The nurse is the "watchdog" for each patient.

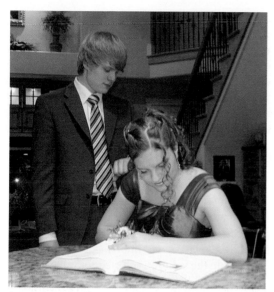

This student LPN has a date to the college prom, but she did not study for her final in medical-surgical nursing. It seems that she forgot the importance of priority setting.

The third primary cause of death in the United States is now attributed to medical errors (Boerner, 2016). The nurse is the person who can assist in prevention of such errors because nurses are there "24/7" to monitor and advocate for the people in their care. You double-check medications and treatments; you observe and assess; and you, as a nursing leader, manage the people responsible for the care.

With downsizing and other efforts at fiscal management, in addition to the nursing shortage, some health-care facilities have fewer licensed nurses on staff. However, recent research has confirmed what nurses intuitively knew: fewer nurses translate into poorer care for patients. Studies have shown that the number of nurses available to provide care has a direct effect on patient outcomes of care (Twigg, Gelder, & Myers, 2015). Your role as caregiver and manager of the care given is critical. The ability to set priorities in your daily position as a decision maker is a powerful tool in protecting the vulnerable people for whom you are responsible.

A simple example of this has to do with medication administration. You have a new order for a medication with which you are unfamiliar. Once again, you are in a rush to give the medications in a timely manner. The new one is just that, absolutely new to you. You are inclined to stay on your time schedule and give the medication without looking it up. After all, the physician ordered it, the pharmacist filled the prescription, and your job is to give it, right? *No,* that is not correct. Your job is to know what the medication is and how to administer it properly as well as to be aware of the side effects that may occur. What do you do?

Your priority is to take the time to read about the medication and be sure it is correct in every aspect. Just guessing or trusting other professionals does not eliminate you from error if your lack of knowledge negatively impacts the patient. Trying to be too quick or too efficient at the sacrifice of attention to detail is very risky for patients who are in your care.

IT STARTS WITH THE ABILITY TO MAKE GOOD DECISIONS

Setting effective clinical priorities begins with the ability to make good decisions. Decision making is a cognitive process used to select a course of action. With the amount of decisions human beings make every day, one would think we were good at doing it! But there is room for improvement for most of us because the demands of making good decisions, when you are dealing with another person's life, are complex. Most people function better when they have a system for making decisions. Some people think that decision making comes naturally, like breathing, but it doesn't. To be a good decision maker, one must be creative, flexible, and willing to take risks. Others think that, with practice, good decisions come automatically. That is not true either. Good decisions, which allow for effective priority setting, require a planned way for thinking and then doing.

There are three basic considerations for decision making:

• First: the decision that can be made based on laws, policy and procedure mandates or decisions for a common problem
• Second: the decision you make in an emergency based on your knowledge
• Third: the decision you have time to process before making it

Identifying your decision in one of these three basic categories will assist you in making the right type of decision at the right time.

REFLECTIVE THINKING

Describe a good decision you made in your life. What process did you use to make the decision? Do you consider yourself a good decision maker? Why or why not?

Making decisions regarding common problems is not as stressful as decisions made under uncertainty and risk. Common problems are just that, common. One example is a medication error. For this common problem, there are procedures and a process to follow. You know that the priority is to notify the physician, carry out any procedures necessary to counteract the impact of the wrong medication, and complete an incident report. Priority setting is not difficult when there are procedures established for managing the situation.

When the decision-making situation is clouded with uncertainty and risk, the challenge is much more difficult. This occurs when the individual or group making the decision does not know all of the attendant risks, alternatives, or consequences of each possible decision. Uncertainty and risk rank high in the complexity of modern health care. Successful decisions and subsequent priority setting depend on the judgment of the person making the decision. That person is you!

Your ability to make meaningful decisions depends on your knowledge base. There is a powerful reason for you to pay attention in class and learn all you can. Be an inquisitive learner who asks questions, reads beyond the assignment, and goes the extra mile to establish a strong knowledge base for clinical practice. Often when a critical decision needs to be made, you have to make it in the moment and there is not the opportunity to review a textbook or ask another nurse his or her opinion. There are some things you simply need to know. Some of these things are policy and procedure of the place where you work as well as laws that impact patient care. You also need a broad knowledge base regarding the care of people who are ill and seeking your services. You need to know how to communicate and process ideas and how to set priorities based on your personal values and mission statement as well as that of the place where you work. When you can do that, you are ready for a leadership or management position.

Not all decisions are made in an urgent or emergency situation, and they all are not made according to policy and procedures that are already established. Often, you will be asked to make decisions and will have time to process the decision you make. When that happens, I suggest you use a modified version of the nursing process. Steps to consider include the following:

1. Define the problem.
2. Determine the most desirable outcome.
3. Research for solutions to the problem that will result in the desirable outcome.
4. Evaluate the alternative solutions for the most effective one.
5. Select a solution and implement it.
6. Evaluate the solution selected for effectiveness.

Using this thinking process will allow you to be thorough in the decision-making process. You will be able to consider all reasonable possibilities and decide on the most viable one.

REFLECTIVE THINKING

Think of a clinical situation you experienced during a clinical rotation when a decision was made. Compare the process you and others used to make the decision with the six-step process listed here. How did the process compare?

Suppose you have a patient with a total knee replacement who simply will not ambulate when the physical therapist goes in to assist him. This man is older and he worked as a farmer and rancher. He obviously is accustomed to being in charge of his life and that of his family, farm and ranch hands, and others. If he doesn't ambulate, he will not develop the range of motion and strength he needs to return to his very busy life.

I am going to use the steps in decision making that will lead me to what I hope will be good priority setting. This is an example of a nonurgent and non–policy-regulated decision.

1. The problem is that this previously active man will not recover from his total knee replacement if he does not do his physical therapy. However, being a nurse who believes in transpersonal caring, I realize there is another problem as well. I "think" it is that he does not like being told what to do, and he does not like to do things on another person's schedule.

This man is very accustomed to regulating his own life.

2. The most desirable outcome is that he regains full use of his artificial joint and returns to his previous lifestyle. This will *not* happen unless he does his therapy.

3. What possible solutions are there? First, recognize that he is accustomed to being in charge, and let him be in charge of all that is reasonable. Next, find an approach to therapy that involves him and his desire to be in charge; give him as much autonomy as possible. Solutions that you know will not work are ordering him or pressuring him to do therapy.

4. I see autonomy as the only possible solution. Along with that is a need for gentle education (information that does not sound bossy or dictatorial).

5. My solution is to make an appointment with him, at a time that he indicates as convenient, and talk to him about his therapy. I will ask him for his desired outcome and simply move from there. I will ask him to set a therapy schedule that will work for him. I will ask whether there is a therapist whom he prefers and arrange for him or her to provide services. I will coordinate his pain medication with his therapy appointments so he will be comfortable while exercising. I will determine whether there are other areas of his recovery in which he needs to determine how or when things should be done.

6. I should know right away if my plan is working because he will be doing or not doing his therapy. I hope he will realize that I respect him by asking his opinion and will be more cooperative. By understanding his objective of the surgery, I hope I also will have identified his motivation. This approach will achieve the priority, which is to send him home with the best possible surgical outcome.

The reason decision making is even discussed is so that you can be the type of nursing leader who can recognize and can meet the priorities of the clinical world.

CONCLUSION

Being able to set and meet priorities in the clinical arena of nursing is critical to being an effective nurse and manager. To be effective in the decision-making role, you need to be clear about your personal values and mission statements as well as those of the facility where you work. The presence of LPNs has been proven to make a difference in the recovery of patients in various settings. Much of that success is based on the ability to make effective decisions that lead to priorities being met. Best wishes with this new challenge. It represents one of the higher level skills in our profession.

REAL-WORLD CASE STUDY

Part A

■ You are taking your leadership and management course and have been assigned to an acute pediatric unit for your clinical experiences. You are very excited because your unit is part of the medical center and you are sure you will see things that otherwise you would not be able to observe.

Your clinical instructor, Dr. Arid, has leadership students on several units, so you don't have her with you all of the time. Instead, she makes continuous rounds and has been very helpful. You are assigned to shadow one of the team leaders, Miss Belay. During report today, you heard about a 6-year-old boy who was on the unit with terminal cancer. His case is unique, and the physicians and medical residents are interested in his process of dying because it will indicate the course of the unusual cancer.

The boy, James, is assigned to your team. When you and your nurse make rounds, you go to James's room last. You wondered why, because you had been taught that the most critical patient should be seen first. However, you are new and a student, so you follow your team leader without question. When you visit James, you are shocked at what you see. The room is larger than most of the rooms, and it is filled with people. There are physicians and residents, pain management personnel, and an EKG tech as well as people you don't recognize. You also see a couple in their 30s holding each other and crying. People are lined around the walls of the room whispering. No one is next to James, and no one is interacting with the parents. Not even your nurse goes over to James or the people you assume to be his parents. You are uncomfortable with what you see and most important with what you don't see.

What are the things you see and feel that are of concern to you? Make a list of possible concerns.

Continued

Part B

■ Your nurse indicates to you that she wants to stay for a while and see what happens. Obviously you need to stay with her. You are uncomfortable but don't know what else to do, so you stay. Within minutes your instructor comes into the room to find you. As she looks around the room you can see, reflected in her face, what you are feeling. Your instructor walks to the middle of the room and says your name. "Ms. Miller, will you please come here?" Everyone looks at her as though she is an intruder. You and your instructor walk to the little boy, who is conscious. She kneels down and gently speaks to him. When she is through, she says loudly enough for everyone to hear, "I expect you to stay this close to him throughout your shift." Then she turns to two medical residents and says, "I need three chairs put here at the bedside. Please retrieve them for me." The residents are surprised at being involved but quickly go out to get the chairs. Her next act was to walk to the parents and talk to them. The mother started crying harder and hugged the instructor. Then they went quietly over to James and kneeled by him until the chairs came.

At about that time, the primary physician, Dr. Carillo, walked toward your instructor, and they go out in the hall to converse. You don't know what was said, but Dr. Carillo returned to the room and asked several of the people to leave. You stay with young James and his parents until his death 3 hours later. During that time your instructor stepped into the room several times to see whether she was needed.

What priorities were met through the behavior of the nursing instructor?

This case study is a real situation. Think through it thoroughly before you answer the questions.

Key Points

- Identifying your values and personal mission in life will assist you in making difficult decisions, both personal and professional. Your mission gives you a foundation for basing your decisions.
- When prioritizing, it is helpful to determine the urgency and importance of the situation. One way to determine priorities is by considering the urgency of the priority. Consider whether the activity is urgent and important or important but not urgent.
- Maslow's and Watson's theories are good examples of a framework that can be used for setting meaningful priorities. This framework reminds managers to keep other individuals' needs in mind and to make caring decisions.
- Knowing the values and mission of a healthcare facility can help you with setting professional priorities.

- Setting effective clinical priorities begins with the ability to make good decisions. When time allows, using a standard process for decision making will assure a better decision.
- There are three basic considerations for decision making: whether the decision can be based on organizational policies and procedures, the amount of time available to make the decision, and whether it is an emergent situation and the decision needs to be made quickly.
- When setting priorities in a clinical setting nurses not only need to work within their own personal mission statement but also need to consider the thoughts and ideas of patients and coworkers. Maintaining patient safety is a major factor when setting priorities.

ANSWERS TO REAL-WORLD CASE STUDY

■ *Part A*

1. Even though the room is filled with knowledgeable people, James is dying alone.
2. No one is acknowledging the grief of the parents. Again, even though the room is filled with people, the parents seem isolated.
3. Death should be a private experience, not a medical "side show."
4. Why didn't you and your nurse visit James first since he is the person under your care who is most likely to die during your shift?

Your list may be different from mine. Be sure to value your own thinking. This is definitely an exercise in critical thinking.

■ *Part B*

1. Although the situation seemed wrong to you, and you felt it seemed that way for your instructor, no one became angry. Your instructor did not criticize anyone or blame anyone (Watson).

2. The instructor was able to recognize quickly that, according to her personal values system and both Maslow's and Watson's theories, the patient's and family's needs were not being met.
3. She addressed James's need not to die alone and scared by inviting his parents to be next to him (Maslow).
4. She addressed the parents' need to be with their son while he died by first, recognizing them and, second, inviting them to be directly with their son (Maslow).
5. Although you sensed she disapproved of the situation, your instructor did not express her disappointment, frustration, or whatever else she was feeling to anyone, especially you (Watson).
6. The instructor role modeled proactive priority setting by making meaningful decisions regarding your learning and the right of James and his family to personal, holistic care.

Again, value your interpretation of this situation. It involved risk taking for the instructor but benefited those who needed care.

REVIEW QUESTIONS

1. The LPN is starting her first job with the hospice agency. She knows she may have to make decisions in difficult situations. Which statement best describes the first thing she can do to help her with the decision-making process?
   1. Write her personal value and mission statements.
   2. Ask other nurses how they approach decision making.
   3. Read several articles about the process of decision making.
   4. Do nothing and just wait until a decision needs to be made and hope she makes the best decision.

2. The LPN is taking care of a patient with diabetes. She has several things she needs to teach the patient. Which item should she address first?
   1. Managing a diabetic diet
   2. Giving insulin
   3. Monitoring carbohydrates
   4. Preventative foot care

3. When making decisions, the LPN likes to keep in mind everyone's self-worth. This is an example of using Maslow's hierarchy of needs as a framework for decisions.
   1. True
   2. False

Continued

REVIEW QUESTIONS *continued*

4. Which of the following are steps in a decision making process? (Select all that apply.)
   1. Determine a desirable outcome.
   2. Evaluate alternative solutions.
   3. Implement a solution.
   4. Evaluate if the solution was effective.

5. Which is the best description of someone who is a good decision maker?
   1. Well liked by coworkers
   2. Competent in her or his job
   3. Willing to take risks
   4. Has several years of experience

References

Boerner, H. (2016). Eliminating harm: How hospital systems are working to reduce medical errors. *Physician Leadership Journal, 3*(2), 30–32.

Twigg, D. E., Gelder, L., & Myers, H. (2015). The impact of understaffed shifts on nurse-sensitive outcomes. *Journal of Advanced Nursing, 71*(7), 1564–1572. doi:10.1111/jan.12616

Web Resources

Decision Making Quiz www.mindtools.com/pages/article/newTED_79.htm

15

Handling Conflict in the Nursing Profession

MELISSA NEVILLE

KEY TERMS

Conflict
Conflict management
Conflict resolution
Distancing
Interprofessional
Patient-centered care
Workplace violence

CHAPTER CONCEPTS

Leadership and Management
Collaboration
Communication
Evidence-Based Practice

LEARNING OUTCOMES

1. Identify the causes of conflict.
2. Summarize communication approaches that can create or enhance conflict.
3. Develop an increased awareness of personal conflict styles.
4. Address communication approaches that can promote conflict resolution.
5. Examine workplace violence in the health-care setting.
6. Describe why conflict can be positive to an organization.

Difficulties are meant to rouse, not discourage.
The human spirit is to grow strong by conflict.

—William Ellery Channing

There are many definitions of conflict. For this chapter, conflict will be defined as real or perceived differences between individuals with differing values, ideas, or goals. Conflict is common in any workplace, and nursing studies have shown it is significant in nursing and that it is a source of job stress and dissatisfaction (Weiss & Tappen, 2015). Two concepts regarding conflict that are important for you to remember: (1) Conflict is inevitable and (2) the results can be constructive if there is resolution of the conflict before it escalates to unmanageable proportions.

Conflict is present in all aspects of life and in all organizations. Because of the complexity and the interactions among the people who work in the health-care setting, conflict will arise. In any organization, nurses encounter varying degrees of conflict, but if handled appropriately, these events can lead to the reordering of priorities and development of a positive resolution. While the presence of conflict can mean that a negative situation exists, it can also provide the opportunity to evaluate organizational processes and reform them. If viewed as a constructive process aimed at transformation, conflict can be a seen as positive motivator for change. To encourage transformation and permanent change, it is important for individuals to see beyond the current cause of the conflict and go a step further by assessing blocks to communication, group dynamics, and the psychosocial climate. It is essential that all managers welcome conflict as a vital force to the organization and develop the ability to keep it from becoming unmanageable.

Poorly managed conflict can create distance and distrust among employees and lead to decreased productivity or less attention to the quality indicators of patient care. In contrast, well-managed conflict can stimulate cooperation, identify legitimate differences and problems in an organization, and serve as a strong motivator for change among employees.

HOW CONFLICT OCCURS

As a reminder, in this chapter we've defined conflict as the real or perceived differences between individuals with differing values, ideas, or goals.

In nursing, conflict occurs as a result of one of the following factors:

1. Competitive or opposing actions of incompatibles
2. Mental struggle resulting from incompatible or opposing needs, drives, wishes, or external or internal demands
3. Collusion

It is important to understand the human dynamics within each of these categories.

Competitive or Opposing Actions of Incompatibles

Conflict that results from competitive or opposing actions of incompatible people or ideologies is a common occurrence in the health-care setting. Some people, groups, or cultures are incompatible. You have heard of family feuds that go on for years. Sometimes people do not recall the original reason for the feud because it was so insignificant in the overall picture. In this circumstance, individuals have chosen to be incompatible by removing respect, caring, and listening from their interactions. Another example is two competent and qualified young attorneys who are seeking the same prestigious position in a venerable law firm. Their competition for the position puts them in conflict with each other.

Mental Struggle Resulting From Incompatible or Opposing Needs, Drives, Wishes, or External or Internal Demands

When individuals or groups of people participate in a mental struggle resulting from incompatible or opposing needs, drives, wishes, or external or internal demands, there is conflict. This type of conflict in nursing is often the result of the unequal distribution of scarce resources. It happens, for example, when raises on a unit are given according to a strict set of instructions or criteria that make the raise difficult to achieve and a competitive item. Nursing faculty members compete for private offices with a window; students compete for 'A' grades; and poor people compete for food, a warm coat, or a bed at the homeless center. Many people want the item that is being sought, but only one or a few can have it.

Nursing conflicts that result from incompatible or opposing needs, drives, wishes, or external or internal demands are natural conflicts that need to be understood by you as a future nurse manager.

As a manager, it is helpful for you to identify the scarce resources that are most desirable and consequently cause the conflict. Then you need to work to increase their availability. The conflict decreases if the resources are not as hard to get.

Collusion

The formation of a subgroup or clique on a hospital unit or floor is indicative of an informal coalition of staff that has formed for the purpose of conspiring, either openly or in secret for the purpose of developing informal power. Workplaces that experience frequent or unresolved conflict are more likely to experience employee collusion. Collusion is a type of power struggle between staff members or between staff and management that creates polarization around charged topics and fragmentation among participants.

This type of group dynamic and acting out may require outside intervention from management or counselors trained in handling these situations. Until the situation has been resolved, it is important for nurses to try to remain outside of the colluding group while focusing on collaboration and patient-centered care. While the situation is being resolved, it is acceptable to seek outside support and counseling from management until the conflict has been resolved.

 ## TYPES OF CONFLICT IN NURSING

Group communication may be defined in a number of different ways, but essentially it occurs when two or more individuals interact with each other on a regular basis. This means that in nursing, the potential for conflict can occur in several different ways, including nurse to nurse, nurse to physician, and nurse to patient. It is important for nurses to become proficient in recognizing and handling conflict in ways that promote understanding and collaboration among members.

Nurse-to-Nurse Conflict

Nurse-to-nurse conflict can arise when different philosophies, professional experiences, collusion, or incivility result in an imbalance of power that interferes with a sense of safety and collaboration. Research related to nursing workplace incivility suggests that incivility can lead to bullying and forms of lateral violence (Croft & Cash, 2012).

Lateral violence generally refers to hostile acts that occur between colleagues. These acts can be covert or overt acts of verbal or nonverbal aggression. Unfortunately, nurses at every level can be impacted by bullying or a hostile work environment. The prevalence of nursing conflict due to intimidation and bullying are largely unknown. However, there are some personnel actions that are indicators of workplace violence or bullying that need to be reported to appropriate levels of management. This might include your immediate supervisor or someone in the human resources department (Box 15.1).

These types of behaviors not only impact the individual but also can impair patient care. For example, if a nurse fails to provide accurate and timely information about a patient or is defensive when questioned about patient information, the licensed practical nurse (LPN) may provide care that is not suitable for the patient. Therefore, it is essential that nurses communicate incivility to personnel in positions of authority who can assist in addressing the issue.

Nurse-to-Physician Conflict

Nurse-to-physician/ancillary provider conflict occurs when a power difference between team members is allowed or is part of the organizational culture. In this type of setting, a power differential can occur. In some instances, one person may view herself as superior to another. Personal or professional acceptance of an imbalance of power

---

Box 15.1 Indicators of Workplace Violence and Bullying

- Verbal and nonverbal attacks
- Information that is withheld or inaccurate
- Hostility directed toward others
- Withholding support needed to do the job
- Public criticism of others
- Complaints about other people without talking to the person first

Source: Lachman, V. D. (2015). Ethical issues in the disruptive behaviors of incivility, bullying, and horizontal/lateral violence. *Urologic Nursing, 35*(1), 39–42.

between physicians and nurses can lead to communication styles that may be condescending, critical, or patronizing.

If this type of communication and conflict is not properly addressed, it may affect employee morale, increase nursing turnover, and negatively impact patient care by inhibiting interprofessional collaboration. Behaviors that create conflict can disrupt the culture of safety and prevent safe patient care because of lack of teamwork and good communication (The Joint Commission, 2015). Fortunately, there is a growing trend in health-care organizations to educate physicians and nurses together about communication, with a goal of interprofessional collaboration and mutual respect. Having a shared goal of patient-centered care that relies upon teamwork and interdependence can improve employee satisfaction and patient outcomes.

Nurse-to-Patient Conflict

The first obligation of nurses is to do no harm by providing safe patient care. Providing competent nursing care includes communication that is patient-centered and therapeutic. When patients and families do not feel they are being heard or are not provided with shared decision-making opportunities, conflict between nurses and patients and their families can arise. Nursing behaviors that have been shown to trigger conflict with patients include not returning pages or calls promptly, ignoring patient pain, not giving medications on time, and communicating in an abrasive manner.

In an effort to improve outcomes, patients and families should be more actively engaged by the health-care team to make decisions about the patient's care and must receive more health information and support from nurses (The Joint Commission, 2015). When patients and families are viewed as partners in decision making, there is an opportunity for improved communication, satisfaction, and patient outcomes.

Staffing

Staffing and schedule negotiation can produce internal and external conflict. Nurse staffing is the process of balancing patient care with the number of available nurses. Several factors affect staffing needs, including patient census (the number of patients), patient acuity (the intensity of nursing care required per patient), seasonal staffing (staffing over holidays), and workload patterns. The amount of change related to staffing needs can lead to considerable conflict for nursing staff, patients, and other team members.

Ideally, nurse staffing should be created with input from floor nurses and should be based on patient number and acuity. Ideally, staffing should also reflect staffing standards from comparable departments during comparable seasons. Unfortunately, nursing shortages and budgetary restrictions don't always allow for ideal staffing scenarios. It is during these times that communication, flexibility, and group decision making should be used to solve staffing dilemmas. Whatever type of staffing is used, transparency, or the providing of timely, honest, and accurate information by leadership, can promote a sense of safety, community, and overall job satisfaction among nursing staff.

REFLECTIVE THINKING

Select two causes of conflict that occur most frequently in your life (personal or professional), and write three strategies for preventing the causes from resulting in conflict in the future. Record your thinking and be prepared to share your thoughts in class.

 ## CAUSES OF CONFLICT AND APPROACHES TO RESOLVING IT

Conflict has many causes. As a nurse, some sources of conflict that you need to be prepared to address include the following:

• Role ambiguity
• Limited resources
• Distancing and unifying mechanisms
• Perceived or felt conflict
• Unresolved conflict

Role Ambiguity

Unclear role expectations are a frequent source of conflict for LPNs. It can be frustrating for the LPN to be assigned a certain set of tasks until a registered nurse (RN) is available. In that case, the LPN is asked to complete additional job assignments and leadership roles that were originally assigned to the RN. This type of scenario can produce role confusion for the nurse, other staff, and patients. This feeling of confusion can be further enhanced when questions arise that only the LPN knows the answer to because of acting in the role of charge nurse. The key to preventing this type of situation from escalating to unmanageable proportions is communication. First, it is important for the LPNs to seek clarification regarding their roles and floor assignments with the unit manager. Through appropriate communication and role delineation, you will be better informed about performance expectations for both patients and among the health-care staff. When the RN returns, express a willingness to report any changes or pertinent patient information that occurred during her or his absence. The next step is to meet with the unit manager and RN together about your understanding of your assigned duties. It is important to remember that in power struggles between staff and management, nobody wins. This type of struggle also places more emphasis on conflict than on patient care. As you resolve role conflicts, it is important to keep the patient in mind! As you work toward open communication and establishing role expectations, your colleagues will respect you and you will be seen as an invaluable team member.

Limited Resources

The second cause of conflict within an organization is limited resources. Limited resources impact budgets for staffing, supplies, room availability, and patient care. Bioethics requires that the unit or facility be fully staffed and prepared for any type of situation that may arise.

As a manager, what do you do? How can you manage the holiday schedule or a high patient census? One option includes allowing staff members the opportunity to coordinate their own schedules, including working half shifts. Another option for managers is to assign work rotations based upon last year's assignments with the newest hires working the less desirable shifts. Another idea is to reward employees with the least amount of sick leave or tardiness or with the highest evaluations with the prime shifts. If any of these options is to work well, leaders must provide transparency in their decision making and seek employee support. To do this, the manager must be proactive by announcing the proposal before the holidays occur, allowing employees time to express their feelings and the manager to address the potential conflict before implementing a new plan.

Distancing and Unifying Mechanisms

Distancing and unifying mechanisms are potential causes of conflict that often are not noticed or understood, so they are ignored. What is the difference? How do you recognize them?

Distancing is behavior exhibited by someone who keeps others at a physical or emotional distance. Perhaps you have an employee who, for a reason known only to that individual, always goes to lunch alone, prefers working with clients independently instead of the team approach used by the rest of the staff, or never participates in staff meetings or comes to staff parties. These behaviors are distancing mechanisms. They are the efforts of a person not to be close to others in the work environment. These efforts often cause other employees to feel discriminated against, left out, or "not good enough" to be a part of the team. Often, the cause for such behaviors is unknown. However, any negative feelings or feedback from staff members needs to be addressed with civility and openness.

This type of conflict requires the manager to ask, clarify, and often teach people about their own and others' behavior. This frequently is a time-consuming problem, but to manage it is much preferred to seeing the personal conflicts and lack of camaraderie that can occur if it is not clarified for all people involved.

Unifying mechanisms are behaviors that bring people "too" close together in a professional environment. It happens when one or more members

Distancing is a mechanism used by people who want to keep others away from themselves, such as this employee eating alone in the hospital cafeteria.

of the work team think of the people with whom they work as family. This concept initially has a positive, caring sound to it, but stop and think. You already have a family, as does everyone else at work. The activities you do with your family, including having conversations, are personal. The functions you do with your work team, including having conversations, need to be on a professional level instead of a personal one. If someone thinks that everyone at work is "one big happy family," personal comments are made that have no place in the work setting. These comments could interfere with other team members' opinions or levels of trust in the unifying person. Most people are uncomfortable knowing personal details about a fellow worker. Sometimes the unifying person takes too much responsibility for the other team member and tells him or her to do something in a certain way that in a truly professional setting would not happen. It can be compared with a mother telling a child what to do. It does not belong at work. The laws and policies on nepotism (members of a family working for the same employer) have a purpose, and it is to prevent unifying behaviors.

The challenge to the manager with employees who exhibit distancing and unifying behaviors is to be sensitive to how people are thinking and feeling and to respect them. The manager must then determine the best way to teach them what is happening and the conflict that can be caused by the behaviors of distancing and unifying. This is a personal challenge for a manager and it takes a great deal of effort. Nevertheless, it is crucial to the process of managing a group of people successfully.

Perceived or Felt Conflict

How conflicts arise and how they are managed have a lot to do with relationships between individuals. Have you ever walked into a room where you sensed the people there were having an argument? You didn't hear anything and didn't see anything that would tell you an argument was taking place, yet you knew one was happening. This is perceived or felt conflict. It also is the feeling you have when you think someone is upset with you. You don't know why or how you know the person is upset, but you do. When people work in an environment where one or more people are causing the feelings that accompany perceived or felt conflict, conflict is inevitable. The feeling of "it is coming" takes a great deal of energy from the person who is experiencing the feeling. It tends to make people uncomfortable, nervous, and edgy.

As the manager, it is important for you to sense when conflict is perceived or felt by others and to seek out the reason for it. This takes personal energy and time, but it is crucial to managing the conflict before it escalates. It is effective to manage this type of situation through one-on-one conversations with people you think may sense the feeling or even be causing it. In a pleasant, caring manner, interview people about what their perception of the situation is. Eventually you will gather enough information to return to the group and share what you have learned. After people are informed about the perceived or felt threat, they can relax and focus on doing their work instead of protecting themselves from something they think is going to happen.

Unresolved Conflict

Unresolved conflict generally occurs when someone is aggressive and devaluing to another person. The offended person is often unable to communicate effectively in the moment. As a result, anger and resentment occur and, over time, can create a negative feedback loop between individuals. The concept of a communication feedback loop is used to describe patterns of communication and interaction between members of an organization. The term *loop* is used to describe communication patterns that occur regularly among individuals. An individual can use negative or positive communication methods to move individuals and organizations toward change.

A negative feedback communication loop occurs when individuals repeatedly seek to correct conflict using negative communication methods such as manipulation, threats, or criticism. Instead of promoting change, this type of communication creates unresolved conflict that if left unresolved can take a physical and emotional toll on the individuals involved. While many individuals seek to avoid conflict or further conflict once it occurs, unresolved conflict can lead to a deterioration of workplace satisfaction and a decrease in productivity (Weiss & Tappen, 2015).

As a health-care leader, you have the opportunity to recognize what negative feedback looks like and promote conflict resolution through the development of positive communication skills, as discussed in this chapter.

ESTABLISHING A CONFLICT RESOLUTION STYLE

For most individuals, the ability to work effectively through conflict is not an innate skill. Fortunately, it has been shown that conflict resolution skills, leadership style, and leadership can be learned and improved upon with time. To establish your own conflict resolution style, I recommend that you observe individuals in your workplace whom you admire and with whom you struggle. Take the time to recognize how a good leader impacts the overall culture and group dynamics. An understanding of what makes groups work and how leaders maximize performance through communication and conflict resolution skills will assist you in becoming a leader who can promote teamwork and collaboration in a variety of settings.

Communication Styles

Communication is a dynamic process in which two or more people create shared meaning using verbal or nonverbal processes. Effective communication is a core skill that must be developed among nurses and nursing leaders.

To obtain an understanding regarding personal communication styles requires a commitment to inward reflection and openness to feedback from trusted peers. Thoughtful self-reflection and a willingness to learn effective communication styles is an important aspect of nursing leadership. Self-reflection can be defined as the honest examination of one's own thoughts and feelings as it relates to life experiences. This type of reflection requires maturity and a desire to gain greater insight into one's behaviors and their impact on others. The next time you are in a group, pay attention to how you act, how you communicate, and how the group responds to you. As you become more sensitive to your own communication patterns and the responses of others, you will begin to be a more effective team member.

While writing this chapter, a reflection regarding my early life experiences related to conflict avoidance revealed one reason for my ongoing struggles in professional communication in the workplace. At a young age, I was taught that as a female, conflict was socially unacceptable. As a result, I learned to manage conflict through accommodation and avoidance. Research has shown that

nurses frequently compromise during conflict through avoidance and accommodation to others' desires (Losa Iglesias & Beecerro de Bengoa Vallejo, 2012). Although learning new communication styles was difficult, I eventually adopted assertive communication techniques and a shared decision-making approach to problems that arose in the workplace. Changing my communication style has allowed me to improve my communication skills.

An understanding of one's own communication styles is essential to individual effectiveness and interprofessional collaboration. Nurses at every professional level are in a position to impact groups in positively in the following ways:

• Develop effective personal communication styles.
• Apply conflict resolution skills.
• Gain insight into others' needs.
• Practice flexibility as a leader or team member of the group.

Collaboration is a vital component to the success of any health-care organization. Patient outcomes are directly dependent upon communication that is open, direct, and timely. Research has shown that the quality of communication between nurses, doctors, and patients has a major influence on patient outcomes (O'Hagan et al., 2013). As a result, the development of communication skills and the ability to manage them are necessities for nurses.

One aspect of communication that is vital for collaboration is positive nonverbal communication. Nonverbal communication is the use of speech tone, facial expressions, and gestures to convey meaning. The positive use of nonverbal communication enhances the sender's message, whereas negative nonverbal communication disrupts the verbal message or conveys a different intent. The nurse leader will need to incorporate consistent verbal and nonverbal messages in all aspects of professional communication and collaboration. It is important to be as mindful of the tone of the message as it is to what is being said. Purposeful verbal and nonverbal communication can convey openness, reduce the likelihood of an escalation of harm, and establish shared problem-solving. Once a message has been sent, it is important to follow up on your communication. Take the initiative to ask whether there are any questions or have the person summarize your message by asking clarifying questions. This type of feedback is particularly critical when it involves patient care.

Another critical component of positive communication is active listening. Being an active participant in communication processes requires giving full attention to another person while he or she is sending a message. Staying silent until the sender is finished delivering the message and using eye contact conveys respect and a desire to understand the speaker. Repeating what the person has said by paraphrasing or restating it will help ensure that her or his message was clearly understood. It also shows the speaker that you care about what she or he has to say. By establishing supportive nonverbal and verbal communication, you can positively impact the culture and more effectively handle conflict when it arises.

 ## THE ROLE OF THE LPN

Some conflict situations may be better managed by an LPN. You may know more about the patients, their families, or the staff members who usually work on the unit. This information can assist you in handling the problems that occur. Because you have this knowledge does not mean that you are the right person to resolve the problem. You need the title and responsibility of being a manager to be involved in the resolution of the problem. Otherwise, you may look like a "busybody" and more conflict may occur.

What is the responsibility of the LPN in terms of resolving conflict? Always report problems to your manager and obtain advice and consultation from that person to integrate with your own knowledge. If you believe you do not have the skills for managing a complex conflict situation, report it to your manager and work with that person to resolve the problem. Do not leave it with your manager to assume total responsibility; work with the person to bring about a positive conclusion. If you do not have a management title or responsibility, avoid trying to resolve the conflicts of other people. Generally, it only causes resentment.

 ## TRANSACTIONAL APPROACH TO CONFLICT MANAGEMENT

Transactional analysis addresses four basic approaches to conflict resolution: win-lose, win-yield, lose-lose, and win-win (Table 15.1). These are

TABLE 15.1 APPROACHES TO CONFLICT MANAGEMENT

Win-Win	Elicits the best in people Based on caring theory No power struggle
Win-Lose	The boss is always right Keeps employees from doing their best work or sharing their ideas
Win-Yield	The boss is always right Employees don't try to resolve conflict Destroys employee initiative
Lose-Lose	Everyone has given up on resolving the conflict Problems do not get resolved

attitudes regarding the process of conflict. Conflict indicates a healthy and dynamic organization. It is something that is going to be a part of your job every day. How do you want to work with this aspect of your job as a manager?

Win-Lose

In the old-fashioned sense of management, the boss was the boss, and all the others did as they were told. This happened even if an employee's idea or solution to a problem was the right thing to do for the situation. If the boss said "no," then "no" was how the idea was treated. Often employees went ahead with instructions given by a boss that they knew were wrong, but they did so because the consequences were severe if they did not. This describes a situation of *win* (the boss) and *lose* (the employee). Have there been times when you didn't even bother to share your suggestion because you knew it would be rejected or ridiculed? Employees know when they are working with a manager who is determined always to be right. This person does not allow anyone else to get credit for good ideas and often uses power and aggressive communication to be sure that the boss is seen as the boss. If you have worked for someone who is a win-lose manager, you know it. Generally, this type of management keeps employees from doing their best work or sharing their innovative ideas because they are never allowed to be the winners. This type of conflict management is destructive to the individual employees and to the entire organization.

Win-Yield

Win-yield is another possible approach to addressing organizational conflict. In this scenario, the manager is the same person I described in the win-lose situation. The difference is that the employees are so discouraged or beaten down by the manager or other negative aspects of the environment that they don't even try to resolve the conflict. That way they never have to lose. They simply do what they are told and don't question or challenge information given to them. This type of organization generally exemplifies a management style that oppresses people and destroys any initiative they may have had previously. It is not a healthy environment for anyone.

Lose-Lose

The lose-lose management style incorporates avoidance and distancing for maintaining the status quo and avoiding dealing with conflict. The consequence of this type of management style is that there are never any winners. Instead, the conflict is always present and active. People are angry and destructive, and problems do not get solved. This type of manager has not accepted the reality of conflict and has ignored the need to develop conflict management skills. This type of management style can produce collusion among employees in which people become hostile and staff turnover is high.

Win-Win

The win-win conflict strategy is also known as the *collaborative* or *problem-solving approach*. It is the approach that elicits the best in people. It is based on caring theory and the desire to assist employees in moving up Maslow's hierarchy of needs pyramid. Problems are viewed as opportunities for collaboration. This means that there is no power struggle, no anger expressed (mainly because you managed the situation before the anger stage), and no passive-aggressive behavior involved in the conflict resolution.

A win-win approach to communication allows conflict resolution to be an opportunity for positive growth or change. As a manager, your responsibility is to assist each conflict to be resolved, with

The objective of conflict management is for everyone involved to have a win-win situation.

everyone feeling good about the situation and its resolution. This approach also allows shared decision making among the involved parties with the goal of creating a resolution that has mutually beneficial results. The goal is for everyone to be a winner, which is a high-level goal.

OTHER IMPORTANT SKILLS

Two other skills that are important to understand and develop in managing conflict successfully are the art of negotiation and skill in managing anger. These skills are discussed briefly in this section. I suggest that you take any opportunity to learn more about these skills as you progress in your career.

Art of Negotiation

The art of negotiation is a critical skill to use when conflict surfaces repeatedly over the same concern or problem. Negotiation is necessary in finding a win-win solution. It may seem easier to tell people what to do and get the work done, but that type of solution is only temporary because the problem still exists and the conflict may resurface. When you have identified the source of the conflict, such as a disgruntled employee, you need to understand the cause of the employee's attitude. How are you going to learn that information? You need to invite the employee into a private area, in a caring way identify what you have observed, and ask for information that can help you understand the situation.

Rule One

The preceding situation is one in which rule one of negotiation needs to be used: Don't take what is said personally! Don't do what comes naturally!

The information you have asked for may be negative about the organization, you as a manager, or your best friend who also works on the unit. Don't take it personally. Just listen and try to identify the core of the problem. Often when people are criticized in an angry manner, it is natural to become defensive and protect their ego, job, friend, or whatever is being criticized. Don't do what comes naturally. Don't get defensive.

Rule Two

If you can listen to what the problem is, you can follow rule two: Identify the need being expressed. Is it a personal need, an institutional need, or a patient need? How can you solve a problem if you don't understand what unmet need (think of Maslow) exists? These two rules are critical to the success of any negotiation. If you are in control of yourself and your feelings and understand the problem, you are ready to negotiate with the disgruntled (or angry) person for a solution.

Rule Three

The third rule for successful negotiation is that both of you need to give up something. Maybe the employee needs more time off on the weekends for the next 3 months. This is a problem in scheduling, but if you agree to do it, the disgruntled person needs to agree that the problem is a short-term one and will not go beyond the 3-month period.

It is hard to give up something. Some managers, if they give up something, think they lose their power base or are seen as a "softie." If you negotiate so that the needs of both are met and no one believes he or she did all of the sacrificing, you should find the opposite to be true. People express commitment to you as the manager; they tell people how fair you are and that you can be trusted. All outcomes eventually should be positive for you, the employees you manage, and the organization as a whole.

Managing Anger

Managing anger is an additional issue that needs to be discussed. I have been in professional situations in which the other person has lost his or her temper. He or she was angry and out of control. How do I successfully manage a conflict like that? In this situation, the possibility exists of being hurt physically or of having another employee or a patient being hurt by someone who is out of control. Do not do what comes naturally, which for many people is to reciprocate with anger. In most situations, returning the anger only escalates the problem. Yelling or hitting back is not professional or caring behavior.

A successful technique for this type of acute problem is to "white out." A person who whites out does not respond to the anger; he or she listens in a polite and respectful manner. This behavior is difficult because of the natural human reaction for fight or flight. I advise anyone in this type of situation to listen to what is being said and try to process what the problem is. Don't respond unless it is to agree, and do not do anything to provoke additional or escalated anger. Just white out: Control your natural reactions, stay put, and listen. Eventually the angry person dissipates the intense

---

 FOCUSED LEARNING CHART

Essential Skills for Successful Negotiation

REMEMBER: The objective of negotiation is a win-win outcome.

1. Negotiate in a private setting.
2. Ask for information from the other person regarding the problem.
3. Listen to what the other person says so you can understand the problem.
4. Do not "do what comes naturally." For example, DO NOT become angry, defensive, or frustrated.
5. Both parties must give up something of value to them.
6. Negotiate so that the needs of both parties are met in the fairest way possible.

anger that is being felt. This happens more quickly when nothing provokes additional anger (that is why you white out). After the anger is at a manageable level, you have to determine whether it is a good time to discuss the problem or to postpone the discussion because the angry person is too fragile emotionally. It takes a great deal of personal strength and commitment to white out and let the problem remain unresolved for a time. You are not losing in this situation; you are postponing the resolution until the other person can participate safely. Don't set an appointment at this time to discuss the problem at a later date. Do not be patronizing or insincere in your comments. Do something caring, such as saying, "I'm sure you are exhausted; why don't you go home and rest?" This person then feels you listened and you care and want to resolve the problem when he or she is better able to manage the situation.

Sometimes an angry person is a genuine physical threat to you, another employee, or a patient. If this situation occurs, for example, if someone has a gun and wants drugs, white out to your maximum ability and give the person what is requested. Simply meet the request and let the person go. After the person has left the premises, call the police, your manager, and the administrator. Your responsibility in a threatening situation is to protect yourself, other employees, and patients and their families. This requires you to cooperate with the angry or aggressive person and hope that he or she leaves quickly without an untoward outburst of violence.

Successful management of conflict is a significant challenge to every manager. Experienced managers and novice managers always hope for a day without a conflict that needs to be managed. In today's modern era of health care, however, that is not a reality. Care is based on costs and efficiency that challenge the nursing paradigm of holistic care. Many nurse managers view conflict management as the least desirable skill, but it is the one that has the most dramatic impact on individuals and the work organization.

REAL-WORLD CASE STUDY

■ You have been the charge nurse on a 12-hour evening and night shift for a hospital-based nursing home unit for the past 6 months. You are comfortable with the job and its requirements and believe that you have grown in your nursing care

skills and management skills. You have had to work with some challenging problems and believe that the staff members have learned to trust you and your managerial judgment.

The unit is assigned a new middle manager who seems uncomfortable in his role. The person is an RN but has not had previous experience in managing. The new manager, Jim, wants to spend time on both shifts to learn about the nursing care process, meet personnel, and evaluate the management styles being used. Last week, Jim worked 4 hours of one of your shifts with you. It seemed that he wanted to be the charge nurse for those 4 hours, and you became confused about what to do to get the work done effectively. Jim told you what to do and reorganized things so that the usual pattern of the unit was disrupted. He made it clear that he was the boss and reprimanded a certified nursing assistant for taking a problem to you. It was an uncomfortable 4 hours, and after he left, the unit was disorganized and the staff members were confused.

Jim plans to work with you again in 2 days. The staff members know he is coming and are complaining about him "interfering" with their work. There are some openly aggressive comments made, such as, "He is so stupid. Did you see how he did the dressing change on Mrs. Lucas?" Other comments are more passive-aggressive and are complaints about having him on the unit watching the staff. You conclude that you are not the only person who is uncomfortable with Jim working with you.

As you see Jim at the change of shift and during report, you notice that his comments to you consistently sound like orders. You find yourself reacting negatively to being talked to this aggressively. Every time you see Jim, you play internal tapes of failed communication, trying out different ways of telling him how you feel about his aggressive communication style. You never share your thoughts or anxiety about working with him again with anyone. You know that you need to do something to make the shift you are going to work with Jim a positive experience for Jim, the staff, and yourself.

1. What is the first critical step you are going to take?
2. What strategies should you use to resolve the conflict?
3. What should you do with any positive results from your actions?

Key Points

- Conflict occurs when two or more individuals have differing opinions, incompatible goals, limited resources, or role ambiguity. It is an inevitable aspect of an organization, particularly in areas of high stress or change.
- The primary types of conflict in nursing are nurse-to-nurse, nurse-to-physician, nurse-to-patient, and staffing issues. It is important for nurses to become proficient in recognizing and handling conflict in ways that promote understanding and collaboration among members.
- Workplace violence can occur between employees (lateral violence) or between an employee and a supervisor; in both cases, the individual feels bullied, afraid, and/or victimized. Workplace violence can occur inside and or outside the workplace or on social networking sites. It may consist of verbal or nonverbal threats, physical assaults, withholding information, making false claims, and public criticisms.
- If handled improperly or ineffectively, conflict can be damaging to individuals, groups, and organizations. However, if handled properly and effectively, conflict can be used to produce positive change and growth.
- Unresolved conflict can undermine workplace morale, increase nursing turnover, lead to legal claims, and, in extreme cases, even result in violence.
- As a nurse, some sources of conflict that you need to be prepared to address include role ambiguity, limited resources, distancing and unifying mechanisms, perceived or felt conflict, and unresolved conflict.
- To establish your own conflict resolution style, observe individuals in your workplace whom you admire and with whom you struggle. Recognize how a good leader impacts the overall culture and group dynamics. Understanding what makes groups work and how leaders maximize performance through communication and conflict resolution skills will assist you in becoming a leader who can promote teamwork and collaboration in a variety of settings.
- The development of communication and leadership skills is vital for nursing students entering the health-care profession. The quality of communication influences relationships, workplace morale, and patient outcomes.
- Transactional approaches to conflict management address four basic approaches to conflict resolution: win-lose, win-yield, lose-lose, and win-win. It is a leadership style that attempts to create win-win situations in which all parties have gained from the transaction.

ANSWERS TO REAL-WORLD CASE STUDY

What you are experiencing is passive-aggressive behavior from the staff toward Jim and perceived conflict from yourself.

1. The critical first step is to recognize what is happening. This means you take some quiet time to process what has happened, comments that have been made, and your feelings and reactions. Taking the time to understand the situation is time well spent because it allows you to identify the problem clearly. Taking time to think about the situation helps you to remember that conflict is inevitable, and the hiring of a new manager means anticipating conflict. After you have determined that what is happening is normal and expected, you can focus on how to keep the perceived or felt conflict between you and Jim and between Jim and the staff from escalating to a major problem.

2. The following strategies should be used to resolve this conflict: Something needs to be done before the shift Jim plans to work with you in 2 days. It is difficult, but you recognize that you need to make an appointment with Jim and discuss your concerns in an assertive fashion. You call and make the appointment for the next day before the beginning of your shift. As you prepare for a successful interview with Jim, you make a mental note that he is an inexperienced manager and a relatively new RN. It is

important that you not threaten him or say things that cause him to become defensive because that would be counterproductive to your goals. Remember that this is not a war scene. It is a conflict that you want to resolve with a win for you, the staff, and Jim. You are excited and nervous about the challenge this presents.

3. You approach your appointment with Jim in a cheerful and positive mood. It would be appropriate to thank him for the time he is spending with you and to tell him how much you respect his efforts to get to know the staff individually by working with them and to learn the organization of the different shifts (if that is a true statement and belief). The next piece of information shared with Jim, or anyone in this type of situation, either can escalate the perceived conflict or can work toward resolving it. You need to depend on your skills and knowledge of working with diverse people to recognize the most meaningful way to talk to Jim. If he seems defensive and is expecting criticism from you, defuse that immediately. Your comments about his time and willingness to get to know the staff and unit should do that for you.

What is said next needs to be done assertively and in a caring manner. It needs to be professional and said with sincerity. Sometimes it is best to be direct: "Jim, I feel there is something amiss between us like a misunderstanding that hasn't happened yet. I don't know where it is coming from or why I feel this way, but I want to talk to you about it."

The response from Jim is hard to imagine. He may look at your sincere (smiling) face, hear your caring (but direct) words, and feel a strong relief that here is someone he can finally talk to about his new job. He also may be a win-lose type of manager and may make fun of you or criticize you because you think there is a problem. You cannot change him; if he is a win-lose manager, you cannot make him into a win-win manager.

I am an idealist, so let it be said that Jim is grateful to you for bringing up the subject, and he is able to discuss with you his observations and feelings about the staff and your management of them. Be open to what is said, and do not do what comes naturally. Merely listen and learn. Respond honestly and with a win-win attitude. Always be assertive in what you say. You should let Jim know that you feel as though you are being given orders when he talks to you. You acknowledge he is the boss, but you are more accustomed to a participative management style. You can then ask him whether he has any suggestions to assist you in supporting him.

Depending on the results of your conversation with Jim, you should take the positive information back to the staff as you go to work. Help them realize that Jim is new and basically wants to do a good job. Share appropriate parts from your conversation with him with the staff, and let them know about his strengths. Your goal is to keep a perceived conflict from escalating into an unmanageable one. By sharing honest and positive information, you can promote the understanding that is required to manage a conflict.

REVIEW QUESTIONS

1. A nurse manager plans to implement a new staffing method for scheduling mandatory shifts during certain times of the year. Senior staff members are in opposition of the change, whereas newer staff members are more supportive. Which is the most effective method for resolving this conflict?
   1. Implement the change immediately following a staff meeting in which the manager provides a detailed rationale for the change.
   2. The nurse manager sends out an e-mail explaining the importance of the on-call shifts and explains that the change will become effective regardless of staffing preference.
   3. Withdraw the proposal based upon negative feedback from the nursing staff.
   4. Plan a meeting to provide time for discussion, communication, and problem-solving among senior staff members, management, and new employees.

2. Following a staff meeting, you and another nurse discuss some differences of opinion regarding a new policy. Which of these would be the best way to communicate in this situation?
   1. Adopt passive and avoiding behavior to calm other people down.
   2. Speak loudly and repeatedly to ensure that everyone can hear your points of view.
   3. Speak calmly, clearly, and state the facts as you see them.
   4. To assert your opinion, stare or roll your eyes at anyone who disagrees with you.

3. Which of these methods is a nonverbal way of showing openness and nonaggression when seeking to resolve conflict?
   1. Standing close to the other person
   2. Listening intently
   3. Frequently looking at an electronic device
   4. Looking away

4. How can a nursing manager deliver a win-win resolution to a conflict situation between a patient and a nurse?
   1. Discuss the situation with the patient until she changes her point of view.
   2. Involve other nursing personnel in the conversation so that the patient is outnumbered.
   3. Refer the patient to risk management to make a formal complaint.
   4. Work with the nurse and patient to achieve a patient-centered outcome.

5. Which of the following statements regarding conflict is true?
   1. Conflict is always bad for an organization.
   2. Conflict should be avoided at all costs.
   3. Conflict can produce positive change.
   4. Conflict is a signal for organizational failure.

References

Croft, R. K., & Cash, P. (2012). Deconstructing contributing factors to bullying and lateral violence in nursing using a postcolonial feminist lens. *Contemporary Nurse, 42*(2), 226–242.

The Joint Commission. (2016, January). "Patient Safety Systems" (PS) chapter as shown in the 2015 Update 2 to the *Comprehensive accreditation manual for hospitals.* Retrieved from https://www.jointcommission.org/patient_safety_systems_chapter_for_the_hospital_program/

Lachman, V. D. (2015). Ethical issues in the disruptive behaviors of incivility, bullying, and horizontal/lateral violence. *Urologic Nursing, 35*(1), 39–42.

Losa Iglesias, M. E., & Becerro de Bengoa Vallejo, R. (2012). Conflict resolution styles in the nursing profession. *Content Management, 43*(1), 73–80. doi:10.5172/conu.2012.43.1.73

O'Hagan, S., Manias, E., Elder, C., Pill, J., Woodward-Kron, R., McNamara, T., & Webb, G. (2013). What counts as effective communication in nursing? Evidence from nurse educators' and clinicians' feedback on nurse interactions with simulated patients. *Journal of Advanced Nursing, 70*(4), 1344–1355. doi:10.1111/jan.12296

Weiss, S. A., & Tappen, R. M. (2015). *Essentials of nursing leadership and management* (6th ed.). Philadelphia: F.A. Davis.

Web Resources

Academic Leadership Support: University of Wisconsin www.ohrd.wisc.edu/onlinetraining/resolution/aboutwhatisit.htm

Association for Conflict Resolution http://acrnet.org

Conflict Resolution Network www.crnhq.org

Healthcare Conflict Management www.healthcare-conflict-management.com

16

Dealing With Chaos

KEY TERMS

Chaos
Newtonian age (scientific age)
Quantum mechanics (new science)
Strange attractor

CHAPTER CONCEPT

Leadership and Management

LEARNING OUTCOMES

1. Describe the basic principles of Newtonian physics.
2. Describe the basic principles of quantum physics.
3. Compare and contrast Newtonian and quantum physics principles as you see them in people's environments and health-care settings.
4. Define chaos theory and the strange attractor principle.

To my mind there must be, at the bottom of it all ... an utterly simple idea. And to me that idea, when we finally discover it, will be so compelling, so inevitable, that we will say to one another, "Oh, how beautiful. How could it have been otherwise?"

—John Archibald Wheeler

More than 40 years ago, I was a student at a 3-year Catholic school of nursing. As a student at St. Benedict's, I did not experience any chaos in my nursing education or professional practice. Things were different then. The physicians and nuns were the power people in my life, and I did whatever I was asked or told to do by them. I felt no hesitation or indecision, and I did not question them. I simply did what I was told with great faith in the person who told me what to do. It was a much easier life.

At St. Benedict's, the students were all female and were required to live in the nurses' dormitory or with their parents. No one lived in apartments off campus, and no one was married, let alone married with children. I lived in the dormitory, and like the other students, if I left the dorm to go shopping, on a date, or for a walk, I had to "sign out" with the dorm mother. Signing out meant that I wrote where I was going, with whom I was going, and when I expected to return. I never questioned this policy.

Nursing school then, as now, was difficult. At St. Benedict's, the nuns strictly enforced curfew and study hours. The curfew was 10:00 p.m. during the week and 12:00 a.m. on Friday and Saturday nights. Study hall was 7:30 to 9:00 p.m. Every student had to be in her room, at her desk studying with the door open, or she had to be in the library where a nun supervised the studying. A second nun patrolled the halls and checked the rooms of the students who did not go to the library. They were simpler days.

When I finished my first quarter of school, the sisters had an elaborate ceremony for us to commemorate our rite of passage from beginning students to more experienced students. During the ceremony, each student had to kneel before a priest in the new chapel and receive her nurse's cap. After all of those hours in study hall, I honestly felt like I had earned that cap twice over! My family members came to the "capping" ceremony, and the sisters served refreshments and made kind comments. I did notice, during the

ceremony, that of the 36 who had started the class 3 months previously, only 19 were "capped." I never asked anyone where my classmates had gone. I simply accepted the fact that they were not there and went on with my education.

The second quarter was filled with intensive and well-supervised clinical experiences in the hospital with "real" patients. Now that we students had earned our caps, we were qualified to give patient care. The hospital was separated from the nursing dorm by a small parking lot. Under the parking lot there was a system of hallways that connected the dorm with the hospital proper and several other areas of the hospital such as the boiler room and the storage area. As a student nurse, I walked that underground tunnel every day as I went to my clinical assignment. It was poorly lit and had a musty smell, but I didn't notice because I was busy praying during the entire walk. I would pray that I wouldn't hurt a patient or make a medication error. I thought about hundreds of things that concerned me as a novice nurse. I wanted to do a great job of giving patient care, and

Capping ceremony, St. Benedict's Hospital School of Nursing, Ogden, Utah.

praying for guidance was not something I questioned. I simply did it.

When it was time for graduation, the entire world seemed focused on the 11 students, the survivors of the original 36 who started in my class. We had a dressmaker who made us matching white dresses. The dresses had long sleeves with cuffs and high necks and were 4 inches below our knees in length. We each had a new starched cap to wear in addition to our blue capes with red lining. Each graduate received 12 long-stemmed red roses to carry. Our parents let us out of their cars almost two blocks from the cathedral where the ceremony was to take place, then went quickly to the street to watch what happened next. The city police stopped traffic from both directions on the street in front of the cathedral. Once the horns stopped honking and the parents were all in place, we, the graduating class of 1967, walked down the middle of the road looking like the revered graduates that we were. When we reached the cathedral, we waited for our family members to enter the chapel and the music to start, and then we marched in to our graduation ceremony.

UNDERSTANDING THE CHANGES

I hope the summary of some of my experiences as a student nurse has been interesting to you. I think that as a person living in a modern and fast-paced world, you may wonder how my friends and I tolerated the organization and control that we experienced at St. Benedict's School of Nursing. At the time, my alma mater was considered the best school of nursing in the state. It had the highest pass rate on what were called "state boards" or the National Council Licensure Examination (NCLEX®). It was not only exclusive and difficult to gain admission, it was also difficult to graduate. I loved being a student there.

Health-care and nursing education have changed dramatically. Most of you have the freedom to choose where you live while going to school. You also can choose to be a married student and when you will study. These are issues of empowerment and are concepts you need to consider.

Your list of personal empowerment concepts could include a wide variety of ideas. Simply think of things you are free to choose to do or not to do or have the strength to determine when and how

you will do them. The following are points of empowerment you have that I did not have when I attended school:

1. Eat and sleep when you wish.
2. Go to the library when you want to study rather than when someone tells you to go.
3. Miss class. (Not a good choice!)
4. Have a family or a job, or both, while attending school.

In the clinical arena, dramatic changes have occurred as well. You need to understand these changes to be effective in your role as a licensed practical nurse (LPN). The changes are often felt by health-care providers as *chaos,* or a general feeling of lack of control. I have a friend who works in a busy intensive care unit. She complains of the chaos with which she has to work every day. The feeling of chaos is an example of changes that have occurred in health care and the scientific world.

The terms *downsizing, re-engineering,* and *capitation* were prevalent in nursing in the 1990s. When the new millennium arrived, a different role was available for the nurse manager because of the impact of such changes. Cost-effectiveness and patient outcomes are the current measures of nursing excellence. These were not the rules when I went to nursing school, but they are the rules now. How can you as a nurse manager work effectively in such an environment? It requires a great deal of creative thinking because doing things in the "old" way will not be successful. As a student of the new millennium, you are being taught in the "new" ways of health care; it will be all you know or have experienced. However, you may be working with registered nurses (RNs) who have been educated and have worked under the old paradigm of thinking. These men and women may be your managers. In another aspect, you will be the manager for nursing assistants who have worked for years or perhaps decades and definitely know the old way of making nursing work. How are you going to work with people who have not made the change from the old to the new paradigm or the scientific age to the new science?

UNDERSTANDING NEWTONIAN PHYSICS OR THE SCIENTIFIC AGE

If you have studied Newtonian and quantum physics, you do not need to read this section. Many of you are saying, "But I don't want to read about physics at all!" I promise it will be painless and even potentially interesting. I am presenting this information because it is important for you to understand that the entire world has changed because of the changes made in science; nursing has traveled along with it. Why such changes have happened is the point I am trying to clarify with this brief discussion of physics.

Sir Isaac Newton was a 17th century physicist who was the chair of the Department of Physics at Cambridge University, Cambridge, England. Newton was a key figure in the scientific revolution. His discoveries were remarkable and changed the world. The Newtonian age brought with it a strong sense of organization. Because of Newton's discoveries, people were able to move into the industrial era. Machines were invented, people became more knowledgeable, and more and more work was accomplished. It was the beginning of the fast-paced life.

Machines were the emphasis because the world shifted to the industrial era. Machines brought more food to the population of the world and improved health simply through improving nutrition. The population increased, and machines provided jobs for the growing number of people. Machines became the essential aspect of most work that was accomplished. Take a moment and consider what machines are like. They have mechanical parts that are crucial for proper functioning. The focus on parts, rather than the whole, is one of the hallmarks of the Newtonian era. If people kept the parts working and in their proper place in the machine, the machine worked, the jobs continued, and people prospered. The point of emphasis was the machine and its parts, not the people.

Newtonian physics dominated the world for 300 years. The world was orderly, compartmentalized, and predictable because everything was mechanized. Now think back to my nursing education experiences. They were orderly, compartmentalized, and predictable. What would have happened to me if I had disrupted the orderliness of school at St. Benedict's? Maybe I would have refused to go to study hall or stayed out after curfew. I have wondered if my fellow students who did not make it to capping or graduation did something like that—disrupted the orderliness of the process. If students did not behave in a predictable way, they were not kept in the system.

That is what Newtonian or mechanistic nursing education looked like for me.

"Newtonian" nursing is orderly, compartmentalized, and predictable. Nurses followed physicians' orders without questioning them. They also followed the rules of the hospital or nursing home without causing any disruptions in the orderly process of delivering care. That is how Newtonian nursing works.

There was a time and place for Newtonian nursing; that time and place are in the past. It was critical that nurses follow the rules and obey physicians while the profession was establishing itself. Now nurses need to learn more and have more diverse experiences so that they can join the new science and become "disorderly, non-compartmentalized, and unpredictable"! Consider the clinical time (school or job) you have spent in a hospital or nursing home. I am sure you noticed the emphasis on long-term and short-term planning. This planning is often seen as goals for the patient, the staff, and the facility. Working toward the fulfillment of goals causes the behavior of people to be predictable. Patient acuity places the person who is ill into a nice, neat, orderly category. It is "almost unacceptable" for a low-acuity patient to have a bleed because that was not predicted. Most decisions are made based on previously determined decisions of a bureaucratic system that exists in the facility. These all are organized and predictable mechanisms for getting the work done in a Newtonian way. See Box 16.1.

UNDERSTANDING QUANTUM PHYSICS OR THE NEW SCIENCE

In science, the beginning of the 20th century marked the end of Newton's domination. Discovery of a strange, new world at the subatomic level could not be explained by Newtonian laws. This discovery opened the human mind to new ways of understanding the universe. Newtonian physics still applies to the world in general, but a new and different science now is required to explain many phenomena—quantum physics or quantum mechanics. This is the world's most successful theory in physics, and it is not orderly, compartmentalized, or predictable. It does not tell us that the universe is mechanistic. Instead, it shares with us a world filled with chaos.

Box 16.1 Newtonian and Quantum Physics Principles

Newtonian

• Scientific age
• Focused on the parts rather than the whole
• Characterized as orderly, compartmentalized, and predictable, with everything mechanized
• Concerned with following rules
• Emphasis is on the process or task, not people

Quantum

• New science age
• The entire experience, relationship, and potential in people are considered
• Characterized as dynamic, chaotic, and unpredictable
• Empowerment, creative problem-solving, and collaboration are encouraged
• Emphasis is on people, not the process or task

REFLECTIVE THINKING

Newtonian Nursing

Have you worked with a Newtonian nurse or in a Newtonian health-care system? If you have, the experiences you had probably validated that you were in a Newtonian environment. Think about your clinical experiences and record three Newtonian experiences in your class notebook. Identify whether the experience was positive or negative for your learning. Were patient care needs met through the process? If you could change the situation, how would you change it? Be descriptive in your responses.

With the scientific acceptance of quantum mechanics, the world ceased to be a machine, and people began to recognize life's dynamic and living qualities. In this new world people look at entire experiences, relationships, and processes rather than just the parts, as was done in Newtonian science. This view makes relationships with all aspects of the world rich, complex, and unpredictable. Physicists urge people to stop teaching facts—"things" of knowledge—and focus instead on relationships as the basis for all definitions. With relationships, we give up predictability for the potential in every person, situation, or environment. Some people want the predictable world. I often have students in my classes who want to know everything exactly: exactly how long to write a paper or exactly how many references to have on the last page. This is not how I teach my classes, and to these students I say, "Write as much as you need to, to learn." That is very challenging for someone who wants predictability.

I do not refuse to give students structure and predictability because I like to see them struggle. I give them such experiences and support them in being successful in such experiences because I want them to be prepared. The new world science demands reaching the potential of every person. People cannot reach their highest potential if they are always given structure, orderliness, and predictability.

Several years ago, I read that elementary particles (the "things" physicists study!) were "bundles of potentiality." I have begun to think of all of us this way, for surely we are as undefinable, unanalyzable, and bundled with potential as anything in the universe. None of us exists independent of our relationships with others. Different settings and people evoke some qualities from us and leave others dormant. In each of these relationships, we are different, new in some way.

An understanding of quantum mechanics provides me with the ability to see the world of nursing in a new and fascinating way. It allows me to focus on the relationship between one person and another rather than the time clock or the acuity levels of patients. It makes the world a much more interesting place; it allows people to be full of surprises rather than predictable. Think for a moment and consider how Jean Watson's nursing theory fits into quantum mechanics. She does not urge predictability, but instead she wants us to consider the individuality of each person we encounter. This type of science also provides people with the opportunity to work toward self-actualization in Maslow's theory. Instead of being stuck somewhere on the pyramid, people can determine their own pace and keep moving to the top of Maslow's hierarchy.

The new science age stresses empowerment for all, creative approaches to problem solving, and collaboration as a team (Curtin, 2013). These are not characteristics of Newtonian nursing. Instead, for us "old" nurses and organizations, it presents us with a new world in which to work, and it often is challenging. The changes brought about by the new science make it necessary for you to be a leader and manager in a different way than those who have gone before you.

New science nursing allows nursing leaders to change the focus from being task-oriented to being focused on person outcome. This means the person—patients, patients' families, or staff—is more important than "getting the tasks done." People are more important than paperwork. This concept fits well because nursing now has a strong emphasis on patient outcomes.

As a student at St. Benedict's, I was required to wear a 100% cotton dress that was laundered and stiffly starched in the hospital laundry. At the end of my shift, I was graded on the number of wrinkles in my dress from sitting. This truly meant that sitting and talking to a patient would negatively affect my grade. It also meant I couldn't sit or sit for very long at lunch or breaks. (Actually, I am sure I never took a break in 3 years!) In new science nursing, personnel are encouraged to sit and take time with patients and families. Nurses do a great deal of teaching and provide emotional

This team of nurse researchers represents quantum physics nursing of the new millennium. The researchers know how to work together as a team and feel professionally empowered through the importance of the data they are gathering.

support that happens while sitting at the bedside. These things were not part of Newtonian nursing because they could not be managed as orderly and predictable events. See Box 16.2.

CHAOS THEORY

The new millennium was accompanied by a stronger presence of chaos in health care. Nurses, as leaders and patient advocates, are in the throes of the chaos, sometimes without even realizing it. Understanding the impact of chaos on nursing is the purpose of this chapter. You need to know what is happening in your profession and have a basic understanding of what has caused it. All of us have experienced chaos in our lives. Sometimes it occurs in our personal lives, at other times in our professional lives. Chaos is the movement away from order or unexpected disorganization (Grossman & Valiga, 2013). Chaos occurs when life does not follow the orderly pattern of Newtonian physics.

Much of the chaos comes from the mix of Newtonian and new science health care practiced by nurses, physicians, and other practitioners. Look around you. Who is Newtonian? Does understanding the foundation for Newtonian behavior assist you in understanding and working more effectively with the person? The same is true of a new science health-care provider. When you give that person a list of things to do, and instead he or she spends most of the morning holding the hand of and talking to a recent teenage amputee, you will understand the behavior.

REFLECTIVE THINKING

New Science Nursing

Have you worked in a new science nursing environment or with a new science nurse? If you have, you have had experiences that clarified for you what new science nursing is. List three new science nursing experiences in your class notebook. Indicate the impact the experience had on your learning and patient care and if there was anything about the experience you would change.

It would be valuable for you to take the assignment you did on Newtonian nursing and compare it with the thoughts you recorded on new science nursing. What are the differences? Does recording your experiences help you to understand the differences in nursing practice in these two science-based concepts? That is the purpose of doing the assignments, so think about them and the work you do in the clinical setting in an effort to define your thinking on these concepts.

Other factors define the chaos in your leadership and management position. An understanding of chaos theory itself helps in understanding such factors. *Chaos* is a scientific term meaning the apparently irregular, unpredictable, behavior of deterministic, nonlinear systems. How does that definition help in understanding chaos? I think we need to work on it.

Clinical Chaos

As a student or employee, have you been involved in or observed a serious emergency, such as a cardiac arrest? I hope that hasn't been a frequent experience for you, and I know that some of you have not been involved in one. Because of the vicarious experience provided by television, however, I assume that you have some idea of what can happen during a code.

Think about a code you have seen (in real life or on television). Was it organized and predictable? Was there a list of tasks to do, and when the list was completed, did the staff members say, "Well, we're done. Pronounce the patient dead"? That is not what I have observed. I see utter chaos. People are doing all kinds of procedures, equipment is flying from one person or place to another, everyone is talking, and there is a blur of movement. If the code is not going well, the chaos increases. Voices might get louder, more procedures are done, and more equipment is used. Whatever the outcome, when the code is over, the room is a mess; the staff members are exhausted from their effort; and everyone recognizes, among other important things, that the code could not have been managed with a list of procedures to follow in an orderly sequence. That is a clinical picture of chaos.

Let's consider the computer you have at your fingertips to be the classic example of an ability to create order out of chaos. A computer can store millions of megabits of information. It can track an entire system, organization, or civilization. With a specific code, the computer can give you, the requester, a small glimmer of light on a screen that is the exact piece of information you desire. That is achieving order out of chaos. Order out of the chaos that exists in health care today is the goal of every nurse manager. The way it is done in chaos theory is by identifying the strange attractor in the chaos and using it. Chaos is here to stay, and you need to know how to identify the strange attractor to make the chaos work for you. (Box 16-2)

Attractor Concept

The chaos of a code in the emergency department is a good way to explain the strange attractor concept. Let us return to the moment the code occurs. You are the nurse in the room. The code is unexpected, the physician is in the next room, and a peripheral intravenous line hasn't been started yet. The RN is walking into the room to do the assessment and is unaware that a cardiac arrest has just occurred. This is chaos! There is not a list in the world that would assist you in saving the life of this patient. Chaos must reign. It is the only way to get the help you need. I am sure you are taught in school not to raise your voice in the clinical area, but you might (and probably should) yell to get the physician who is next door into your room. In addition, the red code button you pushed should bring the others who are needed in this critical situation. As people come into the room, they are not going to grab a list and follow it. No, they are going to get involved in any way they see would be effective. Two people may start doing the same thing; that is better than no one doing anything and is part of the chaos. Chaos is the final state in movement of a system, team, or person away from order. The code, a highly charged situation, certainly qualifies.

Perhaps your morning before coming to class one day this week was a "movement away from order" for you. There are mornings when a child is crying, no one told you there was no milk for breakfast, and the car does not start. I would consider that chaos.

Box 16.2 Leadership Based on Theories of Quantum Mechanics

- Empowerment of others
- Collaboration as a team
- Promotion of other people's potential
- Building of relationships that nurture others
- Creative approach to problem solving

The code patient in the emergency department could not have been saved through an orderly process. Most crying children I know would not respond well to a list of prepared, orderly, predictable statements. When you are working a chaotic shift, you need to recognize it for what it is, chaos—the movement away from order—and look for the *strange attractor* rather than a list of tasks to complete.

STRANGE ATTRACTOR

Not all systems, shifts, or mornings before school require a strange attractor because they all are not chaotic. When a system is dislodged from a stable state, it moves into a period of oscillation where it (or he or she) moves back and forth from order to chaos. If the system moves from the state of oscillation, the next stage is chaos. This is a place where total unpredictability exists. It is the opposite of the place where most people start, and it is often stressful because it is a dramatic change. In this realm of chaos, where everything should fall apart, the strange attractor comes into play. It is the phenomenon of natural organization. Think back to the code experience; the chaos did self-organize. The team of people managing the code does not stand around wringing their hands saying, "I don't know what to do!" Instead, they get in and "do" in a self-organizing way.

Consider chaos at work. The patients are not neglected. No one dies as a result of the chaos because the staff somehow self-organizes to make things happen as they should. The same is true of your hectic morning getting to school. Perhaps you

These firefighters are first responders to many emergencies. The work they do to assist others is an example of people self-organizing into strange attractors.

called someone to help with the car, and a neighbor took your crying baby for a few hours while you are in class. Somehow, when you were experiencing utter chaos, your system self-organized, and you made it to school, albeit probably late.

To accept the reality of strange attractors, you need to accept the concepts of quantum mechanics. Do you remember that the theories of quantum mechanics brought forth the concepts of empowerment for all, collaboration with others, and dealing with people's potentials? You need to have faith in the strange attractor theory. Yes, people in chaos self-organize. It happens every time. Perhaps it does not happen the way you would have designed it, but it happens.

You know it will happen because, as a new science nurse manager, you believe in the potential of others. You provide empowering environments for people so that they can do their best work, you design opportunities for collaboration between nurses and other disciplines, and you embrace chaos as a mechanism for accomplishing the tasks of modern nursing.

As a manager, you are responsible for defining and sharing the expectations of acceptable behavior and providing people with the opportunity to empower themselves. Not every day or shift will be chaotic, and not every person will want to give up his or her "list" when chaos occurs. Chaos will occur, however, and the strange attractor principle eventually will enter into the chaos. The strange attractor is the symbol of self-organization that eventually changes the chaos. It allows people to be their best when the situation is the most chaotic.

In "my" nursing era, no one knew about the strange attractor theory. When chaos occurred, management people, symbolically, just kept making more lists. No opportunities for empowerment or self-determined behavior existed. There was no self-organizing behavior. We all had the symbolic list and followed it without question. That is why my friends and I did so well at St. Benedict's School of Nursing; things were not chaotic, and we followed our lists without question. I am so grateful nursing has changed.

The physics lesson is over, and I know that you have had to read more about physics than you ever wanted to do. Did it help you understand people and their behaviors better? Are you now willing to look at chaotic situations and watch for the strange attractor to surface? I am counting on you to make this way of thinking a part of you.

FOCUSED LEARNING CHART
Living With Chaos

As nursing has progressed, it has moved toward more chaotic environments. The move toward chaos is referred to as new science nursing.

UNDERSTANDING THE STRANGE ATTRACTOR THEORY

1. The normally organized system becomes dislodged from its stable state.

Example: A community is hit by a devastating tornado.

2. A period of oscillation occurs. This is where the situation moves back and forth from order to chaos.

Example: There is a tornado warning that starts the oscillation; then the tornado advisory is lifted; then announced again. During this time, the emergency departments are working to assist people, which is part of the oscillation.

3. If there is no resolution (the tornado does not pass them by), then chaos occurs. This is a time of total unpredictability.

Example: The tornado hits!

THEN when everything should fall apart

4. The strange attractor principle surfaces as people self-organize.

Example: Neighbor helps neighbor; other communities send emergency services people to assist; FEMA begins to deliver food, water, and blankets. Many other acts of caring occur as people are attracted to resolution of the problem.

REFLECTIVE THINKING

My Observations Related to Physics

Give a brief response to the following in your class notebook. It would be interesting for you also to discuss your responses with a colleague or friend.

1. Identify a person from a clinical setting and determine whether the person is old or new science in behavior. Do not list the person's name but do list the characteristics you identified as old or new science.

2. Identify an environment where you spend a great deal of time. Is it old or new science? List the characteristics of the environment you identified.

3. Think for a moment about what you need to feel empowered in an environment. Do you have a place where you really feel empowered? Record the factors you need to feel empowered in a clinical situation.

ARE YOU READY?

Health care is changing at a rapid pace. The result of the change, some of it with instruction and some of it without instruction, is chaos. You are a nurse manager or soon will be one. In that role, you have a tremendous responsibility. Whether or not you can embrace the chaos is a critical criterion for success.

I hope you feel you can go to any unit on any shift, and when chaos strikes you will swell with pride because you are ready to embrace it. Such behavior means you have faith in the strange attractor theory, you feel good about providing empowering environments for staff, and you believe in staff and interdisciplinary collaboration.

It is important that modern-day nurses understand modern-day theories of science and nursing. This chapter has reviewed basic concepts of Newtonian physics and quantum mechanics as a way to contrast two ways of thinking. The new science or quantum mechanics approach is best adapted to current health-care settings. That means one must embrace the chaos that occurs every day in clinical settings.

REAL-WORLD CASE STUDY

■ You just completed your first 3 months on a surgical floor in a large metropolitan hospital that uses nurse–certified nursing assistant (CNA) dyads for care. Your probationary evaluation was excellent, and your nurse manager thought you were now ready to be the leader of your own dyad.

When you walked on the floor at 5:30 a.m., you found the entire unit in utter chaos. The night nurse was angry and impatient with everyone, and the day RN was a new graduate who looked horrified at what she saw the day would be. A physician at

Continued

the end of the hall was talking loudly to another nurse, and a family group in the meditation room was crying and hugging each other. When you looked at the assignment list, you noted that you had four very ill patients with complicated treatments and a CNA who was new to the unit. Today was only the CNA's third day. You smiled confidently and went to report.

The chaos seemed to be increasing, as report was 20 minutes late because of the attitude of the night nurse and the unavailability of the nurse patiently listening to the physician who was so upset. While you were waiting, you introduced yourself to the new CNA. What else could you do during the 20 minutes while waiting for report that could serve as the strange attractor for behavior on your part? How would you involve the CNA in what you were doing? Remember that your responses will differ from my case study answer. Value your own thinking.

Key Points

- The Newtonian age allowed people to move into the industrial age, which focused on machines and the benefits brought by mechanization. This brought a strong focus on how the parts of a process worked rather than a focus on the process as a whole. The world became orderly and predictable because everything was mechanized.

- Using the concept of quantum mechanics, a nurse can better focus on the needs of the whole patient instead of on the required tasks. Providing care to the patient as a whole individual assures better patient outcomes.

- The new science age stresses empowerment for all, creative approaches to problem solving, and collaboration as a team. The focus is now on empowering people to solve problems on their own and to work together to improve performance.

- According to Newtonian physics, chaos occurs when life does not follow an orderly pattern. In health care today, much of the chaos comes from the mix of Newtonian and new science health care practiced by nurses and other health-care providers. Some individuals

follow a list of steps that need to be completed when providing care to patients whereas others continually assess the ongoing needs of the patient and provide care based on the evolving needs.

- Creating order out of the chaos that exists in health care today is the goal of every nurse manager. By providing an empowering environment so staff can do their best work, allowing opportunities for collaboration with other disciplines, and providing necessary resources needed to get the job done, employees will be able to self-organize to handle the unexpected issues that arise.

- When chaos occurs, strange attractors come into play to provide natural organization. In nursing, the strange attractor might be the extra nurse who is called in to work to care for the recently admitted residents. Or it might be the new committee that is formed to address an ongoing employee concern. Strange attractors are those things that provide more organization and stability to the nursing unit or organization as a whole.

ANSWERS TO REAL-WORLD CASE STUDY

During the 20 minutes I was waiting for report, I would spend approximately 10 minutes with the CNA explaining to her the apparent challenges of the day and assessing her skills in handling the situations that might occur. I would determine her skill level by asking her questions and having her demonstrate handling of some equipment, such as the automated vital sign machine. I would assess how comfortable she feels with the routines and physical layout of the unit. Can she find things on her own? Does she know when vital signs are due? Does she understand that she is working with you as a team member and she should do only the things that you have delegated to her after assessing the patients?

Then I would take 10 minutes and make "quick" rounds on my patients. I would take the CNA with me and introduce us as a team to the patients. I would determine whether the patients would be safe and comfortable while the CNA and I got report. While making "quick" rounds, I would determine with which equipment the CNA was familiar and which

she didn't know how to use. Then we would go to report.

After report, I would pass medications and do anything else that urgently needed to be done. Then I would sit with the CNA and delegate the responsibilities I wanted him to assume. I would clarify anything that was confusing to the CNA and teach him any skills that were necessary for the day. The most important thing I want him to know is that we are a team, and when we work together, the chaos will abate and the patient care will be done in the way it should, with high-quality technical skill on a foundation of caring behavior.

REVIEW QUESTIONS

1. You are working a day shift on a surgical floor with multiple admissions. Things are quickly getting out of control. Which best describes how you might handle the ensuing chaos?
   1. Begin to panic and develop a list of tasks that need to be completed.
   2. Continue doing what you can to manage until things slow down.
   3. Encourage the nursing assistants to work harder.
   4. Call the OR department and ask them to stop sending patients.

2. You are a nurse leader and want to lead using the principles of quantum mechanics. Which of the following best describes your approach? Select all that apply.
   1. Provide opportunities for staff to collaborate on patient care.
   2. Allow staff the ability to make decisions.
   3. Recognize the potential of each individual.
   4. Develop a plan that people need to follow.

3. Nurse leaders need to embrace chaos to be successful in their careers.
   1. True
   2. False

4. You are on your way to the cafeteria for lunch. A man in front of you drops to the floor. The person with him starts screaming for help. You stay calm and begin assisting the individual as others arrive to help. The person is transferred to the ER in a timely manner. What could have been a chaotic situation is managed well. What best describes this concept?
   1. Chaos theory
   2. Strange attractor
   3. Quantum physics
   4. Newtonian physics

5. As an LPN you know that health care is continually changing. Which best describes how to adjust to the dynamic health-care environment?
   1. Become a lifelong learner.
   2. Understand that change is constant and embrace it.
   3. Change professions to one that is more stable.
   4. Continue to change clinical specialties until you find a more stable environment.

References

Curtin, L. (2013). Quantum leadership: Upside down. *American Nurse Today, 8*(13). Retrieved from https://americannursetoday.com/quantum-leadership-upside-down/

Grossman, S. C., & Valiga, T. M. (2013). *The new leadership challenge: Creating the future of nursing* (4ed). Philadelphia: F.A. Davis.

Web Resources

Chaos Theory https://www.youtube.com/watch?v=JnlkKdDXk-I

Quantum Leadership https://americannursetoday.com/quantum-leadership-upside-down/

17

Ethics and Law in Nursing Management

KEY TERMS

Bioethics
Deontology
Ethical principles
Ethical reasoning
Regulatory laws
Utilitarianism

CHAPTER CONCEPTS

Ethics
Legal
Collaboration

LEARNING OUTCOMES

1. Discuss the differences between the words *ethical* and *legal*.
2. Explain the difference between deontological and utilitarian ethical theories.
3. Define one's personal values.
4. Illustrate how the following ethical principles apply to nursing practice: beneficence, autonomy, nonmaleficence, veracity, justice, and fidelity.
5. Describe how ethical decision making can be applied to the field of bioethics.
6. Describe the importance of the nurse practice act and its governing body, the state board of nursing.
7. Define statutory law, common law, criminal law, and civil law.
8. Describe how the following legal principles apply to nursing practice: duty to seek medical care for the patient, confidentiality, permission to treat, informed consent, defamation of character, assault and battery, false imprisonment, advance directives, negligence, malpractice, and fraud.

Ethical knowledge does not describe or prescribe what a decision should be; rather, it provides insight about which choices are possible and why.

—Chinn & Kramer

Ethics is a branch of philosophy that examines ideal human behavior. Think back to the things your parents (ideally) taught you. Most parents teach their children that lying, stealing, and cheating are wrong. Such behaviors are unethical. But what about the ethics of telling a "small" lie to save a friend from embarrassment? Is the character Jean Valjean in Victor Hugo's classic novel *Les Miserables* unethical because he stole bread for his starving sister? Is it ethical to allow a friend whose child's illness prevented her from completing her homework to copy yours? Such questions are ethical dilemmas—situations that result in a conflict of two or more fundamental values. They are complex problems, and their solutions are not apparent. By its nature, ethics is an unclear realm of philosophy. It requires critical thinking and an understanding of the situation before a meaningful ethical decision can be made. The struggle for ethical behavior is a constant one.

PERSONAL VALUES

Last night I planned to treat myself to a night of mindless television. Instead, I watched a documentary about the treatment of women involved in the suffrage movement in the United States. These women had strong feelings regarding the value of voting rights and wanted to participate in the democratic process. Unfortunately, during that time the general consensus was that women needed to be taking care of things in the home and not concerning themselves with other affairs. These women organized themselves to express their opinions, march in groups, and gain recognition for what they felt was their right.

The local governments did not appreciate the large showing of support, and many women were arrested, imprisoned, and mistreated. Some women were left in small cells with no toileting facilities, no water, and no food. Other women were degraded by being placed in cells with very little clothing, and most of the women were not allowed to speak to family or friends. Health care for injuries suffered was not offered, and many of these women suffered with residual effects of the imprisonment for the remainder of their lives.

Examples of unfair treatment abound in the movie *Titanic,* which tells the dramatic story of the sinking of the ship and the deaths of 1,500 passengers. The one small slice of the story I would like to share with you is when the lifeboats were being filled. The British, in their customarily proper fashion, called for the women and children to board the lifeboats first. Because there were not enough lifeboats for everyone, it meant that the women and children would be saved and the men would die. This privileged treatment of women is in sharp contrast, in terms of values, to the treatment of the women featured in the documentary I saw. Yet it also is a type of discrimination. How would you have decided who would go into the *Titanic*'s lifeboats? This is a classic ethical dilemma.

Why am I describing these two situations for you? It is not to be critical of the people during the suffrage movement era. I am simply sharing my television viewing experiences to point out that the standards of ethical behavior differ depending on the era, culture, or setting, and the individuals. For example, if men in the United States today started jailing women for organizing and expressing themselves, it would be stopped very quickly. The courts would prosecute the men for abuse of authority and the country would be shocked. The difference lies between values that prevailed then and values that prevail now.

What about the lifeboats on the *Titanic*? As a woman, I might think that the system the British used in 1912 was justifiable! As a woman of today, however, I have to admit that saving the women and children and sacrificing the men is a biased system and one that would need to be reviewed if a similar situation occurred today. Please note that all of my thoughts are based on my values.

Personal values are the underlying principles of ethical behavior. *Values* are the personal beliefs about the truth, thoughts, and behaviors of a person. Some nurses willingly work in women's health clinics that perform abortions because of their value and belief that women have the right to decide what happens to their bodies. Other nurses choose to work in clinics that would not place them in a position to assist with abortions because they believe in the right of a fetus to be born. These two examples are not ethical but rather personal values. However, the ethics and values of a person are intertwined and determine behavior.

Different societies and cultures have different ethical standards. Such differences should be respected. It is important for you to identify your personal ethical standards. Have you ever walked out of a store without paying for a package of gum or candy? If the clerk gives you too much change, do you return it? Ethical considerations also relate to your clinical practice as a nurse. Do you take the time to give transpersonal caring? Do you look up medications about which you are unsure? Do you double-check orders that are unclear? Do you call in sick when you are not ill? Such situations relate to your own ethical standards.

As previously noted, when you are faced with a conflict between two or more fundamental values, you are facing an ethical dilemma. What makes ethical dilemmas so difficult is that the conflict is between two fundamental values, not something evil and something good.

REFLECTIVE THINKING

What are your three top personal values? Based on your commitment to getting into nursing school, I would think success in school or getting an education is one of them. What would be the other two? Love of family? Living a healthy lifestyle? Adhering to the values of your religion? Saving money for later years or having fun while you're still young? Love of country? I don't know what they are for you, but it is crucial that you recognize them for yourself. Take some time and think about the question, "What are my strongest personal values?" Talk to others close to you to get input and gain understanding. For most people, this is not an easy assignment, but commit yourself to identifying your values. Then list them in your class notebook. Determining your personal values also will provide the foundation for developing your personal philosophy of nursing.

Now that you have listed your values, what will you do with them as a student and a future LPN? A great deal, I hope.

UNDERSTANDING ETHICS

Most nurses I talk to about ethics do not express concern over being able to make ethical decisions. I applaud them for their strength. When I ask them how they make their ethical decisions or what

process they use, many of them seem surprised that I would ask. It is as if ethical thinking processes were private and not to be shared. That is not true. We all are accountable for our decisions, and when ethics are questioned, we each need to be able to define how we came to our decisions.

The most common answer to my question, "How did you make that ethical decision?" was "My gut." Another common response was "It just felt right." A third response was "It seemed like the right thing to do." These responses demonstrate decisions made by intuition.

Intuition is the feeling that you should or should not do something, and yet there is no reason for having the feeling. Intuition develops through years of practice in making decisions. Research indicates that nurses have confidence in the feelings described as intuition and have described it as helping them to pay more attention to patients when needed (Hassani, Abdi, Jalali, & Salari, 2016). I believe in intuition and have found it helpful in my nursing career. It is a valuable part of each of us, but it is not an acceptable way for a novice nurse to make an ethical decision.

When you are in the hospital, nursing home, or some other care environment caring for people, administering medications, and performing multiple and complex procedures, you need a framework for making ethical decisions. Licensed practical nurses (LPNs) face ethical dilemmas every day. You need to decide how soon to give a pain medication, or whether you should call the physician even though it is 2:00 a.m. Nursing puts you directly into the intimate and critical aspects of other people's lives.

Ethical Principles

Nurses are considered trusted and ethical professionals (Gallup Organization, 2015). When a nurse is faced with a difficult patient situation and decision, thinking and reasoning from a moral framework are required. Moral development begins in childhood and involves learning what is considered right and what is considered wrong. Although morality is considered a personal standard, it becomes part of ethical decision making in the workplace. It is important to understand basic moral and ethical terminology as you move forward in your nursing practice (Box 17.1).

Box 17.1 Ethical Principles

1. *Autonomy:* The right to choose one's own actions
2. *Beneficence:* Do what is good for the patient
3. *Nonmaleficence:* Do no harm to the patient
4. *Justice:* Being just, impartial, or fair
5. *Fidelity:* Faithfulness to promises or agreements
6. *Veracity:* Being truthful and honest

Autonomy

Autonomy is defined as "independent functioning" (Venes, 2016, p. 238), or the right to choose one's own actions. As nurses, we respect the rights of the patients under our care to make choices regarding treatment. Consider medication administration. If you enter a patient's room with medication to be given at certain time, that individual has a right to refuse to take the medication. Even if this impacts the outcome, it is still the right of the patient to refuse. You may need to talk with the patient to discover why the refusal occurred, which will assist in future instances. As a nurse manager, you will also see autonomy as you allow individual nurses to manage their own time during each shift. Not all nurses want to do the same things in the same order, but as long as patient care is not affected, individual time management should not be a problem. Autonomy can have different meanings in other cultures, so become familiar with cultural standards when working with someone from a different background.

Beneficence

Beneficence is a "principle that emphasizes doing what is best for the patient" (Venes, 2016, p. 274), doing good, or showing kindness. An example of an action that would benefit a patient is the discovery of a high pain level during a routine assessment and administering pain medication before continuing other activities, such as walking. As a nurse manager, you could benefit the patient, family, and nursing staff in this situation by assisting the nurse to obtain an order for pain medication if one is not in the chart.

Nonmaleficence

Nonmaleficence is similar to beneficence, but refers to "the principle of not doing something that causes harm" (Venes, 2016, p. 1633), not to inflict harm on purpose, or rather, to do no harm. Consider the situation of a patient who has been losing weight and needs to increase oral intake. You are assigned to assist in the feeding, but as you enter the room you notice the patient is having difficulty breathing. Do you insist that the patient eat for calories? If you decide to feed this patient, you could cause harm if the patient inhales any of the food while trying to breathe. As a manager, you will also have opportunities to do no harm to those with whom you work. There will be times that a staff member will not be able to work because of an injury, such as a sprained wrist. So as not to cause further injury, you would allow this individual to stay home for recovery rather than insisting this person report to work because of already limited staff on duty.

Justice

Justice is an obligation to be impartial or fair, and implies all patients will receive equal treatment (Wilkinson, Treas, Barnett, & Smith, 2016). This is an important concept when working with multiple patients during the day. There may be some patients who are time-consuming and difficult, whereas others are talkative and interactive when you are in the room. It would be easy to spend more time with the talkative patients, but for fairness, you divide the time as needed for each patient, and you do not base it on how much you like being with certain patients. Patient care is also an area in which managers can practice justice as work assignments are made for the shift. A fair manager would divide the workload evenly among the staff and not give all the difficult patients to one staff member and all the easy patients to another staff member.

Fidelity

Fidelity is the concept of faithfulness or keeping promises or agreements (Wilkinson, Treas, Barnett, & Smith, 2016). What if you were checking on each patient before beginning a difficult dressing change and discovered one of the patients wanted pain medication? You tell the patient you will get the medication and return in 5 minutes. To be considered faithful in your promise, you will need to have the medication to the patient in that 5-minute time frame. Honoring requested time off from employees is a way that managers display fidelity. I remember needing to go in to work for meetings on days I had requested off and being approached by a manager to work because I was already at the facility!

Veracity

Veracity is an obligation to tell the truth, or truthfulness (Wilkinson, Treas, Barnett, & Smith, 2016). This involves being honest with patients when questions are asked. I can remember times that I was passing medications and one of the patients wanted to know what every medication was and why it was being given. It would have been so easy to give only minor details so I could get on with my work, but to practice veracity, I needed to give all the information that was requested. Managers can also practice being truthful with employees by discussing the needs of the facility regarding budgeting, staffing, and other needs. It would be much easier just to tell an employee to stay home, but the manager who discusses patient loads and facility needs garners greater respect from the employees.

Ethical Issues

Ethics is a part of nursing. In your work you will encounter ethical situations and problems on a regular basis. The decisions you face may not simply be a choice of what is right or wrong from a personal viewpoint, but will need an understanding of the issues from multiple views. It will be important for you to have a basic understanding of some things that not only have presented health care with wonderful opportunities, but have also raised some questions that require the use of ethical principles and ethical reasoning to obtain the best answers. Genetics has provided us with an opportunity to discover what diseases individuals may encounter during their lifetime. In stem-cell research, which offers hope to repair or grow tissues, ethical questions have been raised regarding how to obtain the stem cells. Bioethics is another area that has given the medical field a vast array of possibilities to improve health for individuals but has also created ethical questions.

Genetics

Imagine being able to identify all the genes that make you who you are. The gene sequences have been identified and can be determined for each individual. This was accomplished in 2003 by the government-funded Human Genome Project that mapped about 25,000 human genes. Gene sequencing provides information about your health and the possibility of planning for the onset of diseases that could affect your mobility, such as arthritis. It can also provide knowledge about possible neurological diseases such as Parkinson's and Huntington's. What a wonderful thing to have to assist with future health decisions! But there are others very interested in this information. Health insurance companies may see this as a way to deny coverage for certain individuals. As a nurse, you may be asked questions about the need for genetic testing, who has a right to the information, and when the patient should tell others about his or her genetic testing. You should have a basic understanding of what is involved. It will also be important for you to explore your personal feelings about issues related to genetic testing.

Stem-Cell Research

Stem-cell research is another area that has offered hope to individuals suffering from conditions in which tissues have been injured or destroyed. Scientists have been able to use stem cells to treat some of these conditions. Think of the joy patients may experience learning about the possibility of having failing health restored through a stem-cell procedure. However, also consider that scientists have encountered questions related to stem-cell research that involve ethical discussions, such as how to obtain the cells. Some research has been based on the use of embryonic stem cells from reproductive technology, which various groups and individuals feel is an improper use of living cells. Research on stem cells is ongoing. To date, research has revealed that certain adult stem cells demonstrate the same properties as embryonic stem cells. These cells may be able to perform the same functions as embryonic stem cells, but ethical decisions about their use will still need to be made. As a nurse, you may be involved in discussions about stem-cell use. Please use the resources at the end of the chapter to help you understand more about this topic.

Bioethics

Bioethics is a new field of ethics that has come about as a result of rapidly expanding knowledge and technologies that are now available. This new knowledge and these new technologies affect decisions about the care of individuals. For example, we have the ability to genetically modify cells. This technology can be used to improve health, such as decreasing the number of children born with inherited diseases. This use of new technology may seem like a wonderful thing to offer to parents who may know that they are carriers of a disease such as cystic fibrosis, but what about the technology being used to determine the color of hair, eyes, skin, or other choices parents may desire in the child? Is it ethical to use this knowledge to design children as requested by parents? The practice of cryogenics (preserving tissue at very low temperatures) carries the possibility of preserving an individual with an inherited disorder who might then be returned to a natural state at a later date when a cure for that disorder is discovered. Is it ethical to preserve individuals who may have funding and not those without the money for preservation? We have technology that can prolong life. Is it ethical to force an individual to use the technology when that person does not desire to have a longer life? There is also the consideration of payment. Should the technology be given only to individuals who are willing and have the ability to pay the high cost of these technologies?

Consider the numerous cases of individuals facing fertility issues. Science is able to offer these individuals options for having a child. One of the options is in vitro fertilization that frequently places more than one embryo in the woman's uterus with the hope that at least one will survive. When more than one embryo maintains viability, the mother is left with a decision about whether to carry all infants or to abort some. This presents an ethical dilemma if the mother does not believe in destroying an embryo. If the mother's health will be put at risk, should the health-care provider insist she have the procedure to remove one or more of the embryos?

Another ethical dilemma to consider is the rights of employees and the rights of an employer owned by a religious organization. Legislation has dictated that all employers are to provide birth control options in the health insurance plans of employees. If the religious organization does not believe in the practice of preventing pregnancy, which party should be granted the right and the ability to observe their beliefs? A decision for the employees would go against the beliefs of the religious organization, but a decision for the religion-based employer would force the employees to access and pay for their birth control.

Bioethics has become an important part of scientific study, and it also raises a number of concerns and questions. You may see or even be involved in stem-cell research, cloning, genetic engineering, euthanasia, and other technologies or medical procedures (Venes, 2016). As a nurse, it will be important for you to be aware of these issues; some of your patients may ask you for information regarding bioethics issues. You may also be involved in the decision-making process related to a bioethical dilemma.

REFLECTIVE THINKING

Review the list of ethical principles. Think of examples of each of the principles and how they relate to your personal or professional life. Include examples for genetics and bioethics. Document your examples for further discussion.

Ethical Theories

There are two predominant ethical theories: deontology and utilitarianism. Their names may be challenging to pronounce, but understanding the theories is important. Sometimes it seems frustrating to have two ethical theories. How do you know which one to use? Is one better for a certain type of situation than the other?

The type of ethical theory you choose to use depends on your personal value system and the value system of the people with whom you are working to resolve the dilemma. This might be a good time to say again that thinking ethically is not always clear-cut. When you know your values, you can move from one concept to another, locating and implementing the best possible solution to the dilemma. It is a challenging way to think. My advice is to learn to value and embrace ambiguity. Show that you are capable of considering alternatives to a problem effectively and within your personal value system. The following descriptions of deontology and utilitarianism are abbreviated but provide you with a foundation on which you can slowly build your ethical knowledge.

Deontology

The word *deontology* is derived from a Greek word that means "that which is obligatory," or one's duty. Duty is what the theory of deontology represents. An underlying principle of deontology is the concept of "to do no harm." Deontological theory, based on the rules and societal norms that determine a person's duty to other people, expects people to feel an obligation to fulfill their duties to one another and to maintain dignity. The concept of human dignity is a strong element of deontological theory (Wilkinson, Treas, Barnett, & Smith, 2016).

How can you apply deontological theory to your personal life? That depends on your personal values. Your values outline what you understand your duty to be. Some people believe their first duty is to their family. Others identify their first duty to be to all of humanity. What could be the difference in the behavior of these two people? Let's look at the example that follows.

There are two men, each of them the hard-working father of three children. As they walk home from work (an effort to save gas and maintain health), they each walk by a homeless person who obviously is malnourished, unclean, and weak. Both of these men are good men. Father No. 1 gives the man enough money for a meal and the address and phone number of the local employment office, then wishes him well and walks home to his family. Father No. 2 sees the man and hails a cab to take them to the local emergency department. There the father arranges to pay for the man's medical bills after he is admitted for malnourishment, even though the hospital bill could be several thousand dollars. He goes to a local store and purchases a new set of clothing for the homeless man and arranges for a work placement counselor to visit him after he feels better.

One may look at father No. 2 in this simple story as the better person. Yet, if you look at each man's personal values, it is clear that both men did what was right for them. Father No. 1 gave the man only what his family could afford to be without. He believes that his family and their needs are his first priority or his highest value. Father No. 2 places his highest value on humanity and did all he could think to do for the homeless man. Two people talking about the same ethical issue could be approaching it from entirely different ways and still be ethical in what they are trying to do. This is how ethics becomes ambiguous and unclear.

To review the deontological theory of ethics, remember it is based on a person doing his or her duty and has a focus on dignity and humanity. The underlying principle is to do no harm to others.

Utilitarianism

The norms and rules for conduct that come from utilitarianism are based on the greatest benefit for the greatest number of people. Decisions made using this theory are based on the utility of the decision or whether the decision is useful to a small or a large number of people. This theory devalues the needs of the individual for the needs of the group (Wilkinson, Treas, Barnett, & Smith, 2016).

Suppose you were a nurse in World War III in the year 2050. You were responsible, among other things, for the one cryogenic machine in your area. A cryogenic machine is a piece of equipment in which people with disease or wounds can be put into stasis until better health-care treatment is available for them. In this case, treatment might be postponed until the war is over or a specialized physician is available. Within an hour, you have two people brought to you to be put into the cryogenic chamber. One is a 97-year-old man, and the other is a U.S. senator on her way to the presidency. If you were a deontologist, you would agonize over the decision and would never feel good about it. If you were a utilitarian, however, there is no question that the senator would be put in the chamber because she has the most potential to impact society.

Utilitarianism is the doctrine that what is useful is good, and the determining consideration of right conduct should be the usefulness of its consequences. In other words, determining what is "right" is based on the greatest benefit for the greatest number of people.

Steps for Ethical Reasoning

There is a basic formula that supports you in making ethical decisions. You need to recognize your personal values and the values of your patient if the situation is a patient issue. Because of the thinking you have done in this chapter, you know whether you are predominantly a deontologist or a utilitarian. When it is time to make the ethical decision, you should use the steps in Box 17.2 for ethical reasoning.

Following this type of thinking process prevents you from following your "gut" reaction and provides you with written documentation of your best thinking regarding the ethical dilemma.

FOCUSED LEARNING CHART:
Ethical Theories
There are two predominant ethical theories used in health care.

DEONTOLOGICAL	UTILITARIAN
Represents "one's duty"	Represents the utility of the decision
"Do no harm"	"Greatest benefit for the greatest number of people"
Based on rules and societal norms	Based on "what is useful is a good thing"
Human dignity and humanity are strong elements	Devalues needs of individuals for needs of the group

---

Box 17.2 Ethical Reasoning Process

1. Clearly identify the problem
2. Identify your personal values as they relate to the dilemma
3. Identify possible alternatives
4. Determine the impact of the outcomes
5. Examine the outcomes as they relate to the listed alternatives
6. Develop a plan of action
7. Implement the plan
8. Evaluate the plan

LEGAL ISSUES

Is cheating on a test at school illegal? You know that cheating on a test is unethical. However, it is not illegal because it is not a criminal act. Police officers do not come storming into the testing center or classroom and arrest students who have cheated.

Compare the idea of cheating on a test with cheating as you administer medications at work. Suppose you are having recurring headaches that interfere with your ability to complete your daily activities. Your physician has prescribed a medication that is ineffective and you want something stronger. You are busy with school and work and don't have time to go back to the physician. A 90-year-old woman with a total knee replacement is on your unit. The woman was admitted in a confused state from a nursing home. You feel sure she would not notice receiving only half a pill for pain rather than the full pill. She regularly receives medication every 3 to 4 hours and you calculate

that you can get at least three half-pills for yourself before your 12-hour shift ends. So you give the woman "half-pills" and take the other halves yourself. Your headache eventually resolves, and you are able to work better for the rest of the shift. You believe that taking some of the patient's medication allowed you to perform your duties better and is acceptable behavior.

I hope you are horrified! What the nurse ("you" in the scenario) did was unethical and illegal. Imagine the pain the older woman experienced because she received only half the prescribed medication. Compound the pain with her preexisting confusion, and it is easy to imagine the nightmare world in which she was forced to live. Which ethical principle or principles did you violate? To place anyone at risk, as the nurse in the story did, is extremely unethical, but let's look at the legal ramifications as well. As an LPN, you are responsible for providing nursing care based on established standards. To neglect to do so is a criminal act. The nurse in this story broke the law and should have been arrested. The tragedy with a confused patient is that the nurse's criminal act probably would never be discovered or reported.

As an LPN, you are responsible for your own ethical and legal behavior. Your legal requirements are essentially determined by the nurse practice act in the state where you practice nursing.

NURSE PRACTICE ACT

Every state has a nurse practice act that governs the laws represented in your licensure and the licensure of other levels of nursing. The nurse practice act in each state provides for the formation of the state board of nursing, the organization that develops and enforces the rules and regulations of nursing practice in the state. The state board of nursing can enforce only the rules and regulations that are in the nurse practice act. The act itself is a set of laws that are determined, written, and changed by the state legislature ("Nurse Practice Act, Rules, & Regulations," n.d.).

State boards of nursing consist of registered nurses (RNs), nurse practitioners (NPs), LPNs, and nursing care consumers. Generally, the governor appoints people to the state board of nursing, although in some states people are elected to the board. The state board of nursing is responsible for nursing practice, nursing licensure, and nursing education for the state.

Another major responsibility of the board is disciplinary action. It is possible for a state board of nursing to withdraw licensure from a nurse, to put a nurse on probation, to require a nurse to be in a substance abuse program before having the license reinstated, and to enact other forms of discipline. Without exception, the state board of nursing is the power organization regarding nursing in every state.

It is crucial that you understand the nurse practice act in the state where you will be working. Nurse practice acts change from state to state, and you cannot assume that the differences do not matter. It is unprofessional and could result in illegal behavior. You cannot be vague about what you can and cannot do as a practicing nurse. When you are licensed, you are totally responsible for knowing and following the dictates of the nurse practice act. Similar to many legal documents, the nurse practice act can be complex and challenging to understand. Check with your instructor to determine whether a copy of the nurse practice act is available for you to review. Perhaps it could be an item of discussion in class.

Generally, the nurse practice act is established into law to assist the nurse to remain within the legal scope of practice *for that state.* It does not provide a list of skills and knowledge an LPN must have to practice. Instead, it provides a framework that the nurse can use along with knowledge, skills, educational preparation, and facility policies and procedures to make legally correct decisions regarding nursing practice.

The nurse *(you)* must follow the law that governs nursing practice. In addition, the nurse must use professional knowledge and critical thinking; this can lead to conflict. The nurse practice act dictates that the nurse has a legal duty to carry out orders given by a health-care provider. As a licensed nurse, there also is a legal and ethical duty to use individual nursing judgment in the delivery of nursing care. How do you obey orders and still act independently? When you believe an order is incorrect, the health-care provider should be approached. If the provider does not clarify or correct the order, the immediate nursing supervisor should be notified. Simply reporting the problem to your supervisor is not enough because the patient still may have needs related to the order in question. Follow through, be a strong patient advocate, and ensure that the order is clarified in the best interest of the patient. A classic example of conflict between obeying the law (the nurse practice act) and being true to your educational and personal ethics follows.

Perhaps the provider orders double the usual dose of a medication. You have had an excellent education and know that the dose ordered is out of the realm of acceptability. You call the provider. She is cross with you for questioning her and tells you to give the medication. The law says you should give the drug; you have a duty to follow the provider's orders. The knowledge and ethical standards you have indicate it is dangerous to give the medication. You immediately notify your supervisor. The supervisor may tell you that the provider is one of the best, and you should give the medication. Is that enough? Should you agree to what the supervisor is asking you to do? I would suggest that you tell the supervisor you cannot, in good conscience, give the medication. Then problemsolve with the supervisor about how to get more information about the drug and its possible impact on the patient. This could warrant a phone call to the pharmacy, or perhaps the supervisor should give the medication instead of you. (This is not a good solution because the patient is still at risk.) The conflicting responsibilities in this situation are serious. You have a responsibility to protect the patient at all costs, but you also have a responsibility to protect yourself and your license. Let me make this perfectly clear: *It does not matter how many people tell you to give the wrong dose of a medication. If it is wrong, you are responsible. Your license and your patient are at risk.*

UNDERSTANDING THE LAW

As a beginning nursing student, you probably are unfamiliar with the laws that will govern your practice. This chapter gives you some basic knowledge that you can build on as you continue your education. Knowing and understanding the law are crucial to your future practice. There are two general sources of law: statutory and common law. Institutional policies and procedures also are discussed in this chapter. There are two classifications of law: criminal and civil. All five items: statutory, common, criminal, and civil law, as well as institutional policies and procedures are discussed in this section.

Statutory Law

Statutory law has two component parts: enacted law and regulatory law. *Enacted laws* are the laws written and passed into law by a formal lawmaking body, such as the state and national legislatures. Enacted laws also can be made by city councils and county organizations. An example of an enacted law that affects each of us almost every day is the speed limit. The speed limit law was made by a statutory body, and official law-enforcement officers are expected to enforce it. An example of a work-related enacted law is the law requiring an LPN to have a license. It is not enough to go to school and be the best in the class. To be an LPN,

It doesn't matter how many people tell you to give the wrong medication. If you give it, you are responsible.

you must pass the licensing examination, pay the proper fees, and receive the piece of paper that states you are an LPN (Wilkinson, Treas, Barnett, & Smith, 2016).

Regulatory laws are made by regulatory agencies to govern according to established rules. Regulatory laws for nursing are the rules and regulations of the state board of nursing. If you were a truck driver, your actions would be regulated by the rules established by the interstate trucking commission. If you were a boxer, the boxing commission would be the governing body. The rules and regulations made by regulatory bodies are the law and are enforced by state or national law enforcement officers. The rules and regulations made by regulatory bodies (state board of nursing) have the same force as enacted law (the state legislature). This fact places a tremendous responsibility on a regulatory body such as the state board of nursing.

Common Law

When an attorney refers to a decision in a previous court case that is similar to the one being tried, he or she is using the principle of common law. *Common law* is based on the common usage, custom, and judicial decisions or court rulings of previous cases. Common law is not as definite or concrete as statutory law. An attorney who uses a previous case is trying to sway the decision of the judge. It may or may not work. Because judges are individuals, each one chooses how to use the common law principle. The decision made by the judge or jury regarding common law is binding.

The previously mentioned situation with the LPN who disagreed with a physician's medication dose is an example of a situation in which common law could be used. Statutory law states that the nurse follow the physician's order. Common law states that the nurse must not act in a way that puts a patient at risk. Common law often is determined by expert witnesses who offer testimony on what they would do in the same situation. An expert witness in the case we've been examining would state the LPN should not give the drug without exploring the reasons for the dose first. Common law is a powerful instrument in making legal decisions (Wilkinson, Treas, Barnett, & Smith, 2016).

Institutional Policies and Procedures

Another type of law, and definitely a consideration when a legal decision is being made, is an institution's policies and procedures. *Institutional policies and procedures* provide guidance to the nurse in how a situation should be managed and the proper course of action. Frequently the court would consider institutional policies as common law. That concept alone is reason enough for an organization to maintain up-to-date policies and procedures that reflect current practice. It also makes it critical that you, especially as a new nurse, know the policies and procedures for the place you work. Because they reflect "common" practice, and you are relatively inexperienced, you need to be sure your practice reflects the common practice of the organization as written in the policy and procedure documents (Rao, n.d.).

Most organizations review the policies and procedures during new employee orientation. This is a time to review them only. It is your responsibility to spend the necessary time to understand what to do in a situation according to the written law (the nurse practice act) and the common law (the institution's policies and procedures). If the policies and procedures indicate that you, as an LPN, can do something you know to be illegal according to the nurse practice act, you must not do it. It does not matter what the common law says if it asks you to break the statutory law. Writing something as a policy or procedure of an institution does not take precedence over regulatory laws (Wilkinson, Treas, Barnett, & Smith, 2016).

Criminal Law

Criminal law applies to laws that affect the public welfare. When a person breaks the law, it is a crime punishable by imprisonment, probation, loss of license, fines, or any combination of these punishments. Criminal laws are designed to preserve society, and punishments are designed to deter people from committing the crimes.

Any violation of a law that governs the practice of nursing is considered a crime (Wilkinson, Treas, Barnett, & Smith, 2016). An example is an LPN who represents himself or herself as an RN. The commission of a crime may be prosecuted even if there was no harm to a patient. It is the act that is wrong.

Civil Law

Civil laws refer to the laws that apply between organizations or individuals. A tort is the violation of a civil law in which another person is wronged. Private persons, groups of private persons, or organizations may request the court to file a civil suit, distinct from criminal proceedings, to be brought against someone or some group. The court generally decides on a plan to correct the wrong, which may include imprisonment or monetary payment for damages or both. Nurses who break the law (generally the rules and regulations of the nurse practice act) can find themselves involved in criminal and civil law cases (Wilkinson, Treas, Barnett, & Smith, 2016).

It is possible for a nurse to be tried in a criminal case and a civil case for the same action. Often, if the LPN is being tried for breaking the law or for damage against a patient, the organization, the RN, and possibly the physician also are being brought to trial.

LEGAL ISSUES SPECIFIC TO NURSING

The law requires nurses to provide safe and competent care. This care is defined as the level of care that would be rendered by a comparable nurse in a similar circumstance and is referred to as a *standard of care.* Every employment environment for nurses should have standards of care. It is your responsibility to review the standards and follow them. Reviewing standards of care is an excellent way to determine whether you are interested in working for an organization. If for any reason you do not think the standards are high enough for quality care to be given, leave the situation immediately. When you do not follow standards of care, you are probably committing a criminal or civil crime. The situations discussed in this section are common problems for nurses. You must be aware of them and thoroughly understand them.

Duty to Seek Medical Care for the Patient

It is the legal duty of the nurse to ensure that every patient receives safe and competent care. The nurse cannot guarantee the patient will receive medical care when it is needed, but it is important that the nurse be a strong advocate for the patient and use every resource to ensure medical care is received. If you determine that a patient in any setting needs medical care, and you do not do everything within your power to obtain that care for the patient, you have breached your duty as a nurse.

Nurses call providers all the time when a patient has a deteriorating condition. This is what the nurse should do; it is an ethical and legal responsibility. Imagine yourself in the following scenario. What would you do?

You have been assigned a postoperative patient who was in surgery until almost midnight. It is now 2:00 a.m., and you note that the patient has experienced a change in vital signs over the past hour. You have continued to take the vital signs every 15 minutes because the patient's initial vital signs were unstable. The patient now has an increased pulse rate and a decreased blood pressure. Although alert when aroused, the patient is restless and pale. The wound has had a moderate amount of drainage, and you have reinforced it once. It is your responsibility to notify the RN about the patient's condition. The RN asks you to call the surgeon to report what is happening. When you make the phone call, the surgeon sounds very sleepy (of course, she did operate until midnight and it is now 2:00 a.m.); however, she gives you an order for a different pain medication and says she will be in early in the morning.

Neither you nor the RN is qualified to make medical diagnoses, but you both recognize that the pain medication will not resolve this patient's problem. It could sedate the patient to the point that it might be dangerous. What do you do? Because you are not a practicing nurse yet, you may not have much experience in solving such problems. You need to start thinking like an LPN, however. This assignment will give you some practice.

Remember the focus in this scenario is your legal responsibility to get medical care for a patient. There are many different actions you could take. Be knowledgeable enough to know what actions follow the institution's policies and procedures and what the standards of care are for the organization. Here is what I would do:

1. I would discuss the phone conversation with the RN. Together we would decide on a course of action. In this situation, I would proceed with the next two steps.
2. I would call the surgeon back and clarify the patient's condition and my concern over the pain medication order. I recognize the second phone call will be irritating to the surgeon, but I have a duty to ensure the patient's medical care. It is hoped that the surgeon will be more alert for the second call (she also may be more irritable, but I can handle that good-naturedly) and will recognize the need to come and assess

the patient herself or ask for another provider to see the patient.
3. If the surgeon does not change her order and my assessment is that the patient's condition is the same or worse, I would call the emergency department physician to come and see the patient. The emergency department physician can assess the patient and then either write more appropriate orders or call the surgeon back and together they can decide what to do.

There are two significant points to remember with the responsibility of providing medical care: (1) You have a duty to do all in your power to obtain appropriate medical care for your patients; (2) you are the patient advocate. No one can do that like a nurse!

Confidentiality

It is a privilege to care for other people. At times, your patients will relate to you in a personal way. One of the outcomes of your relationship is that you may be told information of a personal nature. In addition to what a patient may share with you, you have access to the person's hospital records. The law requires you to treat all such information with strict confidentiality. This is also an ethical issue. Unless a patient has told you something that indicates danger to self or others, you are bound by legal and ethical principles to keep that information confidential (American Nurses Association, 2015).

Does confidentiality mean you do not report areas of concern to the RN or provider? No, you need to share the information with anyone who is part of the care team, but that is all. You don't share patient information with your roommates or family members, the nurse with whom you go to lunch, or the person you ride with in the elevator. Another important concept regarding confidentiality is to share patient information with the right person in the right place, which means a private place.

Let's assume you are working in labor and delivery as part of your clinical experience. Today you are working with a mother who is going to have twins. One of the twins is very small, and the sonogram has caused the obstetrician and pediatrician to be concerned that the smaller twin may have serious complications. You have worked most of the morning with this mother and really feel a commitment to her and her babies. It also has been exciting to work with the RN to prepare the room for a possible "bad" baby. Your excitement carries over when you go to lunch with a school friend who is working in the nursery. It seems normal to tell your friend about the concerns over the one twin and then discuss the different scenarios you and the RN are prepared to manage if a problem occurs. It is an animated conversation. When you leave to put your tray away, however, you turn and recognize the twin's father sitting behind you. It is obvious that he has heard everything you had to say, including some personal things his wife had confided in you. He looks horror stricken and angry.

REFLECTIVE THINKING

In the scenario described, you did breach patient confidentiality. What can you do about your behavior? Make a list and be prepared to submit it to your faculty person. I have made my own list as a way of helping you think about a situation like this one. It is difficult to know exactly what to do when the situation is not real, but, theoretically, the following could be done:

1. Immediately report what you have done to your instructor.
2. The instructor will have you immediately report your behavior to the charge nurse. Follow the directions of the charge nurse. The charge nurse may have you fill out an incident report. A decision would need to be made about whether you would continue to care for the patient. Your behavior could result in dismissal from the nursing program. It may also result in a lawsuit that includes you, the instructor, the charge nurse, the nurse with whom you were working, and the hospital.

What did you do that was a breach of confidentiality? You shared confidential information in a public place with someone who did not have the right to receive the information. In addition, the information was overheard by a family member and others in the cafeteria. What you have done is unethical, and you could be held liable for your actions. *Liability* is a term used to describe the legal obligation a person has to make compensation for an action. If someone stole money, that person could be required to return the money or an equal amount to the person from whom the money was taken. In this instance of breaching confidentiality,

you could be held liable and be sued for breach of privacy and confidentiality.

Permission to Treat

When people are admitted to hospitals, nursing homes, and home health services, they sign a document that gives the personnel in the organization *permission to treat* them. Every time the nurse provides nursing care to a person, however, permission must be obtained. The courts have ruled that people are expected to have some understanding of basic care, which means the nurse should explain briefly what he or she is about to do. The concept of permission to treat should be in your mind as you give nursing care. For example, most personnel who pass food trays automatically ask, "Are you ready to eat?" When preparing to ambulate a person, it is common to ask, "Are you ready to go for a walk now?" These automatic questions actually are permission-to-treat questions. When you are giving medication, you may say, "Here are your pills," or "Here is the new medication the doctor ordered for you." If the patient takes the medication, he or she has given you permission to treat.

The critical aspect of permission to treat is that every person has the right to refuse the treatment or care; they have the right to be autonomous. There are many reasons why a person might refuse treatment or care. It is your responsibility to honor the wishes of the patient. Within that responsibility, you also must try to explain to the patient everything about the treatment or care so that the person will have enough information to consider seriously whether or not to receive the treatment or care.

Do not harass or punish the person in any way, but instead quietly and competently discuss the treatment or care, explain what it is, how it will be done, and the reason it is important. It is not acceptable to say, "Okay, we won't do that treatment," or, "Well it's been 5 days since Mr. Harris had a bath, but he just keeps refusing to take one." It is expected you will do all you can do to promote compliance in a patient while respecting personal wishes. It is a challenging part of the job. In some cases, you may find yourself in conflict between the ethical principles of autonomy and beneficence. It is important to allow Mr. Harris his autonomy by letting him refuse his bath. However, in order to provide good skin care, making sure you are doing

This older woman, who has congestive heart failure, has the right to refuse treatment for her illness.

good for the patient, it is important that Mr. Harris bathe on a regular basis.

There are special situations that relate to permission-to-treat issues. How do you make decisions to treat when working with a child, an elderly person with dementia, or someone with a severe mental illness?

When working with a minor, it is common to have the child refuse treatment such as an injection. The medication (an antibiotic), however, is crucial to the child's recovery. It is hoped that a parent is present and has given you permission to give the medication. Keep in mind that permission from 100 qualified people will not change the reality of you giving an injection to a child who is crying, screaming, and overall terrified. There is nothing transpersonal about this scenario, even though you are acting in a legally and medically responsible manner. My suggestion is to try another approach to give the injection to the child. Following are things I would do to try to administer the medication with the least possible distress and discomfort to the child:

1. Stop the process! The child is overly stressed, and there is simply too much negative energy in the room. You can give the medication late rather than give it under such stressful conditions.
2. Ask the mother or father to hold the child and rock or sing to him or her. This helps the child

and the parent relax. You can give the medication when the child has relaxed.
3. Develop an approach to giving the injection based on what you know about the child. Don't use bribery (remember the ethical principle veracity) but think of something that would intrigue the child so the focus is not on the injection. Some ideas are (a) let the child give his or her doll a pretend injection before you give the real injection; (b) use the old standbys, such as picking out a colorful Band-Aid or the right flavored lollipop; (c) if there is a pet or stuffed animal on the pediatrics unit, let the child hold it while being given the injection. Develop a plan, then if it works, write it on the care plan and share it in report so the patient won't have to be so upset again.

A loving, laughing, diversional tactic generally works with elderly patients with dementia. The key to being successful with someone with dementia is to remember that the person does not have short-term memory. If there is a problem, you can go back in 10 minutes and try something new because the person may not remember you or what happened previously.

Trying new approaches is the key to obtaining cooperation from minors, persons with dementia, and persons who may be mentally ill or developmentally challenged. In these situations, the person probably has a legal guardian. For the child, it generally is the parents. For the person with dementia and the mentally incompetent person, the legal guardian is appointed by the court and often is a family member. Consent for all procedures must be obtained from the legal guardian. Simply having the consent is not enough. It is a skilled and caring nurse who can elicit cooperation from patients so that the treatment and care can be given in a pleasant and meaningful manner.

A final thought about the concept of permission to treat is that any person at any time can change his or her mind and stop the treatment. Perhaps someone is halfway through a liter of intravenous solution and tells you he wants it stopped. You have a legal responsibility to stop the solution. I hope you will try some intervention tactics first, however!

Informed Consent

The concept of permission to treat is closely tied to the concept of informed consent. The law states persons receiving health care must give permission to treat based on informed consent. The principle of *informed consent* states that the person receiving the treatment fully understands the possible outcomes, alternatives to treatment, and all possible consequences.

The health-care provider is responsible for obtaining informed consent for complex medical procedures, such as surgery, chemotherapy, or electroconvulsive therapy, whereas the nurse is responsible for obtaining informed consent for nursing procedures. Check with your institution and review the forms available for informed consent.

Surgical procedures commonly require informed consent. Although the law states that either verbal or written consent is acceptable, most institutions require written consent because it is the most legally binding. It is the provider's responsibility to give the surgical patient the information necessary to meet the requirements for informed consent. It is also the responsibility of the provider to obtain the patient's signature on the consent form. What is your responsibility if the patient asks you questions that indicate to you that he or she does not have the full and necessary information to have the surgical procedure? First, do not have the patient sign the form. (Do not say anything that would be slanderous, such as "Didn't the physician explain that to you?") Then go to your instructor if you are a student or to your charge nurse if you are an LPN, and tell him or her about your perceptions. The person you report to may want to verify what you have said. Do not be offended if that happens. If the patient is found to be lacking in necessary information, the provider should be notified and asked to come in and explain things in more detail to the patient. In this situation, you would not be held legally accountable for the patient not having informed consent, but ethically you are accountable for what happens to every patient in your care.

Defamation of Character

Whenever you say something or share information that is detrimental to another person, you could be held liable for defamation of character. *Defamation of character* is the act of sharing information that is malicious and false. It often is shared during angry moments. There will be times when you have negative feelings about a patient who is noncompliant, vulgar, or hostile or exhibits other behaviors that make him or her difficult. It is

inappropriate to act angrily with such a person. You are the health-care provider, and your responsibility is to manage problems, not add to them.

A negative or hostile verbal remark about anyone in your care is defamation. When the defamation is written, it is called *libel*. Libelous defamation is seen most frequently on a chart when inappropriate comments are made about a patient or the patient's family. When the defamation is oral, it is called *slander*.

The legal concern over defamation is one that you might misinterpret as a reason not to report other professionals for misconduct. If you follow the institutional policies for reporting misconduct, you are not committing slander or libel. When you are in the hallway or even a more private place and are complaining about the poor-quality work of another nurse or physician, you are committing slander. Venting your negative emotions in an improper place is not the professional or legal thing to do (this is the negative communication style called *passive-aggressive behavior*). All problems should be reported to your nursing supervisor, who theoretically will take the problem up the administrative hierarchy for resolution.

Advance Directives

Although the Patient Self-Determination Act was passed by the U.S. Congress in 1990, it was not implemented until 1992. The act states that all health-care institutions are required to give clients or patients an opportunity to determine what lifesaving measures or life-prolonging actions they want implemented. This requirement applies to all hospitals, long-term care facilities, and home health agencies and is to be done at the time of admission. The institution is required to give adequate information to the person and assist in completing any forms. In most situations, the nurse is responsible for educating patients if there is not enough information to make an informed decision.

The purpose of advance directives is to give the person an opportunity to make decisions regarding health care before an illness or a need for treatment occurs that would prohibit making such critical decisions. The major decision made is in regard to resuscitation. Does the patient want cardiopulmonary resuscitation done to prolong life? Other issues to be addressed are use of antibiotics and nutrition. A patient who is legally competent can make all advance directive decisions. These decisions should be discussed with the physician, family members, and significant others so that these individuals have full information about the situation.

Some people have assigned a durable power of attorney to someone they trust to make health-care decisions in their stead. Often, people designate on their advance directive a person assigned to sign consent forms and make other decisions about the welfare and treatment of the patient. It is important for you to know about these details regarding a patient.

Negligence

The law requires nurses to provide safe and competent care. The measure of safe and competent care is the standards of care discussed earlier in this chapter. A standard of care is the level of care that would be given by a comparable nurse in a similar situation. *Negligence* occurs when a person fails to perform according to the standards of care or as a reasonably prudent person would perform in the same situation.

Requirements to Establish Negligence

There are four legal requirements that must be met for negligence to be proved:

1. A standard of care exists.
2. A breach of duty or failure to meet the standard of care has occurred.
3. Damage or injury has resulted from the breach of duty. (This could be commission of an inappropriate action or omission of a necessary or appropriate act.)
4. The injury or damage must result from the nurse's negligence.

I have never met a nurse whose goal was to be negligent, but it does happen. Examples of negligent acts are (1) leaving a patient's bed in high position with the side rails down and the patient becomes confused during the night and falls out of bed; (2) committing medication errors of either omission (not giving the drug) or commission (giving the wrong drug); (3) breaking sterile technique when changing a dressing, with a resultant wound infection; or (4) mistakenly ambulating a patient who is on bedrest.

Nurses are not supposed to make mistakes, yet even the best-educated and well-intentioned nurse can. To avoid neglect, you need to pay attention to the details of your assignment and focus on managing your workload efficiently. It is important to practice such skills now while you are a student and have an instructor to help you determine the most effective way to get your work done.

As previously noted, to be sued for neglect, all four of the listed criteria must be proved. That is easy to do when the damage is obvious, as in a patient who has a fractured hip. But, it is more difficult to prove neglect when the damage is emotional suffering. What is most important for you is to learn the skills and knowledge you are being taught and to implement those things to the best of your ability so that neglect is not a part of your practice.

Malpractice

Malpractice is a term used for negligence. Malpractice specifically refers to negligence by a professional person with a license. You can be sued for malpractice once you have your LPN license. If you are a nursing assistant right now, you may be negligent, but it would not be malpractice because you are not licensed.

Fraud

Few cases of fraud exist in nursing, but it does need to be mentioned. Fraud is a deliberate deception for the purpose of personal gain and usually is prosecuted as a crime. For example, if you applied for an LPN position, stated on the application you were an LPN, reinforced that you were an LPN in the interview, but you had not taken your National Council Licensure Examination for Practical Nurses (NCLEX®-PN) examination yet, then you would have committed fraud. You can complete school and be a graduate practical nurse, but you cannot practice as an LPN unless you have the proper license. In this situation, you intentionally deceived the potential employer for personal gain (the LPN salary), and you could be arrested for fraud. Most courts are harder on cases of fraud compared with cases of negligence or malpractice because fraud is deliberate and results in personal gain.

Assault and Battery

I find that most nurses do not understand the definitions for assault and battery. It is important to your practice that you do understand them. The following definitions are from *Taber's Cyclopedic Medical Dictionary* (Venes, 2016):

- *Assault* is the threat of unlawful touching of another; the willful attempt to harm someone.
- *Battery* is the unlawful touching of another without consent, justification, or excuse. In

legal medicine, battery occurs if a medical or surgical procedure is performed without patient consent.

In both situations, it is not necessary for harm to occur. The events simply need to happen. If you understand and practice the caring and empowering concepts shared in this text, you should never have to be concerned about assault and battery.

Assault can be verbally threatening a patient. Rather than threaten a patient, you need to use your creative tactics to assist the patient in whatever is his or her choice in the matter at hand. By definition, giving an injection or starting an intravenous line when the patient does not want it or simply kindly touching a person who makes it clear the touch is unwanted constitutes battery. You do not have to hurt the person. If you practice transpersonal caring, however, you should not have to be concerned with these legal issues.

False Imprisonment

Preventing movement or making a person stay in a place without obtaining consent is false imprisonment. This can be done through physical or nonphysical means. Physical means include using restraints or locking a person in a room. In some unique situations, restraints and locking patients in a room are acceptable behaviors. This is the case when a prisoner comes to the hospital for treatment or when a patient is a danger to self or others. In these situations, be sure you know the standards of care and the institution's policies regarding physical restraints. To restrain a person is a serious decision. It requires a physician's order and permission of the patient or the patient's family members. Restraints should be used only in the most dire situations and then only if everything else has been tried.

It used to be common practice to use restraints on nursing home residents who wandered or exhibited other behaviors that were difficult to manage. This is no longer an acceptable standard of care. Most nursing homes now have areas for people to wander in safely. Staffing patterns have changed so that residents can have the same freedom as other people. These changes were created by a legal act of the federal government called the Omnibus Budget Reconciliation Act of 1987. The act implemented numerous laws focusing on long-term care and making powerful positive changes for elderly people. The Joint Commission also has guidelines for use of restraints in acute care settings (The Joint Commission, 2009).

Confining a patient by nonphysical means is more difficult to identify. One example is threatening to sedate a person if he or she doesn't stay in his or her room. Another is to take away patients' or residents' clothes to keep them in the facility. These efforts at imprisonment are illegal and unethical. If an individual needs to be confined for safety or healing reasons, you need to talk to the person and explain the situation repeatedly, if necessary. If the patient is not competent, you need to contact the legal guardian or person with durable power of attorney to discuss the situation. Always include the physician in such discussions and obtain the necessary medical orders. Restraining someone is a medical order, not a nursing order. Always refer to the institution's policies and procedures before confining anyone in any manner.

AMA is an acronym used for leaving *against medical advice*. It is the right of every patient (unless they are legally confined, such as a prisoner or someone who has been legally deemed incompetent) to leave the facility at any time. If the patient is competent, just have him or her sign the paperwork. It is hoped that you can spend some time teaching the person about the illness and the treatment that was planned. Sometimes when the nurse does not argue with the patient leaving AMA but follows through on the process, the patient changes his or her mind and decides to stay. Be sure to notify the appropriate people of what is happening and chart everything carefully.

A situation in which the person is not mentally competent is challenging because you have a responsibility to safeguard such individuals. Know your institutional policies regarding this situation and be prepared to call your supervisor, family members, and the physician. You must chart everything in detail. The record is an important part of all legal decisions made regarding health care. There are specific laws regarding the confinement of psychiatric patients who are involuntary admissions. Know the policies and follow them.

The best approach to avoiding a charge of false imprisonment is to work closely with patients who seem at risk for confinement. Talk to them, do an ongoing assessment, assign extra staff to assist the person, or implement some other creative way to manage the problem. To resolve such complex issues is truly practicing the art of nursing.

SAFEGUARDS

Guidelines for Preventing a Lawsuit

Even an innocent mistake could result in a lawsuit. You need to protect yourself from being sued. You can do this by carefully adhering to the following three guidelines:

1. *Knowledge:* Know your patients and their needs and wants. Know your institutional policies and procedures. Know the standards of care for the clinical area where you are working. Know how to give excellent nursing care by applying what you learned in school.
2. *Record and report:* The record you make in the patient chart is a legal document that can be summoned to the court for review or evidence of what happened. Be sure what you record is the truth and is an objective record of events. Do not state your opinion. When you encounter a problem with any patient or the family, you need to report the situation to every appropriate person—the charge nurse, nursing supervisor, physician, and other family members as appropriate.
3. *Question, question, question:* As a new graduate, it is crucial that you ask questions so that you can determine the right approach to resolving problems. Don't assume that you know all there is to know. Remember the principle of being a lifelong learner.

REAL-WORLD CASE STUDY

■ You are a new LPN graduate who just passed your NCLEX®-PN examination. You are working on a medical floor of a large medical center, and you are excited about your job. The patients you care for are interesting people with complex illnesses, and the nurses seem supportive of you as a new nurse. It is a dream job. You have just finished your 1-month orientation and now are working on the 12-hour evening shift from 7:00 p.m. to 7:00 a.m.

This is your first night working after orientation. You are disappointed that the usual RN, the one who oriented you, called in sick and a float RN from labor and delivery is working as the charge nurse. As you take report, you notice that things seem disorganized from the previous shift. You merely see it as a symptom of how busy the shift must have been. You are surprised when you are assigned 14 patients with a nursing assistant to assist you because it is your first "real" shift, and the patients seem very ill according to report.

From the beginning, things don't go well. You recognize as you make your rounds and do your assessments that you have the 14 most ill patients on the floor. You are concerned about the situation. By 10:00 p.m. (3 hours into the shift), you recognize that you are not keeping up with the workload in terms of passing medications on time or giving pain medications in a timely manner. You also have two major dressing changes that need to be done. When you went to the float charge nurse (the labor and delivery nurse), she did not offer any help or solutions and seemed stressed over her own assignment.

1. What are the legal issues that are at risk in this situation?
2. What can the LPN do about the situation?
3. Write the solution to the case study on a separate piece of paper to submit to your instructor.

Key Points

■ Personal values are individual beliefs regarding truth, thoughts, and behaviors. They are the underlying principles that guide ethical behavior. It will be important for you to identify your own personal values and ethical standards to develop your personal philosophy of nursing and decision making.

■ Ethics is a branch of philosophy that examines ideal human behavior. When a nurse is faced with a difficult patient situation and decision, ethical reasoning from a moral framework is required. This framework is guided by principles of autonomy, beneficence, nonmaleficence, justice, fidelity, and veracity.

■ Bioethics is a new field of ethics that has come about due to the rapidly expanding knowledge and technologies that affect individuals, families, communities, and health-care institutions.

Bioethical decisions may be involved with certain medical procedures, treatment, or care.

■ Deontological ethical theories are based on rules and societal norms. They represent the idea of doing one's duty and doing no harm. Human dignity and humanity are strong elements of this principle. Utilitarian ethical theories are based on what's useful. They represent the usefulness of the decision and focus on the greatest benefit for the largest number of people. In this type of ethical theory, the needs of the group are greater than the needs of individuals.

■ Every state has a nurse practice act that governs the laws represented in your licensure. The nurse practice act was established as law to assist the nurse to remain within the legal scope of practice *for that state.* It is crucial that you know and follow the nurse practice act for the state in which you are working.

■ There are two general sources of law: statutory law and common law. An example of statutory law is the required nursing license for practice, whereas common law comes from customs and usage. There are two classifications of law: criminal and civil. Criminal laws apply to laws that affect the public welfare, whereas civil laws refer to the laws between organizations or individuals. Nurses who break the law (generally the rules and regulations of the nurse practice act) can find themselves involved in both criminal and civil law cases.

■ Nurses are governed by rules, regulations, and laws. As an LPN, you are responsible for providing nursing care based on established standards. To neglect to do so is a criminal act.

■ It is the legal duty of the nurse to provide safe and competent care. The employment environment should outline these in the standards of care confidentiality. These include the duty to seek medical care for the patient, confidentiality, and permission to treat.

■ Legal actions that could be taken against a nurse include negligence, malpractice, fraud, assault, battery, and false imprisonment. To safeguard your nursing practice, know your patients, policies and procedures, and standards of care; record patient care and report situations as needed; and ask questions to clarify.

■ The law states persons receiving health care must give permission to treat based on informed consent. The health-care provider is responsible for obtaining informed consent for medical procedures, such as surgery, whereas the nurse is responsible for obtaining informed consent for nursing procedures. Check with your institution and review the forms available for informed consent. The patient should also be given the opportunity to make decisions about lifesaving procedures in the form of advance directives.

ANSWERS TO REAL-WORLD CASE STUDY

There definitely is risk for negligence and malpractice by the LPN and the RN. If medications and dressing changes are being done late, legal problems already have started.

■ *Possible Solutions to the Problem*

Talk to the float charge nurse again. Locate a quiet place where you can get her attention so that she will focus on the problems. Explain your concerns and that you feel you could be negligent in your care.

If all goes well, the RN will agree with you, and together you decide to call the nursing supervisor to ask for more licensed help. If the supervisor has no one else in the hospital who can assist you, the RN needs to call the nurse manager

for the medical floor and tell her that the two of you need more help to give safe and prudent care. This may be upsetting to the nurse manager, but it is much less upsetting than coming in the next morning and finding that there have been serious incidents involving patients.

Any court would find the RN and the LPN guilty of malpractice if something happened to a patient on that shift because they were not practicing in accordance with the standards of care. It is unreasonable for a labor and delivery nurse and a new LPN to manage the care for 14 acutely ill patients. No institution would have a standard of care that approved that staffing situation. Because the RN and LPN are licensed personnel, they are responsible for changing the situation.

REVIEW QUESTIONS

1. You are a nurse on a busy medical unit of a facility and have been assigned six patients. The patients require hourly checks and one of the patients has complained about being cold. On your second round, this patient specifically asks you for an extra blanket. You tell the patient you still have two more patients to check and then you will get the blanket. When you return in 20 minutes with the blanket, you are following the ethical principle of:
   1. Justice.
   2. Beneficence.
   3. Veracity.
   4. Autonomy.

2. A nurse working in an oncology unit has admitted a patient in a great deal of pain. The physician orders do not include any prn medications for pain management. It is late at night and the calls to the physician have not been returned. The nurse tells you she is just going to borrow some pain medication from one of the other patients because she knows what the doctor will order and she can return the medication to other patient's stock. This is an example of:
   1. Standards of care.
   2. Malpractice.
   3. Fraud.
   4. Duty to treat.

3. A nurse is preparing pain medication for a patient and notices the dose listed is higher than recommended for the patient's weight. What would be the best thing for the nurse to do in this situation?
   1. Call the pharmacist to discuss the dosing.
   2. Administer a smaller dose to the patient.
   3. Call the provider to verify the order.
   4. Refuse to give the medication until the order is changed.

4. A patient has been acting out and threatening the nursing staff. A medication is ordered to help calm the patient. When the nurse enters the room, the patient tells the nurse to stay away. The nurse continues into the room and gently guides the patient to the bed, lifting the gown and giving the medication by injection despite protests from the patient. The family learns of the incident and accuses the nurse of which of the following?
   1. Negligence
   2. Slander
   3. Assault
   4. Battery

5. The nurse practice act in each state provides:
   1. Standard nursing care plans.
   2. Licensure to all nurses.
   3. Rules and regulations of nursing practice.
   4. Certification in special organizations.

References

American Nurses Association. (2015). *Privacy and confidentiality: Revised position statement.* Retrieved from http://www.nursingworld.org/MainMenuCategories/EthicsStandards/Ethics-Position-Statements/PrivacyandConfidentiality.html

Chinn, P. L., & Kramer, M. (2014). *Knowledge development in nursing: Theory and process* (9th ed.). St. Louis: Mosby/Elsevier.

Gallup Organization. (2015). *Honesty/ethics in professions.* Retrieved from http://www.gallup.com/poll/1654/Honesty-Ethics-Professions.aspx

Hassani, P., Abdi, A., Jalali, R., & Salari, N. (2016). The perception of intuition in clinical practice by Iranian critical care nurses: A phenomenological study. *Psychology, Research, and Behavior Management, 2016*(9), 31–39.

The Joint Commission. (2009, October). Retrieved from www.jointcommission.org

Nurse Practice Act, Rules, & Regulations. (n.d.). Retrieved from https://www.ncsbn.org/nurse-practice-act.htm

Rao, P. (n.d.). *The policy and procedure manual: Managing "by the book."* Retrieved from http://www.asha.org/slp/healthcare/policy_procedures/

Venes, D. (Ed.). (2016). *Taber's cyclopedic medical dictionary* (23rd ed.). Philadelphia: F.A. Davis.

Wilkinson, J. M., Treas, L. S., Barnett, K. L., & Smith, M. H. (2016). *Fundamentals of nursing: Volume 1. Theory, concepts, and applications* (3rd ed.). Philadelphia: F.A. Davis.

Web Resources

National Council of State Board of Nursing https://www.ncsbn.org/index.htm

International Council of Nurses Code of Ethics www.icn.ch/about-icn/code-of-ethics-for-nurses/

Bioethics http://osp.od.nih.gov/office-clinical-research-and-bioethics-policy

Genetics https://ghr.nlm.nih.gov/

Stem-Cell Research http://stemcells.nih.gov/info/basics/Pages/Default.aspx

18

Understanding Use of Power

LEARNING OUTCOMES

1. Discuss positive and negative approaches to the use of power.
2. Differentiate among the common sources of power.
3. Identify effective power-based strategies for the LPN.
4. Describe and differentiate empowerment for self and others.
5. List five characteristics of powerlessness in people and describe possible interventions.

Things that matter most must never be at the mercy of things which matter least.

—Goethe

The use of power in health care takes on many different forms. One is the power of a large organization to buy and manage smaller hospitals, nursing homes, or home health agencies. Another is the power of a manager to alter work schedules and assignments, control pay raises, and empower or oppress fellow workers. The most critical aspect of power is the power each person possesses on a personal level. It is the power to give or not to give safe and effective nursing care to patients. I am referring to situations in which health-care professionals abuse or take advantage of vulnerable patients. Society knows about and fears the stories of abuse to dependent people in health-care settings, such as nursing homes, state institutions for the developmentally disabled, and state psychiatric hospitals. These incidents do happen in the health-care system, and they show the individual power one person can have over another. Not all use of power is abusive, however.

Personal power in clinical practice allows for the art of nursing to be practiced. The intentional use of what Dr. Jean Watson refers to as the *caring, healing moment* is what I view as the hallmark of nursing. The personal power to design and give care that shows the art of nursing is the greatest privilege of a nurse. Some people use that power to desecrate the foundation of the profession; others use it to make a profound difference in the lives of people, one at a time over a lifetime. From all the information you will read in this chapter about power, the most

The greatest power of a nurse is to participate in caring, healing moments with other people.

important is the awareness of the meaning of personal power in your relationships with other human beings. This power is used by professional nurses at the bedside, chairside, and curbside of humanity while truly practicing the art of the profession.

WHAT IS POWER?

When thinking of power, what thoughts and feelings come to your mind? Many people respond that thinking about power makes them uncomfortable. Some of the phrases that come to mind when considering power are as follows:

• Power play
• Power dress
• Power lunch
• Power deal
• Power talk
• Power hungry
• Power struggle
• Power move

Do these concepts seem unfamiliar to you or even undesirable? This list of phrases shows why some nurses often avoid power situations. This is a new arena for many nurses, who also are predominantly female and frequently not socialized in the use of power. Clinical nurses often are so focused on the daily work of patient care and responsibility that they do not think about "power dressing" or planning a "power lunch." These considerations are not a part of the day-to-day world of nursing practice unless that nurse is a manager. In management roles, nurses are forced to move beyond their personal power skills to power skills and knowledge that affect many people in a dramatic way.

What is power in the management sense? There is not total agreement on what power is for nursing. It is seen, however, as the broader concept under which authority and influence are listed. This is an uncomplicated definition that I like to use: *Power* is the ability to influence others through the use of energy and strength (Weiss & Tappen, 2015). This definition could conjure up thoughts of big, mean bullies who can overpower anyone because of their physical strength. The use of power is quite different from that for most nurses.

Power is something that needs to be developed as a skill to be used and understood. Some people reading this book may think, "I have never had to worry about power in my job before, so why do I have to worry about it now?" This type of comment or thinking indicates a need for more understanding of power.

Take some thoughtful time to look around the organization where you work and identify the power people. In most situations, the administrator or president of the organization is powerful. If that person is not powerful, your organization is in trouble, and you probably can see where the major problems are.

Ideally, the nurse manager at the highest level in your organization is someone who is familiar with the use of power. Does the top nurse manager sit on important committees? Is that person someone whose ideas are listened to by other department heads? Are problems resolved in an efficient manner when the nurse manager is involved? I hope the answers to these questions are yes. If not, again I assume the nursing department in your organization is in trouble, and you can feel it or recognize it.

As you follow the traditional "chain of command" (which also can be referred to as the chain of power), it is important to look at your immediate supervisor or manager. Does that person have power? Does the unit or team run smoothly? Are the supplies you need there for use? Do you and the employees feel confidence in your manager? A "yes" response to these questions indicates that the manager has the power to connect with other departments and to have the work environment conducive to meeting the goals of the team. A positive response also indicates that the manager has the ability to influence others (including you) to work toward the overall goals of the unit or team to get the outlined work done.

You, as the licensed practical nurse (LPN), are the next person in the chain of power, if you have assumed a management role. What power do you have, and what are the most effective ways to use it? One of the purposes of this chapter is to assist you in recognizing these crucial concepts.

TYPES OF POWER

Power does not come in one pretty package conspicuously marked with a bright red bow (notice that the color of the bow I picked was a strong power color) so that you are always able to use it in a variety of ways. It is important to understand the different types of power so that you can identify

Six bases of power.

them in yourself and others. Power types also are referred to as *bases of power* or the *source* from which the power comes (Focused Learning Chart). Power bases are divided into two categories: soft and harsh (Box 18.1). The category a power base represents is determined by how positive or punitive the power base is perceived as being (Mittal & Elias, 2016).

Expert

Expert power is the strongest power base for nursing. One reason you are in school is to become an expert at being an LPN. If you take additional courses, the desire to be an expert at some other aspect of nursing probably is the motivator. Remember our discussion about novice and expert nurses? To whom does the novice nurse go for information or assistance in problem solving? It

---

Box 18.1 Bases of Power

Soft

• Expert
• Legitimate
• Referent
• Informational
• Reward

Harsh

• Coercive
• Reward—if used in a negative manner

Source: Mittal, R., & Elias, S. M. (2016). Social power and leadership in cross-cultural context. *Journal of Management Development, 35*(1), 58–74. doi:10.1108/JMD-02-2014-0020

FOCUSED LEARNING CHART

Bases of Power

It is important to identify the different power bases commonly used by others.

EXPERT POWER

Strongest power base

Positive and nonaggressive way to have power

Requires hard work and an increased level of ability

Genuine power; work hard to earn it

Example: You are seen as "the best" in clinical arenas.

REWARD POWER

Strong power base if not misused

If you use this base, BE FAIR!

Often is used as manipulation

Example: You can give weekends and holidays off and control salary increases.

LEGITIMATE POWER

Person is assigned the power necessary to do the job

Based on knowledge, hard work, and ability

Real power that comes with a title and backing from administration

Example: The chief nursing officer or director of nursing has legitimate power.

COERCIVE POWER

Unhealthy power base

Generally this person does not have the leadership ability necessary for the job

Focus is to hurt and punish others

Avoid this power base

Example: "If you start both of my IVs today, I'll ignore the fact you were late again." *Note:* This person not only does not have leadership skill but also lacks the clinical expertise (expert power) to start her own IVs.

INFORMATIONAL POWER

Genuine source of power

Do not gossip

Accurate information empowers everyone.

Nurse managers have access to a great deal of information!

Example: Nurse manager spends time in meetings with top administrators.

REFERENT POWER

Caring power

Uses the skill of networking to get to know these people

Successful people who are willing to assist others

Example: "I am having dinner with our nurse manager tonight. I will share your great idea with him."

should be to the expert nurse instead of another novice nurse. This is an important concept to keep in mind if you are responsible for the schedule. It is not wise to put novice nurses on the same shift the same day. An expert nurse needs to be there to mentor, support, and teach the novice nurse. If you were in trouble with a patient and wanted another nursing opinion about how to manage the situation, who would you seek out? It should not be another novice nurse.

Being an expert is powerful. It also is a positive, nonaggressive way to have power. Managers

This hospital specializes in treating children and is recognized throughout the western United States. Nurses who work here have expert power, the most important power a nurse can have.

with power based on expert knowledge do not have to engage in power struggles or other types of power battles because when one is an expert, that is an obvious fact not to be questioned. It is a fact that others know because of the expert work of the person with that type of power. It is always noticed. I am sure you can identify the experts in your work area. They don't wear signs or different (power) uniforms; they simply are the experts, and their power is noted by others.

Not everyone can be an expert at every aspect of the profession. I suggest you determine an area of interest and become expert at it. The area could be in administering medication, giving pressure ulcer treatments, making fair schedules with the right mix of people, or effectively managing groups of employees and patients. Expert power is the strongest power base; it is one you should learn to recognize, respect, and develop within yourself.

Reward

Reward power derives from an interesting power base. The person with this type of power has the ability to give rewards to others. Anyone reading this book who has been a parent probably has had experience with reward power. An example is allowing a child to go to the movies with a friend if the household chores assigned to the child are completed. The parent has power over the rewards given to the child.

Nurse managers also have a strong reward power base. A middle manager is responsible for the schedule and with that power determines who gets weekends and holidays off duty. The manager has power over vacation leave and salary increases as well and is the person responsible for the employee's evaluation. This is a strong power base.

Compare the reward power base with the expert power base. The person with an expert power base generally does not or cannot use it to manipulate other employees. It is possible, however, for the person with reward power to do just that. Not everyone who has a reward power base uses it to manipulate people, but it is possible and does happen occasionally. The concept of giving and receiving rewards often alters a person's behavior. The manager may identify and reward favorites or "pets" with the preferred schedules. This type of power also can cause what is referred to as "brownnosing," which is employee behavior performed to receive the most desirable rewards. You can quickly recognize when reward power people are manipulative or are being manipulated because conditions in the work environment are unfair. You feel it, people complain about it, and the possibility for conflict is high.

Not all reward power–based managers use their positions to manipulate others. Many are fair and committed, giving rewards to people who have earned them while using the possibility of a reward to motivate someone else to change behaviors that are undesirable. When you have reward power, which should happen during your management career, keep in mind the importance of using the rewards carefully and with fairness as a mechanism to support the work of the team's responsibilities.

Coercive

The *coercive power* base is exactly what the manipulative use of reward power turns into, coercion. It occurs when someone has reward power and uses it specifically to treat employees negatively. The focus of coercive power is not to assist others to improve or contribute more to the work team but instead specifically to hurt and punish others. This manager has reward power but chooses to use it in a negative manner.

A nurse manager who has coercive power may give a formal reprimand when a quiet teaching moment would have been more effective, may assign undesirable jobs to a nurse who is showing creativity and initiative at work, or may hold the threat of being fired over people who question the manager's thinking. This is an unhealthy power base and must be avoided by nurse managers who wish to be successful.

Information

By virtue of being alive and able to converse with others, you know about *information power*. The person with the most information is listened to and respected. This happens even when the person is sharing information that is not accurate and could be considered gossip. There is something psychologically comforting about getting information even if it is not the truth. You need to determine whether legitimate information is coming from the person who is sharing it. Be discriminating about whose information you value.

Often the nurse manager has a reason to know important information because of work on committees or meetings with other department heads and the administrator. The information that comes from someone in a management position should be valued and recognized as a source of power as opposed to information from someone who does not have a legitimate right to the knowledge.

Knowledge as a power base is a genuine source of power and generally comes with the job of manager on many levels. If you are working with a manager who is not informed or who has information and does not share it with you, you quickly recognize that you have a management problem.

Legitimate

I jokingly refer to *legitimate power* as the power that accompanies the three-line nametag. The inference is that the more lines on a person's nametag, the more responsibility the person has and the more legitimate the power. This person has earned the power that actually accompanies a job and its responsibilities.

REFLECTIVE THINKING

If you had 1 hour to talk to Dr. Jean Watson in her home, what would you say? Stay focused on the topic of power and its use by nurses. Make a list of questions or concerns you would like to discuss with her and record them in your class notebook.

A nurse with the title of nurse manager, head nurse, team leader, charge nurse, or others that are similar has major responsibilities and, theoretically, the power to do the job required. The power

is based on the authority that someone higher in the power chain has given to the nurse manager. That nurse manager has a position in the hierarchy of the organization. Legitimate power is real power, earned by the person who yields it. It is based on knowledge, hard work, and high-level ability.

Referent

Referent power is a caring type of power that many people use but do not recognize as a formal power base. It develops from feelings of admiration and respect for another person. For example, if you knew Dr. Jean Watson personally and shared her views from your personal conversations with her in class, I think you would quickly develop referent power. People would respect you because you had a relationship with such a significant person.

Sometimes people want advice on personal or professional matters. Generally, they seek out someone they admire or who has referent power. Referent power people often do not recognize that they have it. They are the type of person who works in a focused manner to do the right things. They usually are successful in their personal and professional lives and emanate self-confidence and integrity. These people have power because of the way they live their lives and their willingness to share their lives with others. It is the type of power you want to work toward developing.

REFLECTIVE THINKING

Identify four power people in your life. List their power base and ways you can work with them more effectively now that you have identified their power base. Write your comments in your class notebook and be prepared to share them in class.

 ## POWER AND THE ROLE OF LICENSED PRACTICAL NURSES

The information regarding the six power bases is important for you to internalize and to use. Think about the people with whom you work or go to school and the legitimate managers at your job and school. Do they have power? What is their power base? Is it easy or difficult for you to identify the power bases they use? Write the names of four "power" people in your life. Beside each person's name, list their power base; then list reasons why working with them can be more effective now that you have identified their power bases. A sample list follows.

1. Sally Fernandez. Sally is a faculty member with expert and referent power. I should consider her as a mentor in locating my first LPN position. Perhaps I could talk to her about my study habits and see whether she has any suggestions. I should make an effort to get to know her better because by genuinely knowing her, I can learn from her and increase my referent power.
2. Joseph Mills. Joseph is a certified nursing assistant (CNA) on the nursing unit where I have been hired as a CNA until I graduate. He has expert power. He is considered the best CNA on the unit, and nurses and patients request him when difficult care needs to be provided. I should talk to Joseph about helping me to become a strong CNA.

You should make a complete list of people you know and their power source for yourself so that you can apply the information given here about power in a way that has meaning for you personally and professionally. The most important person to look at carefully regarding power is you. Because you are an adult, you do have power of some type. Take the time to examine your power bases and clarify your thinking about how you use the power you have. It also is important to think about the type of power you want to have in the future as an LPN. Think clearly about the types of power you want to develop and the reasons why. This type of early planning can assist you in your role as a nurse manager (Box 18.2). It can give you purpose and focus in the development and use of power.

 ## POSITIVE AND NEGATIVE USES OF POWER

Power can have dramatic effects on the lives of people. It is a resource that can take many shapes. Money is power; use of the media also qualifies. The power of an idea is a concept most people recognize. For example, a 30-second commercial during a widely viewed televised sports event can cost almost $5 million. This amazing example combines the power of money, the media, and an idea all into one powerful, 30-second commercial.

Box 18.2 Leadership Roles Associated With Power

1. Understands the appropriate use of power
2. Uses referent power to develop respect
3. Builds strength in others when possible
4. Role models an empowered nurse
5. Maintains small power gaps between people
6. Wisely uses legitimate power

Source: Adapted from Marquis, B. L., & Huston, C. J. (2015). *Leadership roles and management functions in nursing: Theory and application.* Philadelphia: Wolters Kluwer Health.

As I explained in the introduction to this chapter, power used one-on-one also is dramatic and meaningful. The same is true of group power, as in political parties or armies of nations. An idea, a moment with another person, or the decision of a military leader all could be used to exert power in either a positive or a negative way. It is important for you to identify not only the sources of power but also its uses.

Some people simply want power without concern for the price that is paid for it. King Henry VIII is an example. He had power but wanted more power to overrule the dominant church in order to marry any woman he wished. He used his power to set his own rules and form his own church and had one of his wives put to death for refusing to give up her heir's rights to the kingdom. That is a negative use of power. When power is used to promote oneself or one's ideas without regard for the larger group, it is being used for negative purposes. Consider the situation in which a group of health-care providers are working together on a hospital unit and a new middle manager is hired. This manager comes from another hospital in the city where he managed an efficient unit but left because of disagreements with the administrator. After 1 month on the unit, the manager decides—without using good change theory—that everyone has to work full-time, and the unit must change back to 8-hour shifts. He makes it clear that those who cannot make the change will have an opportunity to apply for positions in other areas of the hospital. The manager has the support of administration because administration desires to support the managers, and there is no apparent recourse to the problem. Within a month, several of the experienced, part-time nurses have left the unit, and others who were in school (because the 12-hour shifts allowed them to go to school and work) either have dropped out of school or have left the unit. The manager has not had any trouble filling the vacant positions, because he can hire former employees from his previous job. He frequently says how he can't work 12-hour shifts because of his pets.

What type of reaction do you have to this scenario? I hope it is a strong one. The manager had the legal right to do what he did. It was, however, a negative use of power because it did not meet the needs of the larger group. Instead, it allowed the manager to surround himself with nurses he already knew, as opposed to nurses who knew the unit, and to work his preferred schedule, not the one that seemed best for the unit. What made this situation worse was that he did not assess to see whether the changes should be made; he simply made them for his convenience.

I hope that you recognize possible ways you could approach this person if presented with such a situation. Assertive communication focused on group needs is appropriate, as is the use of other people on the work team as a source of power. At this point in the book, you also have knowledge about conflict management. This knowledge may be helpful to you in working with this situation.

Almost everyone can describe a person who uses power for personal gain. However, somewhere in your memory banks are scenarios about people with power who used it for positive outcomes. An example is the manager who uses power within the context of the principles taught in this book. The caring and professional application of management theory is the positive use of power. It allows for people to be cared for on a higher level, it encourages thoughtful change, and it brings together forces to support the human potential. Power dressing, power lunches, and power moves are positive concepts when they are used to promote and influence the greater good personally or professionally (Box 18.3).

Another negative use of power is the *power struggle*. This struggle occurs when two people want opposite outcomes and refuse to cooperate with each other. You have witnessed power

> **Box 18.3 Developing Personal Power**
>
> - Learn to compromise and be flexible
> - Take care of yourself to maintain your energy
> - Continually contribute to your organization
> - Present a positive self
> - Obtain additional education and certifications
>
> *Source:* Marquis, B. L., & Huston, C. J. (2015). *Leadership roles and management functions in nursing: Theory and application.* Philadelphia: Wolters Kluwer Health.

struggles or perhaps participated in them. They never are pleasant. There is only one definitive thing to say about a power struggle: *No one wins!* Both people in the struggle come out as losers. As the wise manager you are learning to become, refuse to get involved in a power struggle. You can postpone the discussion until a later date, which gives people time to reevaluate the situation, or you can excuse yourself and walk away. If you choose the second option, make it clear that you are willing to discuss the issue again when you both are able to negotiate a win-win conclusion.

EMPOWERMENT

Empowering Self

Self-empowerment may be something you haven't considered as you have worked through school and its many demands. If you haven't thought about it before, now is an appropriate time. It is essential for a manager to understand the importance of self-empowerment and the ability to support self-empowerment in others. Self-empowerment should be considered first. For the purpose of understanding how to develop self-empowerment, I'll refer to the *self-empowerment ladder* (Box 18.4). It begins with feeling self-confident. For some people, that is a real challenge. You may ask, "How can I feel self-confident when I am still a student, a novice nurse, or a person without much experience in life?"

Self-confidence is one feature that a person truly has to develop from within. Contributions

Box 18.4 Empowerment Ladder

1. Have self-confidence
2. Be able to control life situations
3. Refuse to be a victim
4. Value self and others
5. Be a risk taker
6. Be creative
7. Resolve conflict
8. Show initiative
9. Become empowered

People who have personal empowerment look that way. This young woman has the glow of self-confidence as she poses for this photograph.

from the external world exist, such as feedback from others, experiences of love and trust, and general feeling of acceptance. These aspects of self-confidence assist in building the inner core of confidence that a person needs to feel self-empowered. The inner aspects of self-confidence come from knowledge, experience, and knowing one's skills and abilities. It is a general feeling of "I know who I am, what I am able to do well, and what I need to learn to meet my goals." It does not call for excellence in any area of your life except understanding self. That is the core of feeling self-confident.

A person who has self-confidence is able to control life situations. This ability comes about as the awareness of self increases and gives the individual the information necessary to say "yes" and "no" at the right time and in the right situations. Controlling your life is a great demonstration of personal power, which gives you the ability to avoid being a victim of situations or people. This ability makes the recognition of your personal power crucial.

When a person has control of life situations and refuses to be anyone's victim (employer, spouse, self), he or she has an attitude change. This attitude change generally focuses on valuing oneself and others. One of the most obvious changes is that negative self-talk stops. Most people experience negative self-talk, for example, "I'm too fat," "I'm not smart enough to understand this content," or "I was stupid to get myself into such a mess."

The attitude change that comes from gaining control of your life situations, based on personal self-confidence, allows you to look at other people and see in them their strengths as opposed to only

their weaknesses. People without self-confidence criticize and see only the negative in themselves and others. You may notice the change in your outlook as you move toward empowerment.

You have reached a fun and exciting place to be when you attain the following rungs of the self-empowerment ladder: be a risk taker, be creative, resolve conflict, and show initiative. It sounds complex, but it is a place where you can experiment with confidence now that you are able to take some risks, such as confronting an aggressive person with assertive communication techniques. You can develop and present a totally new idea and be capable of working with people who need to understand it. You are able to embrace conflict and participate in win-win resolutions, and you show initiative by moving forward. You may recognize that you are on these rungs right now because you have the initiative to go to school, to study this book, and to master the skills taught here. You also may be using initiative in your personal life that brings a great deal of creativity to what you are doing.

All of these behaviors bring you to a state of "becoming"—becoming empowered. A self-empowered person has self-confidence, is able to control life situations, and refuses to be a victim. This person recognizes the strengths of others and of self, and because of an awareness of these strengths, an empowered person becomes a risk taker. These skills and experiences take one to the state of being self-empowered.

Why is self-empowerment important? Self-empowerment is essential for successful adulthood. It allows a person to create a life instead of merely existing. It places personal power where it belongs—in the hands of the individual. As a nurse manager, self-empowerment is crucial to being effective in the role. A manager who is not empowered simply follows directions instead of creating a direction. In this democratic society, you have the right to manage your own life and responsibilities. Self-empowered people are successful at living. Your success involves providing successful experiences for others.

Supporting Self-Empowerment in Others

It is not enough to find empowerment for yourself. An inherent responsibility is to assist others in finding it as well. Research shows that when nurses work in environments that promote empowerment, they are more effective in their jobs and have higher job satisfaction (Read & Laschinger, 2015). As a nurse manager who practices under a caring mantle and as a professional who understands and applies the principles of Maslow's hierarchy of needs, you have a responsibility to support empowerment in others as part of your job.

An autocratic manager is not concerned about the empowerment of others because that manager wants only people who follow orders without question. An autocratic manager does not want to encourage independent thinking, self-esteem, or other measures of personal development that lead to creativity, ability to manage conflict, or development of personal and professional initiative. These are characteristics that indicate movement up Maslow's pyramid. They represent needs that go beyond survival and safety. Empowerment of others is a strong caring behavior and a strong motivator to move upward on the needs pyramid. An autocratic manager does not care about these things.

A laissez-faire manager may think that empowerment has been given to all employees because the manager "doesn't get involved" and "lets them work things out themselves." You now know much more about empowerment than the laissez-faire manager does. You know that you have to work in stages to support empowerment of people and give them self-power only when they are ready to assume its responsibility.

As a participative manager, you start the development of an empowering environment by providing opportunities for the employees to develop self-confidence. Employees you are working with on empowerment need to go through the same stages that you do to be truly empowered. Movement upward on the empowerment ladder is the focus of the manager who is trying to empower employees. Similar to so many of the skills you have been asked to learn and implement, this one also takes time and focused attention.

When you identify one person for whom you are responsible as a manager to work with on the process of empowerment, you become empowered yourself. Work with the person to help her or him move up the ladder of empowerment. The first step is to assist the person in developing increased self-confidence. With that self-confidence, the person has more control over life situations. Consider a novice CNA who has been certified for only 3 months. Perhaps to assist the CNA to improve self-confidence, you teach him or her skills that the CNA is now performing in an unpolished or unsure manner. When those skills are retaught or reinforced, the nursing care on your unit improves, and the CNA is on the way to increased self-confidence.

As another example, perhaps there is an LPN you think may resent that you are the charge nurse

Supporting self-empowerment in others begins with building self-confidence. This requires "nonbusy" caring time with the other person.

instead of her. You think this may be the case because there is some aggressive communication from the other LPN toward you on a daily basis. If you role model caring behavior and spend some time alone with this person sharing your observations (aggressive and hostile communication), you can work out an understanding of valuing for each other and a healthy pattern of communication. The LPN immediately has more self-confidence because she understands that you value her skills and decision-making abilities. The LPN's effectiveness as a nurse increases because she spends less energy being angry with you. Also, the fact that the two of you worked out your conflict and now are working as a team contributes to improved nursing care on the unit and to self-confidence for both people. When self-confidence improves for a person, the other rungs of the empowerment ladder fall into place as long as you, as the manager, maintain a caring and supportive environment.

Assisting people, one at a time, to become empowered is good for them, good for you, and good for the patients for whom you are responsible. Empowerment enhances everyone. Try it, talk to people about it, be sure that you are empowered, and then go out and change the world for the rest of us!

POWERLESSNESS

This chapter would be incomplete without a discussion of powerlessness. Powerlessness is a sense of helplessness. Have you ever watched a burning building and been able to do nothing or attended the death of a beautiful teenager who was far too young and unfulfilled to die? These feelings of powerlessness are removed from your personal power base because they are occurrences you can do nothing to stop. Personal powerlessness, however, is a personal nightmare. It brings about feelings of frustration that generally lead to anger; it saps energy levels and leaves the person in a constant state of exhaustion from fighting to alter the balance of power; it defeats the spirit and soul of a person.

Characteristics of personal powerlessness are listed in Box 18.5. I don't believe that they need to be discussed in detail because they are self-evident. If you recognize that you are experiencing the behaviors on the list, you need to stop and reevaluate your life. Consult your mentor, talk to

> ### Box 18.5 Characteristics of Personal Powerlessness
>
> 1. Being threatened by the competence of others
> 2. Accepting a job without sufficient training or experience
> 3. Depending on others to meet own needs
> 4. Transferring feelings of inferiority to others while demanding perfection from subordinates
> 5. "Nitpicking" over small things
> 6. Wanting to keep things predictable
> 7. Being trapped by roles and stereotypes
> 8. Devaluing the group process
> 9. Protecting his or her own turf
> 10. Blaming others to protect self
> 11. Taking all the responsibility
> 12. Resisting change

your manager if the relationship allows it, or seek professional counseling. A person who is exhibiting powerless behavior is someone who needs immediate attention. You need to recognize these behaviors within yourself and find a method for changing them. If you observe them in the people you manage, you need to do a reality check, discover what is causing the behavior, and assist in resolving it. Powerless people do not function well in their jobs, they lose their motivation and drive to do well, and they are a negative influence in any work environment. Such people should not be eliminated from the environment; they should be assessed and worked with in an effort to alter the situation.

Take note of these symptoms of powerlessness and constantly look for them in yourself and in people you manage. If these symptoms occur, take action through any of the previously suggested mechanisms that seem meaningful to you.

CONCLUSION

The management of power in any of its forms is a major responsibility. Some skeptics say that an LPN is not capable of management on such a critical level. I do not agree. In my clinical practice in nursing homes, I see LPNs on a daily basis working wonders with the people in their care and the personnel they manage because of their personal empowerment. These men and women allay any concern I have over an LPN's ability to work with the power shifts and pulls of nursing care. The information in this chapter can assist novice and expert LPNs to use power in their practices. Read it, try it, ask a mentor how it went, and then do it all over again. Do you remember how many times you had to practice to insert a bladder catheter with perfect technique? This is simply a new skill. If you study and practice it, you can incorporate the skill successfully into your professional personality.

REAL-WORLD CASE STUDY

■ You are on a shared governance committee for a hospital nursing unit. The chairperson of the committee, Lucas, a registered nurse with an associate degree who has been out of school for only 3 months, has made a decision for the committee that is unpopular. Lucas has decided that all charge nurses (you are in this group) are to work 6 days on and 2 days off with a 3-day weekend once a month. He makes the decision without using group process, which is how shared governance is designed to work, and he is adamant that this decision is not negotiable but is his right as chairperson of the committee. Lucas seems to be authoritarian in his use of formal power (he is,

after all, the chairperson) and is unwilling to listen to input or ideas from you and other members of the committee.

To accept his scheduling plan would be a serious problem for you and one other charge nurse because both of you are in school and need set days off each week to attend classes. You know that another charge nurse has set a schedule because she tends her grandchildren every Friday and to change that for her would be a serious alteration in her life. As you observe Lucas refusing to listen or discuss his plan, you recognize that he is showing intolerance to the comments being made. He states that the decision has been made and that, as professionals, everyone needs to adjust to the new scheduling pattern. Then the meeting is terminated.

After the meeting, you observe that the charge nurses are angry and stay in the room to complain about Lucas in negative and hostile terms after he has left the room. Several subgroups are complaining about what has just happened. You are not willing to participate in the subgrouping, so you leave the room. At the nurses' station you observe Lucas, who appears angry. He is sharp in his comments with the unit secretary, he is scowling, and his entire body looks tense.

1. What assessment do you make of this situation?
2. What plan can you formulate for dealing with the situation?

Key Points

- In management roles, nurses use power skills and knowledge that affect many people. The use of power is a skill that nurse managers must develop and use wisely because power can have dramatic effects on the lives of others.
- Nurse managers need to understand the various types of power and the effect each type of power has on others. Power is divided into two categories: soft and harsh. The category a power base represents is determined by how positive (soft) or punitive (harsh) the power base is perceived. The management of any type of power is a major responsibility.
- There are six types of power that a nurse manager might use. *Expert power* is the strongest power base and requires an increased level of

ability. *Referent power* is referred to as the caring power and is demonstrated by successful people who are willing to help others. *Reward power* is a strong power base if it is not misused, but it is often used as manipulation. *Legitimate power* is power that comes with a specific title or job. *Informational power* is a genuine source of power used by people who have access to a great deal of information. *Coercive power* is an unhealthy power base generally used by a manager who does not have the skills to do the job.

- As an LPN, you need to determine the power bases you have in your current position and how you use that power. It is also important to determine the types of power you want to develop in the future and the reasons why. This type of early planning can assist you in developing the power you will use as a future nurse manager.

■ The positive use of power is demonstrated when it is used in a caring and professional manner. Positive use of power encourages thoughtful change in an organization and brings people together for the greater good.

■ A negative use of power is a power struggle, which occurs when two people want opposite outcomes and refuse to cooperate with each other. Nurse managers with power based on expert knowledge do not have to engage in power struggles.

■ Self-empowerment begins with feeling self-confident. Once you have self-confidence, you can continue up the self-empowerment ladder. As you work toward empowerment, you will learn to value yourself and others and have a better ability to control life situations. You will be more confident in showing initiative, taking risks, and resolving conflicts. These are important skills for an LPN as well as nurse managers.

■ An inherent responsibility of a nurse manager is to assist others in developing self-empowerment by increasing their self-confidence, knowledge, and skills. When nurses feel self-empowered, they perform at a higher level and provide better patient care.

■ Effective power-based strategies for LPNs include understanding personal power and how it can be used to provide safe, effective patient care, understanding how the various types of power can be used in a positive manner when working with others, and understanding the importance of self-empowerment and supporting self-empowerment in others.

■ Individuals who feel powerless may exhibit some or all of these characteristics: being threatened by the competence of others, transferring feelings of inferiority to others, resisting change, devaluing the group process, and blaming others to protect themselves. When a nurse manager identifies characteristics of powerlessness in an employee, the manager should assess the individual to determine what is causing the behavior and assist the individual in an effort to alter the situation.

ANSWERS TO REAL-WORLD CASE STUDY

This situation is a power struggle that is going to have serious negative effects on the entire staff. The charge nurses are upset, and their passive-aggressive behavior may carry over to others on the staff, and soon everyone may be involved.

1. Your assessment could follow the following format:
   • **Assessment of Lucas**
     It is crucial to try to understand people who attempt to exert power over you. It is important that you spend time to understand Lucas and his behavior. He is a novice nurse with an associate degree. He did pass his National Council Licensure Examination for Registered Nurses (NCLEX®-RN), but he has had little experience in management. Because he has been a nurse for such a short time, you wonder whether he has the experience or theoretical background for his position. His management of the scheduling

change indicates that he does not because of his lack of change theory skills. His presentation indicates an assumption of power that he hasn't earned yet. You identify the situation as a power struggle and want to use your knowledge and skills to resolve it without damage to anyone involved. You perceive that Lucas needs to establish his power base and is using the scheduling plan to do so. It is important not to compromise him while seeking a solution to this problem.
   • **Assessment of the other charge nurses**
     It is clear that the charge nurses as a group are willing to engage in a power struggle with Lucas. This is not a good idea because no one can win. You are not sure the other members of the charge nurse group recognize that fact. You observed passive-aggressive behavior immediately after Lucas left the room and

Continued

are concerned that it may transfer to the entire staff. The members of the charge nurse group are angry and feel powerless. You sense that any progress the group had made in developing empowerment as individuals has been destroyed by this arbitrary decision made by Lucas. You are concerned about the overall functioning of the group and how they may handle this immediate problem.

- **Assessment of yourself**

  This decision has a negative impact on you and your plans for school. You also recognize it as a power move by Lucas and a potential power struggle that could be devastating to the group. You recognize that you feel angry and imposed on by the decision and how it was implemented. Your goal is to resolve the situation with a win-win approach by using your own power base and knowledge.

- **Possible solution**

  You are not the nurse manager for the entire unit or an administrative person. You cannot resolve this problem independently because you do not have the formal power to do so. You recognize that if you take the problem to the nurse manager for the unit, you may be committing the ultimate passive-aggressive "crime"—that of "tattling" to the boss. You are not willing to do that. You recognize that your strengths are the following: (1) You believe you understand the situation, (2) you want a win-win solution, and (3) you have the respect of most of the members of the charge nurse group because of your ability to use management skills and your expert nursing skills. What plan can you formulate with the information you have identified?

2. One possible plan follows. You may have devised a plan different from the one shared here. Many possible approaches would be effective. Examine yours carefully to determine whether it correctly uses the principles of communication and power.

- Informally talk to each of the charge nurses and discuss with them the need for a win-win solution to the problem. If you are comfortable, let them know that passive-aggressive behavior cannot resolve the problem, and show support for Lucas as a nurse.

- After you have communicated with different members of the charge nurse group, you should find that they are still talking about the problem but in a different way. The people in the group are intelligent professionals, and perhaps they needed to be reminded of information (win-win) they had learned previously, or they needed to be taught the concept. The discussions that occur should be less angry and more focused on the solution to the problem.

- When the group as a whole has shown that it is interested in a win-win solution, it is time to approach Lucas. You or anyone from the group can do this; however, it must be done well. Remember this is a nurse who does not want to be told he is a novice. The objective in talking to him is to ask for another meeting to discuss the scheduling format before it goes into effect. Do not make threatening comments like "We have a problem to discuss with you." That may bring out the fear in him and cause him to act in a more autocratic manner. Instead, try this approach: "Lucas, there are some details of the new scheduling procedure the charge nurse group needs to have clarified. Could we have a meeting to clarify them?"

- The meeting should be friendly and have the spirit of cooperation. Lucas should not be threatened. Think of how to support his self-empowerment, which begins with developing his self-confidence. Someone should be prepared to point out the positive aspects of his plan. There are some because, after all, he is not stupid or uneducated; his goal was to bring about an improvement in the scheduling process. Next, someone should identify the problems, one at a time. A barrage of problems should not be presented, but one person at a time should voice concerns until they all are verbalized. Then Lucas can recognize that no one is trying to take away his power or be hostile with him (the group is being nurturing by trying to support him), and he may join in the spirit of cooperation.

• If someone begins to exhibit behavior during the meeting that is not win-win, a member of the group needs to point that out. It is acceptable to say, "The goal of this meeting is to resolve the problem so that everyone is a winner." By showing that professional spirit of working together for one another's good, the problem can be resolved. Often give-and-take is needed to resolve such situations, but that goes with belonging to a group and working successfully within it.

REVIEW QUESTIONS

1. An LPN who has worked at the facility for 10 years is mentoring the new LPN. What type of power is the mentor using?
   1. Legitimate
   2. Coercive
   3. Expert
   4. Referent

2. The LPN is asked her opinion by other nurses about how they can improve their professional practice. What type of power is the LPN demonstrating?
   1. Legitimate
   2. Expert
   3. Informational
   4. Referent

3. Understanding the use of power is important for all nurses.
   1. True
   2. False

4. Which of the following would a person who is self-empowered say?
   1. I can take that challenging patient today.
   2. Are you sure you want me on the committee?
   3. I need help with this patient.
   4. Let's ambulate this patient together.

5. Which of the following best reflects power-lessness? Select all that apply.
   1. Threatened by the confidence of others
   2. Blames others to protect self
   3. Devalues the group process
   4. Requires perfection from others
   5. Takes a job without sufficient training

References

Marquis, B. L., & Huston, C. J. (2015). *Leadership roles and management functions in nursing: Theory and application.* Philadelphia: Wolters Kluwer Health.

Mittal, R., & Elias, S. M. (2016). Social power and leadership in cross-cultural context. *Journal of Management Development, 35*(1), 58–74. doi:10.1108/JMD-02-2014-0020

Read, E., & Laschinger, H. K. S. (2015). The influence of authentic leadership and empowerment on nurses' relational social capital, mental health and job satisfaction over the first year of practice. *The Journal of Advanced Nursing, 71*(7), 1611–1623. doi:10.1111/jan.12625

Weiss, S. A., & Tappen, R. M. (2015). *Essentials of nursing leadership and management* (6th ed.). Philadelphia: F. A. Davis.

Web Resources

Forms of Power https://www.mindtools.com/pages/article/newLDR_56.htm

19

Motivating Employees

LEARNING OUTCOMES

1. Describe intrinsic and extrinsic motivation.
2. Identify the characteristics in nursing of oppressed group behavior and codependent relationships.
3. Use David McGregor's theory X and theory Y when managing staff.
4. List the characteristics of the two factors in Fredrick Herzberg's theory of motivation and indicate the importance of each factor.
5. Discuss ways to create a motivating environment.

Leadership is the art of getting someone else to do something you want done because he wants to do it.

—Dwight D. Eisenhower

Have you given much thought as to what motivates you? It is an important concept to understand about yourself, and once you understand it, you can apply it to your work with others.

Motivation is the general desire to do something or behave in a certain manner. Motivation can be divided into two types: intrinsic and extrinsic. Intrinsic motivation is motivation that comes from within a person to do something because it is rewarding to them. Extrinsic motivation is driven by external rewards such as money or praise (Todde, Routasalo, Helminen, & Suominen, 2015a). Let's consider two nurses recently hired in a skilled nursing facility. One loves working with older adults and sees this as a good fit and is excited to start working with the residents. The other nurse prefers working with children and only took the job in the skilled nursing facility because she needed a job and this was the first job she was offered. The first nurse is intrinsically motivated to take the job and will most likely engage fully in the activities related to the job. The second nurse is extrinsically motivated to take the position and will most likely perform the job at the minimal expectations and move on to a different job when possible. In some situations, motivational factors may be generational. An older nurse who has worked as a unit manager for several years may

decide to step down from her position to work part-time. She is motivated to give up her high-paying administrative job (extrinsic) to work fewer hours and spend more time with her grandchildren (intrinsic). In comparison, a younger nurse may be interested in becoming a unit manager (intrinsic) so she is willing to further her education and work hard to meet her goal.

What motivated you to go to nursing school? It is challenging to become a licensed practical nurse (LPN) in 1 year or less. What motivated you, intrinsically or extrinsically, to do it? Many of you reading this book are in school and working simultaneously. Perhaps you have families for whom you are financially responsible. Perhaps you just enjoy taking care of people and see nursing as a rewarding profession. The motivation you experienced when you entered a nursing program may or may not be clear to you, but it does exist. It would be good for you to clarify for yourself what it is.

All people are motivated to perform the activities of their lives. Remember Dr. Abraham Maslow? Why did he spend most of his adult life designing and researching the needs hierarchy pyramid? He is deceased, so I cannot ask him that question, but I am sure he knew what his motivation was. What motivates you to eat, sleep, or swim to shore instead of drown in a body of water? Why do you take time to talk to people you like and avoid people you don't like? The reason is behavioral motivation.

REFLECTIVE THINKING

Consider what motivates you to perform well in your current job. Make a list and share it with your classmates.

 ## MASLOW'S HIERARCHY OF NEEDS REVISITED

Maslow's work was focused on what motivates people in terms of their desire to meet their needs. He designed a pyramid that clarified levels of needs for people. Why do people eat? They eat because they are hungry, are nervous, or desire something that has a particular taste. Without food, people die; the survival needs, such as food and oxygen, must be met first. The motivation for satisfying survival needs usually is easy to identify; it is basic to the survival of every living thing. The desire to live runs deep in every species; the desire

There has to be a strong motivation to remain in school. Many student LPNs have families and jobs in addition to the demands of school. What is the personal motivation for choosing this lifestyle?

for a pretty dress does not take priority over the need to eat to appease hunger.

Because basic survival needs are easy to recognize, people are more tolerant of them than of other needs. A crying, irritable child who is hungry is tolerated by parents. After the child is fed, the assumption is that he or she will no longer cry. A crying, irritable child who is not hungry, cold, or in pain is not tolerated well. This child is expected to function on a higher level when basic needs are met. The parents may be embarrassed by negative behavior that does not have an apparent cause. Parents generally are critical of this behavior and reprimand or punish a child who exhibits it. Why crying and irritable behavior are acceptable in some circumstances and not in others is related to the tolerance of people for the motivation of the behavior. Perhaps a child who is not hungry is crying because he or she becomes afraid of a store mannequin or feels the emotional need to be held and hugged. Because these needs are not visible or as easy to recognize and identify, they sometimes are not respected by others.

If people who are assumed to be higher on the hierarchy pyramid (they are people with more needs met) act like people on the survival level, there usually is little tolerance for that behavior. An acutely ill, dying patient who is swearing and rejecting others is more likely to be tolerated than a patient well enough to go home who acts in the same way. Why? Because the motivation of the terminally ill patient's behavior is recognized by the staff. The patient is acting out because he or she is in pain and is dying. People can understand that. A higher level of functioning is expected of a person well enough to go home.

Consider for a moment that you are caring for a patient who is acting out and appears to have no reason for pain medications and yet asks for them aggressively and frequently. The patient looks healthy and ambulates without assistance but complains of pain and whines a great deal. There would be minimal tolerance for the patient's behaviors by most staff members. Why? Because the staff might see this person as someone who is higher on the hierarchy pyramid, and they would expect better behavior. Don't misunderstand me; staff members would not be standing around saying, "Well, he is on the third level of the pyramid, so he shouldn't be acting this way!" Instead, people have an expectation based on intuition and life experience about

where someone should be functioning based on what is known about the person.

The reason Maslow's work is being revisited is to clarify an issue regarding motivation that has to do with the imperfections we have as human beings. Many (actually most) humans feel capable of placing people on the needs hierarchy even if they have never heard of Maslow. An 18-year-old mother who can tolerate crying from a hungry child but not from a child without any apparent need to cry is an example. It is possible this mother has never read about or studied Maslow's theory, yet she is acting on a rudimentary understanding of it. That basic reaction to another person is a testimony to the truth of Maslow's work, and presents an opportunity to explore it further.

The larger picture of the theory is that every behavior has a cause. When a child cries or a patient frequently asks for pain medication, we as nurses may not understand the need that motivates the individual, yet it is our obligation to accept it. Why? Because whether we know what it is or is not, the behavior is motivated by an unmet need. The need simply may not be obvious to us. It is egocentric (self-centered) for any nurse to assume he or she knows what motivates every behavior seen in people who are ill; that is impossible. The most professional approach is to recognize that all behavior is motivated by a need. The nurse's responsibility is to identify the unmet need and attempt to meet it in an acceptable manner. It is not the nurse's responsibility to assume knowledge about patients and label them according to one person's or one team's opinions. Whatever you or your team says, the need that motivates the behavior is still the need that motivates the behavior. The fact that you mislabel it does not change the motivation felt by the person. The truth is you, as a nurse, can never understand the many needs that exist. Yet it is your responsibility to work with the unidentified, unmet needs of the people in your care instead of judging them for acting on their unmet needs.

Maslow's hierarchy of needs is an excellent tool but is a concept that no one should assume can be used without truly understanding the person expressing a need—whether employee or patient. I am making an argument against labeling people based on their behavior and then acting on that label. I am suggesting that, as an effective manager, you cannot assume anything about other people that classifies them or labels them. You should apply concepts taught to assist you in understanding human behavior, you should ask the people involved if your concepts are valid, and you should test assumptions that seem clear to you. What you should not do is label and stereotype a person, because it prevents the reality of that individual to be recognized.

To take this concept to the management arena is a critical move. As a nurse manager, you work with many people from diverse backgrounds, experiences, and educational levels. It is apparent that they have many different needs and sources of motivation. To be aware of this extensive diversity and need for individual acknowledgment is one of the most demanding responsibilities of your management job. Managers who (1) assume they know where people are on Maslow's pyramid or (2) label behavior they don't understand and then (3) place someone on the pyramid in a convenient slot are unable to understand individual employee motivation. Without understanding, you are unable to motivate the people who work with you. The result is that the individuals and the organization lose.

When employees are not motivated, the work of the unit or organization gets done, but it does not get done at the optimal level. People are confused about what is asked of them because it does not affect their motivational reasoning. The result often is mediocre work performance. Another aspect of this situation is the loss of motivation for the individual. These people do not reach their potential because they have no reason or motivator to move them there. Often such employees move on looking for a more satisfying position, one that motivates them and really gets them excited. The inability to have an impact on the personal motivation of employees is a losing situation for the people involved and the organization. This is not the type of manager you want to be.

You can avoid this losing situation through learning and using motivational theories, avoiding judging or labeling people, and embracing the diversity of your staff. With motivation coming from so many different sources, you can maintain a great deal of excitement in your work environment. People are eager to work with change, to resolve conflict, and to focus on the goals of the work setting because their own needs are met.

OPPRESSED GROUP BEHAVIOR

Oppressed group behavior is one of the reasons the nursing profession is not always successful in understanding motivation as Maslow expected it to be understood. This is one of the major reasons why nurses find it easy to label people instead of understanding their motivation. It is one of the principles that prevent the nursing profession from achieving its greatness. Finally, it is a critical concept for you to understand.

Oppressed group behavior is part of the history of nursing. Nurses always have been obedient to other forces (Roberts, 2015). Only more recently has their behavior begun to change. Historically, physicians were the leaders and decision makers, and nurses were the handmaidens to the physicians. Early nurses in the United States were educated to do what they were told without questioning their instructions. They were required to be morally clean, plain looking, and willing to work all week with one afternoon off duty. They were expected to live in the nurses' home located near the hospital, and their life commitment was expected to be to their role as caregiver. This scenario is our history, our roots, and our beginning. Only the future can be changed.

Dramatic changes have occurred in the process of nursing throughout the past 100 years, and most of them have taken us to a higher place of functioning. This is good for individuals and the profession overall. Similar to all people, however, we still have our roots with us. I will explain that statement and then apply it to your personal and professional motivation. Groups that are oppressed in different ways, such as by physical violence, financial inequity, or being silenced, express their anger in different ways.

Lateral Violence

One of the classic behaviors of members of an oppressed group is lateral violence. I am confident about the existence of the oppression of nurses across the United States, and I am sure you have witnessed this, perhaps without knowing what it was.

Lateral violence occurs when nurses do not support one another on issues, when nurses talk about one another in passive-aggressive ways, or when nurses refuse to join their professional organization because, subconsciously, they see it as a noncohesive organization without power (Roberts, 2015).

Many nurses educated before the 1970s were educated and employed in an oppressed group behavior mind-set. Notice the seriousness of this nurse and her patients. It is behavior typical of the era.

The phrase "nurses eat their young" is commonly heard in nursing environments. It is the classic oppressed group behavior. Nurses who have been oppressed (older nurses) oppress those who come behind them (younger nurses). The reason is often stated, "I had to do [or learn] it the hard way, and so do they!" I am hopeful you recognize that this attitude does not contain any concepts from caring theory and does not assist anyone to move up Maslow's pyramid. It is destructive, mean, and clearly oppressive.

Do you remember the last time you experienced or observed two or more nurses acting out with passive-aggressive behavior toward another nurse? If you are actively involved in a work setting, it probably was not long ago. Passive-aggressive behavior is one of the most subtle forces of oppression. This behavior does not allow anyone to feel safe, and it does not promote productive teamwork. Definitely not a caring behavior, it promotes the oppression of others in the group (individuals being bashed by a passive-aggressive conversation).

If a physician (male or female) is standing in the hallway of the unit where you work, yelling and shaking a fist at another nurse, do the other nurses on the floor come to the assistance of the abused nurse? I have never seen this happen. Generally, the response to such a horrible situation is for the other nurses to leave the environment or go "to get help." They do not intervene when one of their own is being verbally attacked. Why is that? I cannot speak for every person, but some common reasons may include (1) belief in the myth that physicians are superior and the nurse must deserve what is happening or (2) the passive-aggressive mind-set that lets another person think, "Good, she

deserves that!" when seeing someone else being abused. There are other reasons, but these are the most common I have observed. When lateral violence occurs in the work setting, it creates the inability for nurses to find support from each other and stand as a united group (Roberts, 2015).

Belief in Lesser Value

Another example of oppressed group behavior is that the members tend to think they can "make do" when there are not enough staff members, supplies, or money for raises. These people feel they are of lesser value than others and need to suffer more or do extraordinary deeds to receive any acknowledgment. Do not accept bad situations as okay. If it is a bad situation, it is just that, a bad situation. Acceptance merely adds to the feelings of oppression. People recognize the devaluing behavior of a manager who allows a bad situation to continue. These people react with less self-esteem, more lateral hostility, or other negative behaviors.

Belief in Superiority of Decisions

Another myth of oppression is that all decisions made at the top are superior to the decisions made by subordinates. This is especially dangerous for an LPN to believe. If only top decisions are valued, where does that place your decisions and thinking? Why bother to be a manager if you cannot make decisions that are worthwhile? That type of thinking places patients at risk because LPNs nationally make millions of decisions a day about patient care. This thinking is a myth; it is not true. You have the responsibility to consider all thinking on an issue, but your thoughts and decisions are as powerful and meaningful as anyone else's thoughts and decisions.

A great deal more information on oppressed group behavior is available, and you should research and study it. For the purpose of understanding motivation in self and others, you need to recognize that oppressed group behavior exists, it is rampant in the profession of nursing, and it has to be managed on some level for nursing personnel to feel motivation in a work environment.

Codependency

Codependency is another aspect to consider as a manager. *Codependency* is the need one person has for the continuous presence and support of another person to accomplish the objectives of the job at hand. Codependency is an unhealthy behavior

FOCUSED LEARNING CHART

Recognizing Oppressed Group Behavior

Historically, nurses have been an oppressed group. To change to an empowering group behavior, nurses need to understand oppressed group behavior.

SYMPTOMS

Physical violence

Emotional violence

Financial inequity

Silencing, where no one listens to members of the oppressed group

Expressions of anger over being oppressed

LATERAL VIOLENCE

Nurses do not support one another

Nurses exhibit passive-aggressive behavior

Nurses do not join professional organizations

BELIEF IN LESSER VALUE

Accept the "make-it-do" mind-set

Not enough staff or equipment

Promotes decreased self-esteem

Increased lateral violence

Lack of trust in management

BELIEF IN SUPERIORITY OF DECISIONS

Myth that all decisions made at the top are superior to yours

This thinking places patients at danger because you do not consider a broad view of thinking on a problem; do not automatically accept the decision from the top

Be sure decisions you make are within your practice parameters

CODEPENDENCY

Need of one person for the continued support of another to meet the objective

Takes away the individual strength of a person

Danger to patients and others because of inability to make decisions alone

---

that takes away the individual strength and motivation of a person. Team building is the topic of the next chapter. Teams that work well together may look codependent to the untrained person because of the smoothness and efficiency of the team. Some teams can work together without even indulging in a great deal of communication. This type of relationship often is based on knowledge of the other team members, their commitment and motivation to do an excellent job, and their practice in working together.

Codependency does not function like teamwork. It occurs when one person on the team cannot make a decision or handle a potentially dangerous situation without the other team member or the codependent partner. This behavior does not allow self-fulfillment at work and is dangerous to patients and others. Someone who cannot work without the codependent partner is dangerous and a liability to the entire team. The manager has the responsibility to differentiate between real team players and codependent members of the team. This can be done in part by understanding the motivation of the people involved.

THEORIES OF MOTIVATION

There are many theories of motivation available to study. Because I am a practical person, I do not expect you to learn them all. Instead, I have selected two that I believe are crucial for you to comprehend. The purpose of understanding theories of motivation is for you to apply the theories when working with your coworkers. With that information, you can manage in a work setting where oppression is low, codependency is nonexistent, and motivation to work together to create a meaningful environment is high because you understand the issues related to motivation of people. The two theories are McGregor's (1960) *theory X* and *theory Y* and Herzberg's (1959) *two-factor theory of motivation*.

McGregor's Theory X and Theory Y

Theory X and theory Y focus on the manager's attitudes about people and are described as two opposite attitudes that a manager can possess. The theories themselves express extreme opposite points of view. McGregor wrote his book describing his theories in the 1960s. He designed theory X after the prevailing management style of that era. The 1960s were a time in the American workforce when taking advantage of workers was common and acceptable. The United States had recovered from the Great Depression and World War II, and promoting the economy was a highly valued concept. This attitude allowed for the emergence of a strong work ethic. People worked hard and expected that of themselves and of others. This was an appropriate behavior at the time and presents the thinking represented in McGregor's theory X. Organizations did not provide day care, stress reduction classes, or health promotion centers for employees. Instead, people were happy to have a job (after the Great Depression, this was the reality) and were willing to do whatever was necessary to keep it. That meant hard, focused work that was not based on a sense of group participation or caring.

The theory X manager is someone who believes that people:

• Dislike work
• Need control and force to make them work
• Like to be directed
• Lack ambition

The underlying belief of this manager is that people are lazy. This manager believes that employees dislike responsibility, prefer to be directed, resist change, and want to be kept safe. Can you recognize how oppressive this management style is? Have you ever had to work with this type of manager? This

person thinks that people work only for money (a survival need on Maslow's pyramid) instead of professional satisfaction, pride, or skill development (higher levels on the pyramid). This manager is identified as oppressive because it is difficult for any employee to move beyond survival needs because of the work situation.

The other motivation this manager believes in is punishment. This is a paternalistic attitude and again indicates oppressive behavior. People who are treated as though the only way they can perform well at work is if they are punished for mistakes think they are in prison. They cannot express themselves freely, make suggestions, be creative, or in any way alter the status quo. The rewards for good work are minimal and seldom given. The work of the organization gets done but on a low level of performance. This lack of motivation causes the manager to be even more oppressive and devaluing of workers, and the negative cycle continues.

I don't like being punished, and I don't like punishing others. I prefer caring theory, in which each human being is treated as a unique person to be valued and respected. I have faith in humanity and the indomitable spirit of people. I believe in discussing problems, clarifying misunderstandings, assertive communication, problem-solving, conflict management, and the excitement of change and diversity. It is fair to say that I am not a theory X manager. What is important for you is to identify whether the theory fits you.

It is important for you, the novice manager, to pick your mentors and role models carefully. Theory X managers still exist in the work environment, and they are dangerous to the human soul. Don't make the mistake of mimicking one. Don't pick one for a mentor. Often this type of manager is older or is someone who has worked with a theory X person and has adopted the traits of that management style. You might have a manager who works under these principles. If you do, you will notice it because you feel oppressed.

If you observe or experience theory X behavior, it is important for you to evaluate the impact it has on others. Generally, such employees have decreased self-esteem, motivation, and respect for the work setting and the manager. This, in a nutshell, is the reason why you cannot afford to be a theory X manager. It labels people instead of assisting them to move up the pyramid, and it is oppressive.

This style of management definitely is a lose-lose approach to working with people.

McGregor identified theory X as the predominant motivational approach of managers at the time. His goal was to change it to allow people to have a more satisfying work environment and to develop a more productive workforce overall. His solution to the problem is labeled *theory Y*. Table 19.1 provides information about the characteristics of theory X and theory Y managers.

The theory Y manager believes that people:

• Like to work
• Can be self-disciplined for objectives to which they are committed
• Accept responsibility

I am sure you quickly recognize that this was a radical approach to management in the environment that existed in the 1960s. Because of McGregor's work, however, it is an acceptable and commonly used managerial approach for the modern era. The critical concept in using theory Y is that people can be self-disciplined to objectives they are committed to—in other words, to objectives for which they are motivated to make a commitment.

Theory Y recognizes the complexity of people. This manager acknowledges the creativity in others and identifies ways to seek out motivation for that creativity. Theory Y managers generally identify the following two items as their responsibilities: (1) to motivate others to higher levels on Maslow's pyramid (2) and to allow for the development of creative

TABLE 19.1 CHARACTERISTICS OF THEORY X AND THEORY Y MANAGERS

Theory X manager assumes individuals:	Theory Y manager believes individuals:
1. Dislike work	1. Like work
2. Lack ambition	2. Are self-motivated
3. Need control and force to work	3. Accept responsibility
4. Dislike responsibility	4. Are creative

ideas and behaviors. I cannot help but think that McGregor's manager must have been a theory Y manager who really stood out in the "forest" of theory X managers at the time. He must have been a creative person who was willing to show that valuing or caring behaviors toward others were motivating behaviors.

This textbook is developed around the philosophy of theory Y people. Think back to previous chapters and recognize the caring behaviors that promote motivation. Assertive communication is an example of theory Y, whereas aggressive communication fits the theory X manager well. The latter person does not allow for the expression of new ideas or another person's feelings concerning a situation. Assertive communication invites dialogue, idea sharing, and elimination of value judgments. Another example of theory Y is conflict resolution. The manager who works to promote conflict resolution is open to the ideas of others and is willing to listen to them. This manager embraces conflict as a means to invite new ideas and promote their growth. The same is true of change theory. Its use in an organization gives employees permission to make suggestions and follow through on their theories and concepts. These and other management characteristics allow for the whole person to be at work on the job. The motivated employee is able to determine priorities for self and the organization. This person is committed to the process of growth fostered under the theory Y management style and is able to take risks without punishment. This type of environment is the most challenging and rewarding to a manager because it deals with energy, creativity, and power. Theory Y management allows for the growth of people and the business.

McGregor's theories do not tell you, as a manager, what motivates employees; instead, it is a theory designed for you in your leadership role. It is a theory about the manager's beliefs that can be used to enhance your choices to motivate and empower the people with whom you work. There is a choice—theory X or theory Y.

Herzberg's Two-Factor Theory

Herzberg first published his motivational theory in 1959. On the inside cover of one book, he wrote: "The managerial choice—to be efficient and to be human." This is a positive statement of what this theory proposes. The assumption is that people who are properly motivated in their work have the potential to be efficient and human. Herzberg's work on motivation is a logical extension of McGregor's definition of managers. This theory applies to the employees of an organization and identifies the factors that motivate them.

Herzberg claims that job satisfaction and dissatisfaction are not opposite ends of the same continuum, but instead they are two entirely different continua. The dissatisfied employee files grievances, calls in sick, and quits the job. This is different from no job satisfaction. The employee without job satisfaction goes to work, but does not contribute in a meaningful way and does not make much difference in the work environment. To be motivated, people need to feel satisfaction at work, not just avoid dissatisfaction.

Herzberg says there are two types of factors that play into the motivation of people, and he developed the two-factor theory of motivation. He refers to these two factors as *job hygiene factors* and *job motivation factors*. Both factors are essential for an employee to be motivated in a job and to remain there; in other words, both factors are essential for the employee to be satisfied. It is important to understand the differences and the complementary areas of these two factors.

Hygiene Factors

Hygiene factors seem to be the hardest for a novice manager to understand, so it is a good place to start. Herzberg says that hygiene factors are the factors that keep an employee with the organization. Without them, no one is attracted to the job. These factors actually have nothing to do with motivation, creative ideas, or high productivity levels. They are the attractors and maintainers of a job. Examples of hygiene factors are insurance, holiday and vacation time, job security, and job status. Other hygiene factors include working conditions, interpersonal relationships, type of supervision, company policy and administration, and salary.

Many people react strongly when salary is listed as a hygiene factor instead of a motivation factor. How do you view this category? I believe that if people were honest, they would admit that an increased salary does not consistently increase their work efforts. What if you received a raise that doubled your salary? Does that mean you would work twice as hard or twice as many hours? I don't find that to be true. People may work harder for a while, which is a nice burst of enthusiasm. Others may maintain their status quo, which is a nice, reliable, and consistent forward movement. Some

This child portrays Herzberg's two-factor theory of motivation. This critically ill baby would not be happy or playful even if she had been given the best and brightest toys available.

people enjoy the status that might come with a raise and slow down because they feel secure now that they have the raise. I do not know anyone who has doubled his or her work effort upon receiving a raise. Because of that observation over time, I agree with Herzberg that salary is a hygiene factor; it attracts people to and keeps them at the job. It does not motivate them.

What do you think about the other hygiene factors? Do you agree that they are not motivators? Instead, they attract and maintain employees. I have known many employees who have changed jobs because the insurance offered at one job was better than that of their current job. Many people leave a job because of the management style of their supervisor or unresolved conflict with other employees. This often is the effect of an environment without adequate hygiene factors (Table 19.2).

Motivation Factors

None of the motivation factors should surprise you because in one form or another each of them has been discussed throughout this text. Motivation factors are the managerial behaviors that bring out the best in people, give them professional autonomy, and allow them to grow. Motivators are growth and advancement in the work setting. People are motivated when they are given responsibility and are allowed to follow it through to completion of the assigned project. Another motivator is the actual work itself; this means the manager has designed workloads and assignments that give people satisfaction in what they do. Motivated people receive recognition for their work and experience feelings of achievement.

TABLE 19.2 HERZBERG'S MOTIVATING FACTORS

Job Hygiene Factors	Job Motivation Factors
1. Insurance	1. Professional autonomy
2. Holiday and vacation time	2. Growth and advancement in the work setting
3. Job security	3. Satisfying work
4. Job status	4. Recognition for a job well done
5. Good working conditions	5. Feelings of achievement
6. Interpersonal relationship with coworkers	
7. Appropriate salary	
8. Effective administration	

Doesn't this sound like a great work setting? It is a place where people can do their work with personal commitment and receive praise for it. This work setting results in feelings of pride in a job well done. If you have experienced that feeling, you know how wonderful it is.

A sense of freedom is felt when working in a motivating environment. The employee is allowed to think, create, and act. When the results of this work are excellent patient care, excellent quality assurance, and excellent management of the diversity in a work environment, it is easy to recognize why employees and organizations benefit from theories of motivation.

CREATING A MOTIVATING ENVIRONMENT

You may think that the motivational theories are interesting but have questions about how to apply them to your management position. When trying to create a motivating environment, you need to remember that motivational factors are personal and vary from one individual to the next. This makes it challenging for nurse managers to decide how to motivate each employee. It is important to consider what factors motivate people both intrinsically and extrinsically (Todde, Routasalo, Helminen, & Suominen, 2015a). Nurse managers who are a positive and supportive role model are better at motivating staff. This can be done by seeking opportunities to have positive interactions with your employees that may involve spending time on the unit, having informal and casual conversations with staff as well as scheduling monthly potluck lunches or other casual get-togethers. Providing a positive work environment is motivating and can be accomplished by asking for feedback, involving staff in decision making, providing job autonomy, and giving positive feedback when the job is done well (Todde, Routasalo, Helminen, & Suominen, 2015b). Box 19.1 provides motivating actions a nurse manager can take.

Allowing lateral violence is demotivating for staff and, if it exists, should not be allowed to continue. Assess your unit for lateral violence and immediately deal with employees who exhibit this behavior. As a nurse manager, you are responsible for providing an environment in which employees feel respected and safe (Armmer & Ball, 2015).

Ensuring employees have the necessary equipment and supplies available to provide good patient care can also motivate employees. It is important to foster growth and development in your employees

Box 19.1 Creating a Motivating Work Environment

To create a motivating environment, a nurse manager should take the following actions:

• Engage in positive interactions with staff
• Involve staff in decision making
• Give positive feedback and praise
• Provide autonomy
• Provide needed resources
• Foster job growth and development
• Provide appropriate rewards and incentives
• Engage with staff

by providing educational opportunities to enhance knowledge and skills as well as opportunities for staff to demonstrate their achievements.

Giving incentives and rewards can be motivating but should be done with caution. Rewards should be given in a consistent and spontaneous manner—not saved until an annual event such as a recognition dinner. Rewards should also be based on individual accomplishments. Giving individual praise to employees can be a great motivator. Giving praise can be as simple as a written personal note or, better yet, telling the individual in person that she or he did a good job. If some of these things sound familiar, it is because they support Herzberg's motivational factors.

Conclusion

I have a commitment to the ideas I have shared with you in this chapter. I have a grave concern for our profession because of the preponderance of oppressed group behavior I see and hear about in all types of professional settings. Florence Nightingale did not foresee the behaviors of modern nurses when she went to the Crimea with her bag of gold under her petticoat. She had hope and optimism for a budding profession. Now, more than 100 years later, I wonder how she would feel if she saw and experienced some of what you and I see and experience. I am sure she would express her disappointment, and then she would devise a plan of action for making dramatic changes.

Gone should be the days of nurses hurting nurses, of patients feeling uncared for and about,

and of employees bickering because of the lack of leadership in their professional lives. People deserve a chance to be great at what they do. Nurses have earned that privilege with their long hours and their unerring fulfillment of demanding emotional and physical tasks. They have earned the privilege of being the star caregiver to others who need their skills and compassion. The only factor that may prevent them from being great is themselves.

I have a great deal of feeling for the new generation of nurses. You are one of those large and heroic groups. The tasks of finishing the job so many of us have started are that of molding nursing into a theory Y profession. The responsibility is yours. Please handle it with care.

REAL-WORLD CASE STUDY

■ Develop and describe your ideal employment environment. The criteria for this setting should be based on describing specific actions on the hygiene factor list and on the motivator factor list. This is an opportunity for you to express your ideas regarding the overall content of this book in addition to your personal concepts of leadership and management. At this point, you have read about the activities and decisions that make an effective manager. The implementation of these skills and concepts should allow you to develop an ideal work situation.

Key Points

- Motivation is the general desire to do something or behave in a certain manner. Motivation can be divided into two types: intrinsic and extrinsic. Intrinsic motivation is motivation that comes from within a person to do something because it is rewarding to them. Extrinsic motivation is driven by external rewards.
- Maslow's hierarchy of needs focuses on what motivates people in terms of their desire to meet their needs. Understanding where an individual falls on the hierarchy can help a nurse manager better understand employee behaviors and determine individual ways to motivate each employee.

- Oppressed group behavior is part of the history of nursing. Until recently, nurses have been obedient to other forces such as physicians and administration but now have opportunities to express their ideas and be recognized as leaders in health care.
- Oppressed group behavior in nursing leads to lateral violence within the profession. Lateral violence is demonstrated by nurses not supporting one another and talking about one another in passive-aggressive ways. These behaviors prevent nurses from developing a sense of unity that is important for the nursing profession.

- Codependency prevents individual self-fulfillment at work and is dangerous to patients and coworkers because the codependent person is unable to make appropriate decisions or handle a potentially dangerous situation. Someone who cannot work without the codependent partner is a liability to the entire team and needs to be monitored by the nurse manager.
- McGregor's theory X and theory Y focus on the manager's attitudes about people and are described as two opposite attitudes a manager can possess. Theory X suggests that people lack ambition and need direction and control for motivation. Theory Y suggests that people are willing to accept responsibility and are self-disciplined to get the job done.
- Herzberg's two-factor theory is a motivational theory based on two types of factors: hygiene and motivation. Hygiene factors include a decent salary, benefits, paid vacation, and a good working relationship with coworkers and managers. Motivation factors include professional autonomy, the opportunity for advancement, and recognition for a job well done. Nurse managers should consider both factors when determining the best approach for motivating employees.
- Creating an environment that motivates employees is an important role of the nurse manager. The nurse manager must be approachable and spend time interacting with the staff on an informal basis and provide positive feedback regularly. The nurse manager must also create a positive, safe, and supportive environment by preventing lateral violence from occurring on the unit.

ANSWERS TO REAL-WORLD CASE STUDY

■ *Instructions*

It is impossible to make a list of all the factors that enhance motivation in the work setting. It also is true that each student doing this assignment may do it differently because it is to be done from a personal perspective. Each person may bring to the assignment personal knowledge and experience. Some students may say, "But I have minimal knowledge and no experience." Whatever your situation is, you have something to contribute to this assignment. It is an opportunity to challenge yourself and focus on integrating the content you have been studying. No other critical thinking assignments are included in this chapter, so you can put all your time into this case study. I compliment you now because doing an integrative assignment such as this one is a high-level challenge. The bringing together of many ideas (many of them new) is definitely high-level thinking. Because you are close to the end of this book and, theoretically, this course, it is a challenge you are ready to assume. Go for it. By trying it, you can learn and grow. I am challenging you to be creative, and I am asking you to assume personal responsibility for this project and to see it through to completion.

■ *Discussion of Answer*

The setting I am choosing to design as an ideal workplace is a 100-bed, stand-alone nursing facility. In developing the ideal work environment, where employee motivation is a priority, I would address the following hygiene factors and would work within the power system of the organization to implement these concepts permanently so that they can be relied on over time by the employees.

■ *Salary*

I would survey most of the nursing facilities in the state to determine the salary scales and benefit packages they offer their employees. Then I would establish the salaries for this facility at 5% above the highest I noted in the state. I would build into the personnel policies and responsibilities a mechanism for merit raises and cost-of-living raises for all employees. Based on my survey of other facilities, I would build into the system a benefits package that would equal or exceed those offered elsewhere. An assignment to human resources would be an annual evaluation of existing benefits packages to ensure that this one is kept competitive.

Continued

ANSWERS TO REAL-WORLD CASE STUDY *continued*

■ *Environment*

The environment at the facility needs to be pleasant and designed to meet the needs of personnel and residents. Some of the characteristics I would build into the construction of this new facility include the following:

- Ample parking space
- No more than two residents to a room
- Rooms with ample square footage to allow for residents' personal items and freedom of movement for personnel
- Each nursing unit with a report room, a room for charting, and a room for private conversations among personnel, families, and physicians
- Modern equipment in the facility with a budget for replacement of worn or broken equipment
- Decoration of the facility to be done professionally with an eye to the needs of chronically ill patients and the staff, with a continuous budget item for remodeling every 5 years
- Suggestions for environmental issues to be readily reviewed by an environmental committee

■ *Management*

The requirements for management positions should be clear and include the following:

- An understanding of Watson's caring theory (videos, reference books, and articles available for study)
- Completion of a facility-based management course to be required of every manager in the facility, not just nursing managers
- Effort to be made to recruit managers who embrace diversity in others
- All managers to be expected to attend a regional or national leadership or management conference annually at the expense of the facility
- Because expert power is the strongest power base, all managers will be assisted in designing a plan for maintaining or enhancing their clinical skills
- Administrator to have an open-door communication policy and to delegate power to committees and other self-designed groups

■ *Job Security*

All employees will be asked to give a 1-year commitment to their job. In return, the organization will define the probation period and its responsibilities, the evaluation process, and the commitment of the organization to employees who rate well on the evaluations. One aspect of the job security program is the public relations department, which is committed to resident recruitment and evaluation of satisfaction. The organization also should be willing to commit scholarship or tuition money to employees who continue their education if it relates to the needs of the facility.

■ *Job Status*

In the overall design of this facility, there will be a center for research and an educational partnership with at least one school of nursing for the placement of students. These are two factors that should attract positive attention to the facility. The public relations department will invite organizations in the community to use the meeting rooms at the facility for their events. All these factors combined should attract others to the organization in a manner that results in valuing the organization and improving its status in the community. Another aspect of job status is that of an employee's personal job. All job descriptions will be clearly written and based on allowing the individual creativity of each employee to be used. All employees will be mentored in the role of teamwork and committee work so that decisions and policy changes come from the employees, not the administration. All ideas will be considered and thoughtfully evaluated by specific committees. These activities give employees the opportunity to contribute to the construction of the work environment and their own job status.

This list discusses ideas for consideration in developing an ideal work environment as it pertains to hygiene factors. You may notice that these designs are costly during the development stage. The cost should be paid back to the organization, however, because employees will remain at their jobs instead of leaving, resident and family satisfaction, adoption of creative ideas to improve the organization, and the overall valuing of the organization in the community. These are the factors that attract and keep people at the job, but remember they are not motivators.

Motivating factors take on a different appearance. The motivating factors I would like to implement into my ideal nursing home follow.

■ *Growth and Advancement*

Employees in this facility should know, through orientation and role modeling, that they are rewarded for designing their own professional growth. Budgets will be designed for attendance at conferences, and tuition reimbursement and scholarships will be available. Another example of self-designed growth would be if someone requested 2 weeks of time cross-training in skills that could be best taught at another facility or hospital; such requests will be evaluated and granted. When growth is stimulated and in progress, advancement generally follows. This organization will be a dynamic one in which conflict is resolved, change is encouraged, and communication is based on honesty and caring. Within that framework, advancement could take many forms. People would be supported in specializing if that were their choice, and management could be done in teams if that were a desire of employees. The key to advancement is to allow employees to define it for themselves in ways that fit with the goals of the organization.

■ *Responsibility*

Because all employees who wish to assume a leadership role on a committee or project should be allowed to do so, there will be a great deal of opportunity to assume responsibility in those situations. People with a good idea should be given the opportunity to process it through a committee and, if it is accepted, to implement it. Because of the management training in the facility, managers should know they are to be mentors instead of "bosses" in these situations.

■ *Work Itself*

An organization with employees who love their jobs is one that has mastered the skills of motivation. When people are excited to come to work and eager to tell others about the positive aspects of their jobs, they are showing motivational behaviors. The design of the work environment should make people feel this way. The most dramatic way to promote these feelings is to assure employees they are not going to be forced to work in an oppressed environment. A commitment by administration to avoid oppression in the work setting promotes the joy of the job for the people working there. The response of employees to "the work itself" is something that should be monitored carefully by the management team.

■ *Recognition*

People need to be recognized for the meaningful work they do. This recognition could be publication of their successes, financial awards (remember, this is a hygiene-type reward), announcements in organizational meetings, and permitting employees to share their accomplishments with others such as at facility meetings or presentations at professional conferences.

■ *Achievement*

Great work deserves great rewards. Does a weekend vacation or a set of excellent tickets to a professional sporting event sound like a reward for achievement? These types of recognition generally result in feeling acknowledged. The complexity of achievement in multiple and diverse employees is based on developing a mechanism that allows the workers to achieve. How is this done? It is based on a focus of providing opportunities for employees to move up the pyramid of needs toward their self-actualization. This is complex and requires many of the mechanisms designed into this dream facility.

■ *Final Thoughts*

I know that most LPNs are not involved in designing an ideal work environment. Nevertheless you need to be able to think through the concepts you have learned from this book; that is the focus of this assignment. I hope your "dream" job has been fun to design and that you may have the opportunity to work in such an environment at some time in your future. Best wishes!

REVIEW QUESTIONS

1. Which statement best reflects intrinsic motivation?
   1. I like my job because I enjoy taking care of older adults.
   2. I perform my job well so I can earn the annual merit raise.
   3. I became a nurse because the pay is good.
   4. I collaborate with my coworkers because it is expected.

2. Which statement best reflects oppressed group behavior? Select all that apply.
   1. The physician I work with listens to my ideas.
   2. The nurses do not support each other.
   3. I wish I didn't have to work with the new hire.
   4. We never have enough supplies but somehow we make it work.

3. The nurse manager believes that her employees are self-motivated, creative, and willing to take responsibility for their jobs. This belief represents:
   1. Maslow's hierarchy of needs.
   2. McGregor's theory X.
   3. McGregor's theory Y.
   4. Herzberg's two-factor theory.

4. When identifying what motivates individuals, the nurse manager should consider both intrinsic and extrinsic factors.
   1. True
   2. False

5. Which statement best describes lateral violence?
   1. It is a symptom of oppressed group behavior.
   2. It is common in the workplace.
   3. Nurse managers do not need to be concerned about it.
   4. It only affects staff and has no impact on patient care.

References

Armmer, F., & Ball, C. (2015). Perceptions of horizontal violence in staff nurses and intent to leave. *Work, 51*(1), 91–97. doi:10.3233/WOR-152015

Herzberg, F., Mausner, B., & Snyderman, B. B. (1959). *The motivation to work*. New York: John Wiley.

McGregor, D. (1960). *The human side of enterprise*. New York: McGraw-Hill.

Roberts, S. J. (2015). Lateral violence in nursing: A review of the past three decades. *Nursing Science Quarterly, 28*(1), 36–41. doi:10.1177/0894318814558614

Todde, K., Routasalo, P., Helminen, H., & Suominen, T. (2015a). Hospital nurses' work motivation. *Scandinavian Journal of Caring Sciences, 2015*(29), 248–257. doi:10.1111/scs.12155

Todde, K., Routasalo, P., Helminen, H., & Suominen, T. (2015b). Hospital nurses' working conditions in relation to motivation and patient safety. *Nursing Management-UK, 21*(10), 31–41.

Web Resources

Staff Motivation www.strategiesfornursemanagers.com/ce_detail/212243.cfm#
https://www.mindtools.com/pages/article/motivating-your-team.htm

Workplace Violence http://www.cdc.gov/niosh/topics/violence/training_nurses.html

20

Team Building

LEARNING OUTCOMES

1. State the importance of teamwork in the current health-care delivery system.
2. List five of the eight characteristics of a high-performance team.
3. Briefly discuss the four stages of team development.
4. Define group norms.
5. Differentiate between functional group norms and dysfunctional group norms.

We are what we repeatedly do. Excellence, then, is not an act, but a habit.

—Aristotle

Why do we, as humans and nurses, feel a need to build or be a part of a team? Professional athletes have perfected the ability to work on teams to achieve victory, fame, and financial success. It would have been amusing for retired basketball star Michael Jordan, of the Chicago Bulls and the Washington Wizards, to say to the rest of the basketball team that he was going to play by himself for the remainder of the season. He would be in a unique situation but not in a successful one. Michael Jordan could not retain his title as a champion if he didn't have the rest of the team playing with him to earn those wins. The same is true of LeBron James, forward for the Cleveland Cavaliers, and all members of the Olympic teams training for their moment to perform before the world.

In many situations, teams work. In health care, they are a method of support and strength for the changes that are occurring in the field. In recent years, the Institute of Medicine and the National League for Nursing have issued statements supporting the importance of team collaboration in providing safe patient care and meeting established outcomes. Teams allow for new ideas to be formulated and plans designed for their implementation because of the diverse skills of the team members. Teams bring people together for a common cause and purpose and allow team and individual growth for the betterment of health care overall.

Teams are not perfect when first put together. I can see someone as a novice sports fan saying, "I want LeBron James, Peyton Manning, and Tiger Woods on my soccer team!" It is amusing to the point of being ridiculous, yet it also happens in the teams we build. Teams need to be put together carefully; they also need to be put together *caringly.* This chapter teaches you how to build a team to enhance the patient care and management roles of your profession. Often this aspect of your management role is done in conjunction with the registered nurse (RN). When you learn how to build and maintain a team, you may be asked to do it over and over again as a nurse manager so that you can do it perfectly. Happy practicing!

UNDERSTANDING CHARACTERISTICS OF A TEAM

To develop and maintain an effective team, it is crucial to understand what makes a team work and what the characteristics of a high-performance team are. There are nine characteristics that you need to learn and perfect so that they can be applied to any team with which you work (Box 20.1). You have teams in both your personal and professional life. The information about these characteristics can translate across those lines and should be important to both types of teams.

Clear and Elevating Goal

The first characteristic is a clear and elevating goal. People in our hectic society do not want to be a part of anything that is not going to be important to

Teams allow for new ideas and plans to emerge because of the diverse skills of the team members.

> ## Box 20.1 Nine Characteristics of a High-Performance Team
>
> 1. Clear and elevating goal
> 2. Results-driven structure
> 3. Competent team members
> 4. Unified commitment
> 5. Collaborative climate
> 6. Standards of excellence
> 7. External support and recognition
> 8. Principled leadership
> 9. Trust

them and a good use of their time. That is the importance of the goal. The goal has to be clear to the potential team members, and it should be elevating and something the participants can take pride in doing. Otherwise the team concept that you are sharing is not desirable enough for people to commit to doing.

It may seem as though every nursing unit throughout the United States is a natural team, but (in my opinion) that is not true. There are groups of people working together in the same space and with the same patients, but do they all exhibit teamwork? I don't think they do. There are many teams, but it is not a natural phenomenon and should not be assumed. We have spent a great deal of time in this book trying to understand people's behavior. Why are they passive-aggressive, passive, assertive, or aggressive in their communication style? Why can't people work without anger and hostility? What causes professional and educated people to be uncooperative or to sabotage one another? Why isn't there more praise for work well done? I believe it is because people may work together, but they do not always work together as a team.

Look around the environment in which you work or have clinical experiences. Can you observe the people working there and determine whether they are a team or just people working together? I think you may be able to do so with this brief explanation. The foremost thing to look for is the clear and elevating goal.

For nursing units in hospitals and nursing homes, it is common to have as the goal "excellence in administering caring nursing care to the patients and residents on this unit." That is an elevated goal, but it is vague. It is the type of goal that needs to be explained further, such as "excellence can be determined by …" This list would need to be specific to each unit. That would make the goal clear and elevating and would be a rallying point for the team members. When a team has a goal similar to the one just described, it often serves as an attractor for other people who want to be on a team with that level of quality.

If the goal is clear (a critical point), people should be able to share it. It would be common for team members to share their goal with others without hesitation or confusion. On the nursing units where there is no goal and no teamwork, people may make nonspecific statements such as, "We give good care," "I like working here because it is fun," or some other comment that does not meet the criteria of being clear and elevating. If there is a goal, people repeat it with pride. That is one of the hallmarks of a successful team.

Results-Driven Structure

For a team to function, it must meet the second characteristic: having a results-driven structure. This is the responsibility of the manager. This characteristic may be retained by the RN on the team and may not be delegated to you. Often the structure is managed by the administrator or a manager higher than the unit manager. This characteristic has a great deal to do with quality assurance checks that provide the team with the ability to meet its goal. It also requires an environment that has the resources, space, and staffing to ensure that the goal can be met consistently. It demands that the team and its performance be constantly evaluated and reordered if necessary. This is done as a method of support, not as criticism or complaint, and is a proactive stance assumed by the manager to see that the team has its needs met and the ability to be accountable for its performance. Results-driven structure fits into the thought circle that plans, performs, evaluates, and changes. This characteristic calls for a team that is dynamic and truly embraces change as a method of improving its service to patients and the organization.

A unit that meets the criteria for this second characteristic is always busy; its energy needs and output are high. The motivation for all that expenditure of energy is to meet the goal and to validate through some process that the goal has been met. It takes focused work and constant support from the administration, team, or personnel. If this characteristic exists in a workplace, you notice it.

Competent Team Members

The third characteristic calls for competent team members. A person may think this is an easy characteristic to meet because of the criteria for employment in most health-care settings. Such an assumption should not be made, however. Because someone is an RN or a licensed practical nurse (LPN) does not mean he or she has the ability to be a team player. Go back again to the sports analogy: Some people are golfers, and other people play on a football team. The differences are in the person's approach to problem-solving, ability to share the satisfaction of goal achievement (some people cannot share it), and willingness to share

Group members should have a high level of expertise, as this nurse does after working for the past decade.

knowledge and expertise. People are successful on a team if they are (1) knowledgeable about how a team works and can work there and (2) an expert in a skill that is desirable to the team and its goal.

On an oncology floor, someone should be an expert in counseling patients and their families in the legal necessities of managing estates of people who are dying, another person should be an expert in administering the specific oncological medications, and another person should be an expert in supporting terminally ill people through the grieving process. These subspecialties of oncology are crucial to the goal (assuming that the goal is excellent care). They are not valuable to the team, however, unless each expert also is good at being a team member. The phrase "a team player" has strong meaning when considering the needed characteristics of a team.

Unified Commitment

Characteristic number four is unified commitment. This characteristic takes us back to the initial goal of the team. It is important to have a goal, but without commitment to it, nothing of significance can happen. Some people live life as a checklist. As far as being a member of a team, they may say, "Let's see, hum, yes, I have a goal. Okay, done,"

then move on to something else. These people do not have a commitment to the goal. I am not bashing people who make lists because I am one. I am saying that a mechanical approach to being a member of a team does not allow for the commitment to surface; the commitment is a requirement of the process. The commitment called for is not your personal, individualized commitment, but it is a unified commitment from the group.

REFLECTIVE THINKING

Write in your class notebook a clear and elevating goal that would draw you to work on a nursing unit. Carefully consider what is important to you. Make the goal easy to understand and impossible to misunderstand. Take some time to think about the goal before you write it in the book. It should be a well-thought-out statement.

An unspoken aspect of unified commitment is the commitment each member needs to have for others on the team. That statement should have flashed across your mind with thoughts of caring, mentoring, nurturing, and role modeling. These are ideas with which you are familiar; now you need to understand that unified commitment is another way to use what you have learned. If there is a unified commitment among the team members, all can focus on the team goal and assist others to achieve it as well. Unified commitment calls for modesty in seeking the rewards of the team's work and a never-ending focus for the completion of the work being done.

Collaborative Climate

The fifth characteristic of teamwork is a collaborative climate. This is similar to working within an environment with a unified commitment. The term *collaboration* relates to the ability to work together. This is a comfortable place to be, where little is threatening or harmful. People have permission to be a learner and a teacher. The art of mentoring is elevated in this environment. Decisions are made as a group and not independently. Generally, people in this type of environment are able to do their best because they feel the empowerment of other group members.

If you notice that people on a team are expressing frustration at being told what to do or not being involved in the decision-making process, the collaborative climate is missing. When power is being used to accomplish the goals of the unit, the environment is oppressive and collaboration does not exist. Some team members express positive ideas about being a part of the team and then eventually admit that they do not have decision-making power. These team members are usually frustrated, and the other benefits of being on a team are lost if this one does not exist.

Standards of Excellence

The sixth characteristic is standards of excellence. If you understand the previous characteristics of a team, you should have no problem with this one. This is more like an outcome of the other characteristics instead of a characteristic itself. It indicates that the goal is met with excellence. If that excellence exists, you can see it, sense it, and feel the atmosphere of a real team working.

External Support and Recognition

Characteristic seven is external support and recognition. The successful team has administrative support. The team knows that support exists and is able to call on that support when the goal of the team or the criteria of excellence are threatened. This characteristic is most obvious in teams that have been in existence successfully for a long time. People in other areas know that the excellent team may be honored, their project may be approved, or their budget may be increased. This knowledge often motivates other teams to strive for a clear and elevating goal and a standard of excellence.

Principled Leadership

The eighth characteristic of a high-performance team is principled leadership. Do you remember the leader discussed in Chapter 10? who had the map for finding the right way through the jungle? This person is *principled,* a term that refers to a variety of characteristics. Some of these characteristics are being focused on the goal. Others are being focused on the members of the team and their needs (could this be caring?), being clear on how best to assist the team, and maintaining high standards for personal and professional conduct. A principled leader is a person with standards of patient care, personal communication, professional behavior, and ability to

discipline self. In addition, a principled leader is an asset to any team and is a team member worth seeking.

Build Trust

The ninth and probably the most important characteristic of a team is trust. Without a foundation of trust, teams are unlikely to be successful. Teams that do not have trust among the members are less productive and do not collaborate well together (Craig & Mckeown 2015). Developing trust in the team leader and other team members is a process that will require time. Some ways to develop trust are getting to know team members on a personal level and developing good interpersonal relationships, giving others the benefit of the doubt, and admitting when a mistake is made. Once trust is established, it is easier to manage conflict within the team and accomplish team goals (MindTools, 2016).

Summary

The nine characteristics of a high-performance team are valuable to you in understanding why a team is working but not performing or why a team is working and performing. The use of these characteristics is similar to making an assessment of a team. Are the characteristics all there? If they aren't, how is their absence affecting the team? How can you as a manager assist the team in acquiring all nine of the characteristics? This method of assessment and level of awareness gives you purpose and focus in working with any team in your work environment.

STAGES OF TEAM DEVELOPMENT

When working with team-building concepts, it is common to learn to identify the four stages of team development originally developed by Bruce Tuckman more than 50 years ago (Tuckman, 1965). (Box 20.2.) The words for these stages are humorous, yet the concept of each stage is significant to the success of the team. The stages of team development unfold as the characteristics of a high-performance team are developed. It is interesting to observe the two processes happening simultaneously. The characteristics develop and strengthen as the energy of the team builds through the four stages. As you review these stages, consider whether you have ever noticed

The four phases of team development: forming, storming, norming, and performing.

the behaviors exhibited by each stage as you work. Then determine what and where you have seen a stage so that it has real meaning for you.

Stage One: Forming

This stage allows the team members time to get to know one another, recognize and value one another's expertise, and work through the need all humans have to develop trust in a relationship. None of this happens quickly or without some sacrifice or pain. It never can happen unless the group is brought together to do the work of forming as a team.

Stage Two: Storming

The second stage is one that some individuals in the group try to avoid. The storming that comes in this normal sequence of team development is often

---

Box 20.2 Building a Successful Team

- Foster a collaborative and trusting environment
- Empower team decision making
- Look for diversity in team members
- Assign responsibilities based on individual strengths
- Allow teams to work autonomously
- Provide continued feedback
- Periodically evaluate team effectiveness

Source: Rao, M. S. (2016). Collaborate to build effective teams to achieve organizational excellence and effectiveness. *Industrial and Commercial, 48*(1), 24–28. doi:10.1108/ICT-01-2015-0010

---

uncomfortable emotionally. People have to work through this stage to move toward the fourth and final performing stage of the team. It is a time when people share their ideas, recognize that the group members have different ideas, and then work out any problems the variety of ideas presents to the team. This stage is challenging, but if managed assertively, it is a meaningful and interesting part of the team-building process. Storming is work that must be done.

Why do people have to have storms or conflict? You have read the chapter on conflict and should recognize that the diversity of the team members and their varying viewpoints bring conflict into the team's work group. This is the time for the group to define roles and objectives, settle philosophical differences, and then move on. The last step is the important one in this stage. After the conflicts have been resolved, keep the group moving toward its overall goal.

Stage Three: Norming

This is an interesting stage of the team's development. The group is together (formed) and has a purpose. It has endured and resolved the team's conflict, and it is working at establishing the status quo or norming for the team. It is difficult for some managers to agree that these stages are necessary and must be given the time it takes to process through them. Teams never get to norming—the process of establishing their work schedule and roles—if they have not been given time to form and storm. This can be frustrating for a manager who wants the work done right now. It is crucial for the leader of the team to provide the time necessary for the team to develop into a healthy work group. This is not the story of Cinderella where mice turn into horses and pumpkins turn into carriages. This is the real world of management, and people need support and time. Providing these crucial aspects of team development is one of the characteristics of a team—external support and recognition.

Stage Four: Performing

This is the time when a team is most productive and the members are able to accomplish their goals successfully. The faltering start and conflict resolution of previous stages do not exist here; there are no impediments to the processes of the team. This is the work time. If a team that has achieved this stage regresses to another stage of group development, you need to assist the members in evaluating

These community health nurses are taking water samples in a community that has reported water contamination. They have achieved the performing stage (stage four) of teamwork.

why that has happened. It often occurs when an established member of the team leaves and someone new replaces the original person. The group needs to learn to work together again without the former person and with the new one. Usually the stages do not take as long as they did originally. The regression also can occur when the goals or the environment change. As a manager, it is your responsibility to recognize the reality of these changes and give support to the team while the changes are in progress. Theoretically, the work output is worth the support and group development time.

GROUP NORMS

An understanding that is crucial to teamwork is based on the concept of group norms. A norm is a common concept in group dynamics. It is something that exists only at the group level; different groups have the potential of having different norms. Are you in class right now? There are norms to your group's classroom behavior. For example, sometimes there is a norm about where people sit in the classroom. Some people like the same seat each week, and their placement in the same chair is seen as a group norm. This type of

norm is obvious when someone new comes into the class and sits in someone else's seat. The group reacts. Another classroom norm could be based on eating or not eating in the classroom or on addressing the teacher. If the teacher is always referred to as Mrs. Fredricks, and a new person comes to class and refers to her as Jean, the group members note the disruption in the norm and generally try to change the behavior of the person who broke with the group's norm of behavior. All groups have the possibility of having functional and dysfunctional group norms.

Functional Behaviors

The functional and desirable behaviors of a group include the following:

1. The ability to welcome new members
2. The willing assistance given to group members who are in crisis
3. A group decision to end meetings on time
4. Attending meetings well prepared
5. A strong attempt to keep group members informed and up-to-date on group happenings
6. The commitment to celebrate special occasions as a group (i.e., weddings, birthdays, and graduations)

Dysfunctional Behaviors

Dysfunctional behaviors cause problems in the group. These behaviors need the skills of a strong manager to resolve them and bring the group back to a functional state. Common dysfunctional behaviors include the following:

1. The demonstration of distrust because of the lack of confidentiality
2. A lack of willingness to take risks
3. Frank comments taken personally by group members (comments being personalized)

Managerial Feedback and Support

The successful manager of a team needs to recognize the functional and dysfunctional behaviors of the group and inform the group of what has been observed and the way it has had an impact on the work of the team. A high-performance team needs this feedback to maintain the performance standards that already have been established.

Sharing observations and expectations is a fair way to manage a team. The other important concept is that teams showing dysfunctional behaviors need time and support to change themselves. An unsupportive attitude defeats the purpose of a team and the effectiveness of having many experts working together to achieve change. Patience and ever-present support are required to allow the team to be successful.

Licensed Practical Nurse Role

The role of most LPNs on a team would not be that of manager. You may be relieved to know this. However, you may be asked to chair an important committee. Being a member on a high-performance team is a demanding position. It requires attention to many details, group behaviors, and personalities. This information on functional and dysfunctional teams is important for you, as an LPN, to note and remember. If you observe dysfunctional behaviors, share what you have seen with other members of the team in an open and caring way. Always be objective and clear in what you are saying, and share your information in an open dialogue in which feedback is permitted. This is a risk-taking role. As an LPN, you are prepared to assume these responsibilities.

REFLECTIVE THINKING

Evaluate your class to determine the class norms. Talk to other class members to identify what is the norm of the class. List the functional and dysfunctional behaviors of the class as a team, as you have identified them. If you have identified a reason for the functional or dysfunctional behaviors, list it.

UNDERSTANDING THE VALUE OF TEAM CONCEPTS

Care and service teams are the new priority in health care. Their effective use is imperative to organizational and individual survival. No longer can one nurse or caregiver meet the multiple and complex needs of today's care recipients. High-performance teams are crucial to the overall effectiveness of an organization because these teams can address the diversity in care that is required while processing and planning additional care needs. That is impossible for a single person to do.

Teamwork is crucial to the quality and level of caring that needs to be given, on a consistent level, to people in the health-care system. Previously, teamwork was not seen as the necessary approach

to work, but in the current health-care environment, collaboration and teamwork are essential to achieving quality patient outcomes and cost control for individuals and organizations. This is an aspect of management that would be easy to ignore, but no manager can afford to do so.

CONCLUSION

It is important to think of the group work you do in school, at work, and in the clinical setting as a student. The application of the ideas in this chapter to real work teams is important. You may find that when you are able to identify teams and their characteristics, their stages, and their skill at functional versus dysfunctional group behavior, you are better able to work in a group. That is the goal. You have learned how to communicate, make change, work with conflict, and motivate employees; now the ultimate test of your skills is to work successfully on a team of high-performance people.

REAL-WORLD CASE STUDY

■ You are the 7:00 p.m. to 7:00 a.m. shift charge nurse in a 56-bed skilled nursing facility. You have been asked to participate on the interdisciplinary team that meets twice a week to evaluate and set goals for residents with resident and family input. This is an exciting invitation, and you are eager to be an active member of the team. You think there is a great deal of information about residents that is identified on the evening shift, and you want to share it with the team members. You believe strongly that it can make a difference in the overall care of the residents. This is your ultimate goal as a nurse in the facility.

As you consider the reality of being on a well-established, high-performance team such as the interdisciplinary team, you have some feelings of anxiety: Will you fit into the team effectively; will they accept or reject you? What do you really have to offer this team of experienced professionals? As these questions come to your mind, you realize that you are not helpless in this situation.

1. How can you learn about teams in general and this team specifically to ease your membership into the group?
2. List at least six strategies that you could use to achieve this goal.

Key Points

- In today's ever-changing health-care environment, working as a team is a critical component to providing quality patient care and meeting positive outcomes. Teams allow for new ideas to be formulated because of the diverse knowledge and skills of the team members. Teams bring people together for a common purpose and allow team and individual growth for the betterment of health care overall.

- High-performing teams must have a clear and elevating goal that is recognized as accepted by all team members. Team members must take pride in the goal otherwise, members will not commit to meeting that goal. Without this unified commitment, the desired outcomes will not be met.

- Teams should be developed with competent team members willing to share knowledge and expertise. Individuals will be successful on the team if they understand how teams work and the importance of being a team player, as well as having the expertise that is desirable for the team.

- The team leader must be focused on the goal, understand team members' needs and how to best assist the team, and always maintain high standards of personal and professional conduct. The team leader should expect administrative support for the team leader role as well as support for the rest of the team.

- When developing teams, it is important to understand the four stages of team development. *Forming* is the stage in which team members begin developing good relationships. *Storming* is the stage in which the team identifies differing points of view and works to resolve any conflicts related to differing views. *Norming* occurs when the team has resolved any conflict and is able to work together as a group to begin working toward the goal. The final stage, *performing,* occurs when the team is most productive and ultimately meets the desired goal. Teams will not always move through the four stages in a linear manner.

- Groups develop group norms that provide a framework for working together. Group norms will vary from group to group and are determined by the group members. All groups have the potential for having functional and dysfunctional group norms.

ANSWERS TO REAL-WORLD CASE STUDY

1. You need to investigate a variety of resources for learning about teams in general and for evaluating this team.
2. Some strategies you may want to implement include the following:
   - Think back to previous group experiences. How did you function in those groups? What information would have helped you then?
   - Talk to a member of the team you know and ask some of the questions about which you have been concerned. This is a good time to get information you need and to see whether the team members are willing to share with and mentor new members.
   - Review a book about team building so that you are up to date with the basic characteristics and stages necessary for a successful team.
   - Go to meetings on time and be prepared with pertinent information about the residents in your care.
   - Remember that it is normal for the team to experience changes in its ability to function when a new member joins. Be prepared to be seen as the new kid on the block and accept the temporary change in team performance.
   - Choose to be a functional, high-level performer.

REVIEW QUESTIONS

1. The LPN has been assigned as the chair for a new committee. Which best describes her role as the new chair?
   1. Support all committee members
   2. Work closely with the administration
   3. Work more closely with members who have the most experience
   4. Take full responsibility for the team's actions

2. Which best describes the characteristics of a team performing at a high level? Select all that apply.
   1. Clear goal
   2. Competent team members
   3. Support from some administrators
   4. Members trust each other
   5. Includes a good leader

3. Working in teams is widely accepted in health care as a way to achieve positive outcomes and provide quality care.
   1. True
   2. False

4. The newly formed wound care team is disagreeing on their goals for the team. This team is in what stage of development?
   1. Forming
   2. Storming
   3. Norming
   4. Performing

5. The nurse manager has a unit team that is demonstrating dysfunctional behaviors. Which statement describes how best to handle the situation?
   1. Disband the current team and select a new team.
   2. Provide time and support until the team works out their issues.
   3. Bring in upper administration to help solve the problems.
   4. Assign a new team leader so the team can be more effective.

References

Craig, M., & Mckeown, D. (2015).) How to build effective teams in healthcare. *Nursing Times, 111*(14), 16–18.

MindTools. (2016). Building trust inside your team. Retrieved from https://www.mindtools.com/pages/article/building-trust-team.htm

Rao, M. S. (2016). Collaborate to build effective teams to achieve organizational excellence and effectiveness. *Industrial and Commercial, 48*(1), 24–28. doi:10.1108/ICT-01-2015-0010

Tuckman, B. (1965). Developmental sequence in small groups. *Psychological Bulletin, 63*(3), 384–399. Retrieved from http://dx.doi.org/10.1037/h0022100

Web Resources

Team Building Techniques www.team-building-techniques.com/index.html

TeamSTEPPS www.ahrq.gov/professionals/education/curriculum-tools/teamstepps/index.html

21

Delegating, Coaching, and Evaluating Performance

SALLY CANTWELL

KEY TERMS

Acuity systems
Coaching
Delegation
Evaluation
Performance analysis

CHAPTER CONCEPTS

Collaboration
Communication
Leadership and Management

LEARNING OUTCOMES

1. Discuss the differences between leadership and management.
2. Apply the three rules of delegation.
3. Identify specific ways to support the empowerment of staff members.
4. Describe appropriate content and documentation for a coaching session.
5. Demonstrate the process of progressive discipline.
6. Describe performance analysis and how it may be used in the work environment.

Alone we can do so little, together we can do so much.

—Helen Keller

To give and receive critical comments, no matter how positively they are intended, is a difficult form of communication for most people. Generally, people do not like to tell others they are doing something wrong, and people do not like to hear that they may be less than perfect. The giving and receiving of constructive feedback is very important, however, to personal and professional growth. In the role of nurse manager, nurses cannot and must not avoid this communication. Stephen Covey's fourth habit in *The 7 Habits of Highly Effective People* is "Think Win-Win." Communicating "win-win" focuses on the idea that all parties can have a positive outcome and that all conclusions through discussion are agreed upon and beneficial for all parties (Covey, 2013). The type of communication just described plays a critical role in each aspect of your career as a nurse, regardless of the position you hold.

This chapter reviews the role of the licensed practical nurse (LPN) in the difficult communication process of delegating, counseling, and evaluating others. In this chapter, you will receive some practical pointers that will help minimize the stress and maximize the positive growth outcomes. Although the process for making staff assignments often is specific to each facility or setting, this chapter also reviews methods to enhance that process.

LEADER, MANAGER, OR BOTH

The role of the LPN in health-care organizations throughout the United States involves considerable responsibilities for leadership and management. Because you are to assume these responsibilities in the practice setting, you need to be prepared to implement them. LPNs frequently are placed in positions to assume responsibility for the care other staff members give to people. You may have certified nursing assistants (CNAs), unlicensed assistive personnel (UAP), technicians, or other LPNs reporting to you. Your role is not simply to tell them what to do. You must be a leader and a manager to get the workload accomplished with caring and excellence. While *management* is the

ability to plan, organize, and manage the resources of an organization, *leadership* is the ability to establish vision and goals and to influence others to meet the goals. You see, although these roles are related, the focus of the outcome differs.

If you are a leader, staff members listen to you and respect what you have to say. You exert an influence over staff members that they may not realize. It has been said that the best leaders are those whose followers do not realize they are being led. As a good leader, you may not receive all the credit when goals are accomplished, but you will have the satisfaction of knowing you set the direction for positive things to happen.

As a nurse manager, you are responsible to work with your staff to accomplish the goals for excellent, holistic nursing care. How do you do this? I would encourage you to utilize an existing tool for writing goals using the acronym SMART (Box 21.1). First, you must work with the staff, the person who is ill, and the family to identify goals that are realistic and achievable. You cannot unilaterally set goals for people (patient or staff) or for your unit. It is essential to use the ideas and opinions of people who are involved in achieving the goals.

For example, one of your patients, Mrs. Brown, needs additional ambulation to improve her walking ability. Without talking to your staff or Mrs. Brown,

---

Box 21.1 Being SMART When Writing Goals

S = Specific: The goal is clear and not general.

M = Measurable: You have established strict criteria for measuring progress of each goal.

A = Attainable: The goals are important to you and not extreme.

R = Realistic: The goals matter and are relevant to the experience.

T = Time-bound: A commitment to a time frame increases the chances for success and establishes a sense of urgency.

Source: Doran, G. T. (1981). There's a S.M.A.R.T. way to write management's goals and objectives. *Management Review, 70*(11), 35–36.

As the LPN, you are often the manager of others.

you tell the CNA that she is to walk Mrs. Brown the length of the hall every day at 2:00 p.m. The next day you find out that Mrs. Brown did not walk the previous day. The CNA says that Mrs. Brown is unwilling to walk. Mrs. Brown says that her favorite soap opera is on at 2:00 p.m., and she does not want to walk at that time. If you had discussed the ambulation goal with Mrs. Brown, you would have known about the soap opera and been able to plan an achievable goal.

After you have worked with the staff and the person who is ill to identify a meaningful goal, your role as a manager is to coordinate the activities to achieve the goal. You may have heard the old adage, "There are many ways to skin a cat." Likewise, goals are achieved in many ways. You do not need to have all the answers. However, you do need to coordinate the many creative ideas of staff members and patients into a workable course of action.

Finally, after establishing the goal and identifying the plan of action, the manager is responsible

As an effective manager, it is important for the LPN to assist others with the basic workload.

for setting up a system of accountability to ensure the actions are taken and the goal is achieved. This system could involve documentation on the part of the staff person or planning a meeting with the patient and the CNA to review progress. The system depends on the needs of the patient, systems currently in place in the organization, and priority of the goal.

What are the three responsibilities of a nurse manager in supporting the successful completion of excellent, holistic nursing care goals?

1. Identify goals that are realistic and achievable.
2. Coordinate the activities that will achieve the goal.
3. Establish a system of accountability to ensure the actions are taken and the goal is achieved.

If the goal is not achieved, the manager needs to determine why. Another important general concept is that you, as the nurse manager, are a role model for others. The way you treat patients, families, and other staff members is a critical factor in how the staff may treat each other, the patient, and the patient's family. The staff members may emulate the way you interact with others. If you are respectful and responsive in your communications, you are showing the staff the way they should act. An example is that in an emergency or when no one else is available, you are willing to answer call lights, empty bedpans, or help with whatever needs to be done. By occasionally helping staff complete their work, you are saying to them that their jobs are important and that no one person is more important than another in providing care to patients.

DELEGATION AND MAKING ASSIGNMENTS

As a nurse, you may have developed excellent bedside and clinical nursing skills. As a nurse manager, however, there are more skills you need to develop. Even if you are "Super Nurse," you cannot be everywhere. To be effective, you must be able to assign responsibilities to other staff members and ensure that those responsibilities are met. This is one of the more critical tasks of a nurse manager, and it involves the art of delegation.

Delegating in Nursing

Delegation is "the transfer of responsibility for the implementation of a task to another while retaining accountability for its outcome" (Nugent & Vitale,. 2014). In most states, LPNs have the authority under the nurse practice act to delegate tasks to others. States have different rules and regulations regarding delegation. It is important to check the nurse practice act in your state for rules regarding delegation as an LPN. Delegation is an integral aspect of nursing practice. The question is not, "Do I delegate?" but "How do I delegate appropriately?" The National Council of State Boards of Nursing (2005) developed the five rights of delegation, which are listed in Box 21.2. In addition to reviewing these five rights, you should review your state's nurse practice act to identify its interpretation of delegation for LPNs. Although it is impossible to make a complete list of which actions can be delegated to a UAP, a list of examples is provided in Box 21.3. You should also check with your place of employment to verify their stance on delegation for LPNs.

Identifying Tasks to Be Delegated

Making assignments involves identifying and delegating specific aspects of personal care to a staff person. You probably will assign the care of several patients to each staff member depending on where you are working. Before you can do this, however, you must know what care each patient requires and the strengths and weaknesses of the staff members. When you have accurate information about the needs of the patients and the skills of the staff, you can match the skills, interests, and needs of the two groups of people effectively. This matching process is essential to providing excellence in care to the patient and maximizing staff abilities and morale.

When you delegate to another person, it is only for a select nursing act on a select patient for that moment (Box 21.4). Although you are

Box 21.3 Tasks That May and May Not Be Delegated to Unlicensed Assistive Personnel

Tasks That May Be Delegated to Unlicensed Assistive Personnel

- Weighing
- Bathing
- Feeding
- Taking of vital signs
- Client transfers and ambulation
- Attending to safety
- Postmortem care

Tasks That May Not Be Delegated to Unlicensed Assistive Personnel

- Assessment
- Interpretation of data
- Gastrostomy feedings in established systems
- Care of invasive lines
- Updating nursing care plans
- Insertion of nasogastric tubes

giving this person the responsibility to perform the task, you are not relinquishing your accountability for how the task is performed and the safety of the patient. Being accountable means you are responsible and answerable for the actions of the individual to whom you delegated the task. This is important for you to understand. When you delegate ambulating a new postoperative patient to a CNA or a UAP, you have done it for *that patient and that time only.* Sometimes nurses become lax in assessing patients to determine whether the CNA is qualified to do the procedure being delegated. Then there are times when the CNA thinks, "Well, he told me to do this with Mr. Johansen, so I will do it now with Mrs. Chen." It is crucial that you and the person to whom you are delegating understand the concept of "one task, on one patient, for

Box 21.2 The Five Rights of Delegation

1. Right task
2. Right circumstances
3. Right person
4. Right direction and communication
5. Right supervision and evaluation

Box 21.4 Three Basic Rules of Delegation

1. Assess the person or situation to determine whether the task can be delegated to another person or whether you should do it yourself.
2. After you have made your assessment, you need to determine whether the person to whom you are delegating has the skills to do the task properly.
3. Do not do all of the work yourself; be sure to delegate.

this time only." Otherwise, serious problems can result.

Delegation is the skill of letting go of some of your responsibilities and gaining the cooperation of others in meeting them. Making assignments, the task done by nurse managers that allows for effective delegation to be made, should not be a problem if the components of delegation are followed.

Effective delegation requires that (1) the task delegated is clearly identified, (2) the patient has a thorough needs assessment, (3) the staff person is capable and empowered to carry out activities to complete the task, and (4) a system of accountability is in place to monitor staff performance. Did you notice that a system of accountability also was on the list for establishing goals? This is a crucial aspect of staff management.

Apply the three rules of delegation found in Box 21.4 to the Reflective Thinking feature that follows.

REFLECTIVE THINKING

Scenario

You are working the evening shift as a float LPN on a high-observation unit (HOBS) that is a step-down unit for the intensive care unit (ICU). This HOBS also gets emergency department admissions who do not meet the criteria for ICU admission. It is a busy unit with a team of registered nurses (RNs), LPNs, and UAPs who work well together. Because of the teamwork that has developed among the nursing staff, more is delegated to the UAPs than you noticed last time you were floated to HOBS. You also noticed that there seemed to be less checking on the work of the UAPs. The situation is causing you some concern.

Remember: You are accountable, in total, for any task you delegate to another person.

You become uncomfortable when you see a UAP getting a patient, who is on strict bedrest, out of bed to ambulate to the bathroom. Fortunately, you were there and were able to prevent what could have been a serious incident. The UAP seemed upset with you for stopping the patient from being ambulated but went on with her work. You have five very sick patients with many parameters of care for you to manage. The behavior and attitude of the UAP do not bode well for the evening. Back to the original question: What are you going to do?

Assessing Patient Needs

An important method for assessing the needs of the patient is walking rounds. Visit each patient at least once a day. Observe how the patient functions physically and cognitively and any unusual problems the patient may have, such as a feeding tube or skin problem. Listen to what the patient has to say about your staff and how his or her needs are being met. If you answer a call light when all other staff members are busy, you have a great opportunity to observe the patients in your care and your behavior shows the staff your willingness to be part of the team. During shift change report, listen carefully for what is said regarding the progress or lack of it for each patient. Ask yourself what you can do to promote healing and which staff person would be best in assisting an individual patient in the healing process.

Another method for assessing patient needs is to refer to the objective assessment measurement used by the facility or organization. Nursing homes use the minimum data set to assess resident needs, including their functional abilities and deficits. Such a standardized assessment form, or the care plan, can provide objective information for each patient on which assignments can be based.

Some organizations use standardized acuity systems to facilitate making assignments. Acuity systems are standardized ways to measure each patient's needs or the nursing tasks that need to be completed for each patient. They allow the nurse to compare patients in terms of the severity and acuity of their needs or the amount of nursing time that may be required to care for them. Most acuity systems measure aspects of patient care needs and group them into categories based on the needs. Each category typically is assigned a name or value that corresponds to the amount of nursing time required to care for the average patient in that category. An example is an acuity system that categorizes people as light, moderate, or heavy care. A person in the light category may need only assistance with activities of daily living, whereas a person in the heavy category may be totally dependent for all activities of daily living, be on intravenous therapy, and be in moderate-to-severe pain.

Acuity systems are used in making assignments by allocating patients by category to each staff member. The number of patients you assign to each staff member depends on the patient-to-staff ratio (the number of patients cared for by each staff member) set by the organization or unit. You may assign each staff person one heavy care patient, two moderate care patients, and two light care patients. If the acuity categories have numerical values, you may allocate a specific number of points to each staff person. If the institution where you work uses an acuity system for facilitating staffing, be sure to ask for a thorough orientation about how the system works and the basis on which the categories are determined.

Providing an Empowering Environment

To gain the cooperation of other employees, which is a necessary aspect of the art of delegation, all involved individuals should be included in the delegation process. In addition, all individuals should be in an inclusive and supportive environment in which they feel safe and can make or strongly contribute to the decisions being made. These are aspects of an empowering environment.

Delegation rules one and two in Box 21.4 have to do with your legal accountability as an LPN. In addition, they focus on the quality of safe and meaningful care given to patients for whom you are responsible. Rule number three

has a different focus. The focus is directly on you. The rule is not to do all of the work yourself; be sure to delegate.

Most people with whom I speak about delegation say somewhere in the conversation that they don't use delegation much because, "I know if I do it, it will get done right the first time." Rule number three indicates that doing it yourself is not a professionally sound practice. It is not emotionally or physically healthy for you, and it definitely is not the type of nursing care that is encouraged.

What happens when you try to "do it yourself"? First, you get tired, frustrated, and eventually angry. The normal emotional reaction to frustration is anger. It is important to protect yourself from frustrating experiences because anger is unprofessional and unhealthy. The second thing that happens when you "do it yourself" is that no one else gets a chance to learn, to develop higher-level skills, to work with a wider variety of patients, or to work with wonderful you! There is a loss all the way around for you, other personnel, and patients.

When you are the nurse manager, you are the person with the higher-level skills. Based on that fact alone, you may think that you should be doing it all. How can you empower staff if you are constantly performing all of the duties, including taking care of the details? Until you give others the opportunity to take on additional responsibilities, you never know what they are capable of. People without knowledge that is rightfully theirs are not empowered. In addition, people who are not given responsibility are not empowered. So take the risk to delegate and then evaluate!

You may find yourself resisting the message of empowerment based on a variety of concerns, including time, a general lack of understanding, being fearful, or having other feelings that lead to a lack of delegating, but the truth is you empower people by teaching them what you know. You share your wisdom and secrets for making things work often without knowing you are empowering others. You give it all away during thoughtfully prepared educational programs or spontaneous teaching moments on the unit. This is the hallmark of a great leader—one who does not hoard information. After you have assessed the people for whom you have delegation responsibility and taught them the things they need to know, you are free to manage rather than do the tasks that rightfully should be assigned to others.

The hands-on caregivers who may be LPNs, CNAs, or UAPs are the experts in the nursing care of patients. They need to be respected as experts, involved in the planning of care, and given permission to make alterations in care, all within their scope of practice and abilities. To support an empowering environment for staff members means that you (1) incorporate their input into aspects of care that involve them, (2) share information with them regarding the care of the patients assigned to them for care, and (3) use staffing models (a process used to determine how nurses are assigned to patients for a shift) that include input from the nursing staff.

Staff members who provide bedside care are experts in knowing the details and idiosyncrasies of patients. Their skills and knowledge are a meaningful aspect of what makes a plan of care significant to the health and welfare of others. That is why their input into the care plan and assignments is crucial. In addition, few people like to be given work assignments without having an opportunity, at some point, to provide input into defining that assignment. Most of us like to be involved in discussing the work we do and suggesting ways, from our perspective, to accomplish the goals of our jobs.

Many ways can be used to solicit staff input in making assignments. Gathering input can range from asking personnel at regular staff meetings what they think of the assignments to having them make the assignments themselves. Although the latter might sound a bit radical, allowing staff members to select the patients they would like to care for is frequently a positive experience for the patients, the staff, and the nurse manager. Staff members also need to have opportunities to provide input during the entire care planning process, from assessment to evaluation.

Another important point regarding rule number three of delegation is that if you live the rule, you should be calling on nursing staff and people from other disciplines to work together. The sharing of knowledge and skills allows for a higher quality of care to be delivered to patients, and it calls on each person who is part of the collaboration to learn and grow simply from working together rather than in isolation. Sharing ideas and learning and teaching together are enriching experiences that staff should not be forced to miss because the nurse manager is unable or unwilling to delegate responsibilities.

SHARING INFORMATION WITH STAFF MEMBERS

To provide the best care possible, staff members must be well informed concerning changes in the patient and the plan of care. Verbal report and walking rounds at the beginning and end of the shift help the staff members and the nurse manager develop a frequent, regular system of communication and provide opportunities for input and feedback. Using the SBAR system and the written care plan are good ways to communicate patient information among staff. Staff members providing the hands-on care need to have ready access to the formal, written plan of care and become accustomed to consulting it frequently. Too often the written plan of care is not a living document that directs the caring activities for the patient; this should not happen.

System of Accountability

After you have become familiar with the needs of patients and personnel, you need a system for holding staff members accountable for the goals and responsibilities of their assignments. Accountability first requires that staff members know and understand what is expected of them. In addition to the plan of care for each of the patients, do they know what other tasks and behaviors are expected? When should they take breaks and where? Do they have other unit assignments, such as ordering medications or putting away supplies? How should they report changes in patient conditions? What should they do when or if they have spare time? These items may be reviewed in a unit orientation, but they also may require review on a regular basis.

An accountability system requires a reporting mechanism. This may be verbal, written, or both. Documentation on flow sheets is a common system of accountability. Flow sheets provide written information that shows whether services were provided. They also may be used to document the outcome of services from the staff perspective. Flow sheets may be used for any aspect of care but are most common for such areas as activities of daily living, mobility, range of motion, vital signs, weights, mechanical measurements, and intake and output.

When you make rounds as the nurse manager, your personal observations may provide feedback for a system of accountability. Take note of particular aspects of the patients' care plans. Does someone who wears glasses have them on? Are residents in a nursing home turned according to the schedules established? Are intravenous lines attended to on schedule and medications given on time? Do patients in the care of you and your team seem content for the condition in which they find themselves? Is holistic care being practiced (e.g., are family members involved in the care)?

When a manager holds staff members accountable for their job responsibilities, it does not mean the manager is correcting them when they do something wrong. It is equally important to commend staff members when they meet or exceed expectations. While making rounds on the unit, be sure to make positive comments to staff members and to point out, in private, areas for improvement. Rewarding positive behaviors is often much more effective in improving performance than punishing negative behaviors. This positive approach to employee management is frequently called *coaching*.

 ## COACHING

Coaching is helping others develop or improve on existing skills, tasks, or behaviors. Think about coaches you have known or have observed on television during professional sports games. What does a coach do? The coach pumps up the team's enthusiasm. He or she commends the players when they have performed well, listens and instructs on how to play the game, and points out mistakes and offers incentives for players to try harder or do better. A manager must do all of these things for his or her employees. The role of the manager in personnel issues far surpasses doling out punishments for mistakes or infractions of the rules. The art of personnel management requires a positive, instead of a punitive, approach to coaching. The aspects of coaching to be discussed in this section are crucial to your success as a manager; they are (1) energizing, (2) providing positive reinforcement, (3) teaching and counseling, and (4) disciplining.

Energizing

As a manager, you have a responsibility to energize the staff members. It is important that you can create an environment in which staff members feel motivated and energized to accomplish the goals of the unit or organization. The first question you need to ask is, "Are you energized?" Do you truly believe in the goals of the unit or organization? Are you excited about your job and the difference you can make in people's lives? In every interaction you have with another person, you can make a positive impression, part of which will be based on your energy.

Second, are you positive in your thinking and your approach to people and the world? Do you view the world as full of possibilities or problems? If you see possibilities, you should energize the staff members to see the same. The power of positive thinking is crucial to the ability to energize others. You must genuinely believe in what you are doing and be enthusiastic about it. Your enthusiasm can be contagious. If you are a naturally shy, reserved person, you may need to put additional effort into creating the energy necessary for success.

Providing Positive Reinforcement

Positive reinforcement or feedback to staff members can be provided on an informal or formal basis. Providing informal and formal positive feedback is an important responsibility for you as an effective coach.

Informal

Informal positive feedback on jobs well done is an effective method of personnel management. The staff members need to hear, on a regular basis, what they are doing well. Immediate, positive feedback reinforces the behaviors you wish to see repeated. As you make rounds on the unit, be attentive to the small aspects of care, to either person or environment, which staff members have done well. Comment to staff members immediately. Although it is never appropriate to offer negative feedback to a staff person in public, commending an individual when others are nearby can be effective. It tells everyone within earshot the behaviors that you, as the manager, value. It also lets people know you think enough of the staff members to take the time to recognize their efforts.

Formal

Formal systems for providing positive feedback to staff members also are important. Does your organization have any formal recognition programs? These may include such programs as "employee of the month" or "caught in the act of caring." The latter is a program for patients, families, or other staff members to recognize an employee who has done something particularly nice. Such formal recognition programs are important to employee morale and provide a means of recognizing valued behaviors of employees in an organization.

I know of an organization where a "caught in the act of caring" program was implemented in the nursing department. It was started by the director of nursing to congratulate staff members formally for doing something special. Examples of the behaviors recognized in this program included volunteering to work overtime for a shift no one wanted, taking extra time with a person who needed patience to be fed, or spending additional time to assist in the orientation of a new employee. The "caught in the act of caring" program can be incorporated into the continuous improvement program for the entire organization. Blank forms should be made available in a variety of locations throughout the facility; completed forms could be deposited in a mailbox outside the nurse manager's office. "Caught in the act of caring" notes should be read daily by the manager, then passed on to the employee and copied for the employee's file. Some organizations have "caught in the act of caring" buttons they give to personnel to wear.

The philosophy behind this program, as a part of the continuous improvement initiative, is that positive reinforcement is an excellent way to perpetuate desirable behaviors. In addition, by publicizing and rewarding such behaviors, in a formal manner, other employees learn the values of the organization and tend to imitate the positive behaviors. If this sort of program does not exist in your organization, it can be started easily by you as the nurse manager who cares about his or her staff members.

Teaching and Counseling

All human beings make mistakes. As nurses, we do our best to prepare ourselves so that those mistakes have minimal impact on the health and well-being of the patients. We must recognize and accept our own human frailties, learn from our mistakes, and continuously strive to improve. As managers, we must create an atmosphere of acceptance for mistakes and help staff members to learn from their own and each other's mistakes.

The primary purpose of counseling is to inform employees that they need to do something differently or that they have done something particularly well. The most common reason for an employee performing inappropriately or making a mistake is a lack of knowledge about the policies and procedures

of the organization. Teaching or providing information is the most effective way to correct the inappropriate behavior or to prevent the error from occurring again. To correct the behavior, however, the employee (1) must be aware of what was done wrong and (2) must know the correct thing to do.

When an employee does something wrong, the first inclination of the manager sometimes is to avoid a confrontation and rationalize with thoughts such as "He's new. I'll give him another chance," or "This is the first time I have noticed this. I'll wait until it happens again." If the employee is never made aware that the behavior was not appropriate and taught the correct behavior, chances are the same mistake will be made again. At the same time, an employee who does something particularly good, but this behavior is never acknowledged by the manager, may think the behavior is not appropriate in the work setting and never do it again.

Session Content

Counseling sessions with employees should be brief and nonconfrontational. In addition, they always should be conducted in private if negative information needs to be communicated. Take the employee aside for a few minutes and discuss the behavior you wish either to change or to continue. A counseling session should include the following elements:

1. Discuss the negative behavior that you wish to change or the positive behavior you wish to continue. For example, "Mary, I noticed today that you did not pass fresh water to the residents in the afternoon," or "I know that Mrs. Brown has been eating poorly, but you took extra time with her today, and she seemed to eat a good lunch."
2. Ask the employee the reason for his or her behavior to be able to elicit the cause. For example, "Were you aware that fresh water is generally passed in the afternoons or did something come up?" or "How did you manage to get Mrs. Brown to eat so well?"
3. If you are trying to correct a negative behavior, discuss the correct action the employee should have taken. If you are trying to reinforce a positive behavior, give the employee positive feedback. For example, in the passing water situation, if the employee was unaware of the policy, you may say, "It is our policy to give fresh water every afternoon. If you run

into any difficulties, please let me know." If the employee says that he or she did not have the time to pass water, you may say, "It is important for the residents to have fluids. Perhaps we can talk about how your day went and how you could organize it differently so that you have the time to pass fresh water." For the employee who did a good job feeding Mrs. Brown, you may comment, "I know you had a heavy schedule today, but I was impressed that you were able to find the time to spend with Mrs. Brown and still complete all of your other work. You did a great job and I appreciate it."

Session Documentation

Counseling is a verbal discussion. It should be documented, however, so that you can remember it when you are ready to prepare the employee's performance review. Different organizations have different policies and procedures related to counseling employees. Some organizations have formal forms called anecdotal notes or critical incident forms on which to record the counseling. Other organizations have no formal method of recording these interactions. All counseling sessions should be documented for future reference. You may keep a card file to record such discussions with employees, or you may make notes in your own file. Be sure to write down the behavior that was discussed and the behavior that was recommended. Include the date and time of the session and the name of anyone else who was present. In most cases, the counseling note does not need to be signed by the employee. It is to remind you of the verbal exchange. Be sure that every employee incident you consider important enough to note for future reference or to include in a performance review has been discussed with the employee. It is not fair or a good management practice to collect notes on poor performance and issue disciplinary actions or poor reviews based on them when the employee was not given an opportunity to change.

Disciplining

An individual who is self-disciplined shows self-control and a sense of personal responsibility for his or her behavior and performance. To be self-disciplined is generally viewed as a positive attribute. To be disciplined by someone else, however, connotes punishment and deprivation. Even the term *discipline* is often avoided in personnel management. Nevertheless, one role of a manager is to ensure that staff members show self-discipline and take responsibility for their actions and performance. At times, this role requires that the manager impose disciplinary actions. A positive instead of punitive approach to this disciplinary process is more effective for all involved.

A positive approach to discipline requires that the manager focus on helping the employee to improve performance and behavior. A punitive approach emphasizes punishment for ill deeds. A positive approach is a problem-solving method that incorporates respect and dignity for the employee and manager. A punitive approach disregards the feelings of either the employee or the manager and requires imposition of sanctions and solutions for dealing with the problem. Despite all preconceived ideas and experiences you may have about the disciplinary process, it can be a positive and motivating force that helps employees do a better job.

Errors

There are several common errors to avoid in implementing the disciplinary process (Box 21.5). Be careful to avoid these when dealing with personnel disciplinary issues:

1. *Ignoring behavioral shortcomings in the hope that the employee's performance may improve with time:* To change behaviors, the staff member needs to be aware of problem areas. Ignoring a performance problem cannot make it go away. It may grow worse, and other employees may begin to imitate the behavior.
2. *Hoarding disappointments and grievances about an employee's work until cumulative irritation provokes a blowup:* In an effort to avoid confrontation, a manager may ignore an employee's performance problem that seems minor. These minor issues can accumulate, however, to the point at which the manager loses objectivity and issues a disciplinary action that is much more severe than any of the issues deserved individually. The employee is baffled that such a small infraction would warrant such a severe penalty and views the manager as unfair and overly strict. Can you blame the employee?
3. *Administering criticism in such a sweetened manner that it is unrecognized by the employee as criticism:* Disciplinary actions can be positive experiences if handled fairly and objectively. The manager should convey clearly to

Box 21.5 Common Errors to Avoid in the Disciplinary Process

1. Ignoring behavioral shortcomings in the hope that the employee's performance may improve with time
2. Holding disappointments and grievances about an employee's work until cumulative irritation provokes a blowup
3. Administering criticism in such a sweetened manner that it is unrecognized by the employee as criticism
4. Administering general instead of specific criticism so that the employee does not know what changes are called for
5. Instituting discipline prematurely and unfairly as a result of faulty interpretation of the circumstances
6. Failing to follow the institution's disciplinary process

Although this course of action may seem expedient at the time, failing to gather all the appropriate information and considering all the facts may lead to an unfair and inaccurate disciplinary action.

6. *Failing to follow the institution's disciplinary process:* Every disciplinary situation should have certain components. If one of these elements is not present, an action other than a disciplinary action may be appropriate. If a standard does not exist, it may need to be developed and all staff members informed about it. If an employee was unaware of the rule, a counseling session may be appropriate. The components are as follows:
   • A rule or standard exists.
   • The employee was aware of the rule or standard.
   • The employee violated the rule or standard.
   • The penalty imposed is appropriate to the violation.

REFLECTIVE THINKING

Review the six errors that are common when implementing the disciplinary process. Pick one that is of particular interest to you; perhaps it is the one you would find the most difficult to do. Document any experiences you have had with the error you selected. Discuss how you would resolve the error in your LPN practice. Add your personal thoughts and feelings as a future manager.

the employee that a particular behavior needs to be corrected. Sugarcoating the discussion may make you as the manager feel better, but if it confuses the employee about the purpose of the discussion, it is not appropriate.

4. *Administering general instead of specific criticism so that the employee does not know what changes are called for:* At the end of a disciplinary discussion, the employee should have a clear idea of exactly what behaviors he or she needs to exhibit or to avoid to correct the problem. Telling an employee, "You need to change your attitude," does not offer specific direction on what he or she needs to do. "You need to improve your attendance" also is general. "You need to be on time every day and you need to call off work at least 1 hour before the shift if you are ill" is an example of a specific direction.

5. *Instituting discipline prematurely and unfairly as a result of faulty interpretation of the circumstances:* Be particularly attentive to gathering all the facts and viewing the whole picture before making a disciplinary decision. In the interest of time, you may want to act quickly and deal with a situation immediately.

Counseling and Disciplinary Interview

Whenever you talk with an employee about a behavior that he or she needs to change, whether it is first-time counseling or disciplinary action for repeated offenses, the following guidelines are helpful:

• Make sure you have the time to spend with the employee. Do not rush the discussion.
• Do not accept interruptions, such as answering the phone. Turn your phone on silent. Devote your full attention to the employee.
• Hold the interview in a quiet place where you can have privacy.
• Open the interview with a few social questions or chitchat to help the employee feel at ease.
• Treat the employee with respect and dignity. Never treat him or her like a child.

The counseling and disciplinary interview should contain the following components; the order in which they are listed is an effective sequence for conducting an interview:

1. Identify the employee's view of the problem. "I understand there was a problem with Mrs. Smith last evening. Could you tell me what happened?"
2. Share the information you have regarding the situation. Keep your communication factual. Do not include your interpretations. "Mrs. Smith complained to me that you refused to give her pain medication when she asked for it."
3. Allow for the employee's response to the information you provided. If information is revealed or other witnesses are identified that you did not know about, you may need to do some additional fact-finding before continuing the interview. If this is the case, tell the employee that you plan to investigate further by talking to the witnesses and reschedule another meeting to conclude the interview.
4. Discuss the appropriate behavior with the employee. Ask what he or she could have done differently in the situation. Be clear on exactly what the expected behavior is.
5. Inform the employee of your disciplinary decision and the type of disciplinary action you are issuing.
6. Review with the employee what the next level of disciplinary action may be if he or she does not correct the behavior.
7. Ask the employee to read and sign the disciplinary action. The employee also may note

comments on the disciplinary form. A copy of the disciplinary form can be given to the employee.
8. End the interview by thanking the employee for talking with you, expressing your interest in helping him or her do better, and offering appropriate words of encouragement for improvement.

Types of Disciplinary Actions

Each organization has its own personnel policies and procedures on rules of the organization and consequences for infractions. These are usually part of the employee handbook. Be sure to refer to these when making disciplinary decisions. In general, however, there are several types or levels of disciplinary action, including the following:

• *Verbal warnings:* If you have counseled an employee previously about a problem, you know he or she is aware of the rule or standard of the organization he or she is breaking. That is the situation that calls for a verbal warning. A verbal warning is the manager's way of letting the employee know that more severe action may be taken if the behavior continues. Even though the warning is verbal, it should be documented on the appropriate form of the organization. You also should have documentation that you shared the rule or standard with the employee in your personnel file. Depending on the policy of the organization, the manager's verbal warnings may or may not need to be signed by the employee and may or may not be included in the employee's personnel file.

FOCUSED LEARNING CHART

Disciplinary Action

When employees do something wrong, they need to know (1) what they did wrong and (2) how to correct the behavior. A disciplinary action should:

Be brief.
Be nonconfrontational.
Be conducted in private.
Explain the problem behavior.
Include a request for the circumstances or reason for the behavior.
Be documented as a counseling session to use when doing performance evaluations.
Follow all facility policies to ensure due process.

• *Written warnings:* A repeated occurrence or a severe violation of a rule warrants a written warning. These always should be signed by the employee in acknowledgment that he or she has received the warning. Written warnings should be included in the employee's personnel file. Some organizations require one written warning and others more than one before progressing to the next disciplinary step. As the manager, it is your responsibility to know what the organization's policies are.

• *Suspension:* A suspension is a specific time period during which the employee is not permitted to work. A suspension may be either paid time or unpaid time. In a disciplinary situation, a suspension is frequently unpaid. A paid 1-day suspension sometimes is offered to employees as a time to remove themselves from the work situation and make decisions or plans related to their performance improvement. A suspension also may be differentiated from disciplinary time off. In this case, a suspension is used as a time for the employee to be removed from the work situation while an investigation of a particular incident takes place. On completion of the investigation, the period of suspension either is paid or remains unpaid, depending on the disciplinary decision. If an employee commits a serious violation that warrants termination, a suspension period for the investigation to take place generally is warranted. A suspension removes the employee from the work situation, allows time for fact-finding, and ensures that the employee is not terminated in the heat of the moment without a thorough review of the situation. Disciplinary time off is a disciplinary action involving the employee's mandatory, unpaid absence from work.

• *Termination:* Except in the most severe circumstances, which generally are defined by the organization, termination of employment always should be preceded by stepwise disciplinary warnings. If progressive discipline is followed, and the consequence of future violations is explained to the employee at each step, termination should come as no surprise to the employee. Most managers find it difficult to tell an employee that he or she is fired. If counseling and disciplinary interviews have been occurring along the way, however, you

as the manager will know you have done everything possible to help the employee improve. Sometimes individuals are not suited for a position and may be happier and more productive doing something else.

REFLECTIVE THINKING

Consider the four aspects of coaching: (1) energizing, (2) providing positive reinforcement, (3) teaching and counseling, and (4) disciplining. As a nurse manager, how will you address these four areas when managing staff? Provide examples for each aspect.

EVALUATING PERFORMANCE

Performance analysis instead of performance appraisal connotes a positive approach to the process of evaluation. Performance analysis is a comprehensive evaluation that promotes communication, provides useful feedback about job performance, facilitates better working relationships, provides a historical record of performance, and promotes goal setting for workplace satisfaction.

Traditionally, either giving or receiving performance appraisals is a cause for considerable stress and anxiety. Approached from a positive perspective, with the major intent of helping the employee improve and develop, the stress involved in the appraisal process can be minimized, and the benefits can be maximized.

A positive approach views the employee as an active agent instead of a passive receptacle in the performance analysis process. Although the traditional view assumes the manager knows best, the positive approach acknowledges that the employee knows best about his or her capabilities, needs, and goals. The role of the manager is to help the employee improve performance and relate personal career planning to the needs and realities of the organization. The emphasis in performance analysis is on the future instead of the past. The manager and employee together establish realistic targets for performance improvement or development and the most effective ways to reach them. Performance analysis is merely a means to a constructive end. The focus is on actions relative to goals as they relate to performance. Personalities should never be the focus.

Why Do We Need Performance Analysis?

Evaluating the performance of an employee serves several important functions. First, they are the basis for coaching and counseling toward improvement. We all have areas in which we can improve. We also have areas in which we excel. A good performance analysis helps the employee identify the weak areas and potential strategies to strengthen them. It also can help the employee maximize positive attributes. A good analysis makes the employee feel appreciated for the valuable work he or she is doing. Second, the analysis is a means of giving the employee suggestions for change. Third, a performance review can provide systematic judgments to back up salary increases, promotions, and transfers. The purpose of an analysis is not to criticize and find fault. It is to help the employee grow and develop.

Pitfalls of Employee Analysis

Performance reviews can fail to serve the purpose for which they were intended—to help the employee do a better job. Employees can be so devastated by a review that their work suffers instead of improves. The following are pitfalls that can lead to failure with performance reviews:

1. The manager does not know the requirements of the job. The performance review should be based on the job description.
2. The manager is not aware of the standards to measure job performance.
3. The *halo effect* is allowing a positive or negative rating on one quality to influence ratings on the other qualities so that they are higher or lower than deserved. For example, the employee is excellent at diabetes teaching but is mediocre at many other professional qualities. The manager bases the evaluation on the excellence in teaching rather than the overall job description performance.
4. *Central tendency* is providing a rating of average or around the midpoint for all qualities.
5. The *recency effect* means ratings are influenced by the most recent behavior instead of behavior that has occurred since the last review.
6. The *strict* or *leniency effect* means ratings are all lower or higher than the expected average. The manager may be unusually lenient in his

or her ratings in an effort to be liked by the staff members and not make anyone unhappy.
7. The *spillover effect* means allowing past performance analysis ratings to influence current ratings unjustly.
8. The *contrast effect* means ratings are made on an employee by comparing with other employees instead of using the performance standards.

Components of Performance Analysis

Performance reviews may contain several types of criteria, including behavioral characteristics, personality characteristics, and goals or objectives. Behavioral characteristics are the activities that employees perform in the course of their job. These are the tasks assigned to them as included in the job description. For a CNA, these behavioral characteristics may include providing restorative care, such as range of motion and walking assistance to patients; communicating with patients; and assisting with activities of daily living.

Goals or objectives are the major components of a performance analysis. These are the specific tasks or accomplishments that the manager and employee agree should be completed during the evaluation period. Emphasizing goals focuses attention on the employee's individual achievements. It motivates the employee to accomplish the goals and measures performance in terms of results. Goals are based on the individual employee's strengths and weaknesses. The number of goals established for any one year may vary considerably based on the complexity and variability of the employee's position. Some employees may identify one or two goals to be accomplished, whereas others may identify numerous projects to be completed. New goals for the next review period should be set at the completion of the performance analysis. In an effort to provide employees with a tool in writing measurable goals, consider using the acronym SMART provided in Box 21.1.

Performance Plan for Improvement

A performance analysis generally is completed on an employee at a specified period after starting a new position. This could be at 3 months, 6 months, or 1 year. This initial review is completed after the new hire probationary period is ended. After the initial review, performance analyses usually are completed on an annual basis. These may be done at one specified time of year or on the anniversary date of the

When you have devised a performance plan for an employee, it is your responsibility to ensure the person has the knowledge necessary to improve job performance.

employee. In addition, an employee who is having considerable difficulty in a variety of performance areas may benefit from engaging in a performance analysis at a time not regularly scheduled.

A performance analysis for an employee with multiple performance problems should include a performance plan for improvement. This plan should detail specifically what the employee needs to do to improve and the time frame to accomplish the improvement. If you have such an employee with multiple performance problems, start by completing a performance review. This identifies the employee's areas of weakness and areas of strength. At the performance analysis interview, review the ratings and discuss ways to improve behavior with the employee. This is the start of compiling a performance plan for improvement. Take notes during this meeting, and at the end set up another appointment to review the written plan. This gives you an opportunity to organize your thoughts and the discussion into a detailed plan.

An effective performance plan for improvement should include the following components:

1. *The performance standards that need to be met:* These are the specific and measurable performance goals that the employee is to meet. They should be observable behaviors that are stated clearly so that there can be no mistake about whether or not the employee has achieved the goal. For example, patients are to be assisted to walk every day, and it is to be documented on the daily flow sheet.
2. *The accountability and time frame for achievement of each goal and for the*

entire improvement plan: The employee should be aware of the time frame that the plan covers. It is reasonable to give a new employee 1 month to improve the behaviors identified in the improvement plan. An employee with years of longevity may need a longer period, however, to change behaviors that have become ingrained over the years. The long-term employee may be afforded 3 months to correct behaviors.
3. *The assistance the manager provides to help the employee reach the goals:* For the employee to achieve the stated goals, you may need to provide some help. Perhaps you need to arrange an education session for the employee to learn a skill that has not been mastered yet.
4. *The guidelines and parameters the employee is being held to:* For the employee to set realistic goals and meet the details of the performance plan, the employee needs to understand what policies and principles she or he is being held to.
5. *The consequence that occurs if the employee does not reach the performance goals in the specified time period:* What happens if the employee fails to achieve the goals agreed on in the performance improvement plan? The consequence needs to be a part of the plan. Does it mean that the employee should be terminated? Should he or she be reassigned to another unit? Should hours be cut?
6. *Signature and date of the employee and the manager:* You also may want the registered nurse supervisor to review and accept the plan.

The performance improvement plan can be a valuable tool in helping employees improve their overall performance. It is important, however, to use it in a positive way and not as a form of punishment. The performance improvement plan should result in a "win-win" agreement for all parties (Covey, 2013).

As a leader and a manager, you may be called on daily to communicate potentially confrontational comments to the people you manage. No one likes to do this. You can make the communication positive, however, by developing the skills outlined in this chapter. Because they are new skills, you may need to practice them on family and friends. It takes experience to be effective in interviewing others. Use the information in this chapter and incorporate it into your management personality. The results will be worth the effort.

REAL-WORLD CASE STUDY

■ You are an LPN recently assigned to work on the skilled nursing unit of an acute care hospital. You are responsible for a team of five CNAs. One of the CNAs has worked in long-term care for many years. She is a caring employee and does a good job, but she does not have a restorative approach. She would rather do for her assigned residents than encourage them to do for themselves. You notice that she does not walk her residents and frequently applies vest restraints to keep the residents "safe."

1. Because you are new and are not sure why the CNA is behaving in this manner, you realize the need to gather more information. You set up a counseling interview with the employee. What should you discuss at this meeting?
2. During the counseling session, the CNA informs you that she does not feel old people should be made to walk. She just wants to keep them clean, safe, and happy. She understands your expectations to help the residents regain function but is fearful to allow them to be unrestrained. She agrees to spend some time in the therapy department, which you arrange, to learn more about restorative care. After a week, you notice that her residents still are not being walked, and most remain in vest restraints during the day. When you ask, she says that there was no time to go to the therapy department as you arranged.

   What is your next step in helping this employee to improve her performance?
3. This strategy is ineffective in changing the CNA's behavior. She is still not using a restorative approach with the residents. In addition, several other areas of her performance are not up to standard. You see the need to develop a performance improvement plan.

   What do you include in the performance improvement plan for this employee?

Key Points

- The role of manager and leader are not the same. Although both involve goal setting, the focus of the manager is on the workplace, while the focus of the leader is on the individual.
- Use the acronym SMART when assisting others in setting goals: The goals should be Specific (clear and not general), Measurable (with criteria established to measure the goal), Attainable (important and not extreme), Realistic (relevant to the experience), and Time-bound (set with a commitment to a timeframe).
- Delegation is an art. It involves assessing tasks, the needs of the patient, and the evaluation of your own abilities. When making assignments, all members of the team should be considered for the benefit of the workplace, the patient, and the employee.
- To support an empowering environment for staff members means that you (1) incorporate their input into aspects of care that involve them, (2) share information with them regarding the care of the patients assigned to them for care, and (3) use staffing models based on this ongoing communication.

- Four primary aspects of coaching are (1) energizing, (2) providing positive reinforcement, (3) teaching and counseling, and (4) disciplining. All of these features are crucial to your success as a manager.
- When coaching an individual, determine whether a formal or informal session is appropriate. Regardless of the setting, be clear on why you are meeting and what the intended outcome will be for both parties moving forward.
- Evaluating the performance of others should be taken seriously. Staff members are vulnerable even when the evaluation is positive in nature.
- When a performance improvement plan is needed to help an employee improve her or his overall performance, follow the guidelines provided by your place of employment. These guidelines are in place for the protection of both the nurse manager and the employee.
- There are several levels of disciplinary action that can be taken by the nurse manager. They include verbal warning, written warning, suspension, and termination. Information regarding

each disciplinary level should be adequately documented and the documentation should be placed in the employee's personnel file.

■ When implementing disciplinary action, the employee needs to know two things: (1) what she did wrong and (2) how to correct the behavior. A positive instead of a punitive approach to the disciplinary process is more effective for all involved and can help the employee to improve performance and behavior.

ANSWERS TO REAL-WORLD CASE STUDY

1. You ask the CNA to see you when she has a few moments available and schedule a time to meet that is convenient for both of you. Meet in private, either in an office or in an area where other staff members cannot overhear. Discuss the behaviors that you wish to change. You want the residents to be assisted to walk or at least to stand every day. You want them to have active or passive range of motion each day, and you want the CNA to use the wedge cushion or other restraint alternatives identified in each resident's plan of care instead of the vest restraints. Ask the CNA why she has not been providing this restorative care. Identify what can be done to help the CNA correct her behavior and begin providing restorative care.

2. Another private interview with the employee is in order. Discuss reasons for the employee's resistance and try to problem-solve to remove those reasons. Give the CNA positive reinforcement for the tasks done well, but emphasize that the skills in restorative care need to improve for her overall performance to be acceptable. Be specific about the behaviors you want the CNA to demonstrate. Inform the CNA that you plan to arrange a specific date and time for her to visit the therapy department. You also arrange coverage for the CNA's residents on the unit. Ask the CNA whether there is anything else you can do to help her improve. Let the CNA know that you consider this discussion a verbal warning and that her behavior needs to change. If it

does not change, progressive discipline should follow.

3. You complete a performance review on the CNA and specifically identify the performance standards she is not meeting. You meet with the employee to discuss the review and identify behaviors that need to be changed, including the need to focus on restorative care. You let the CNA know that although this is not the usual time for a review, she has areas in which she is particularly strong and other areas that need improvement. The performance review and the compilation of a performance improvement plan give the CNA specific ideas on what needs to be done. Together you discuss what should be included in the plan:

   • Determine the performance standards the CNA needs to meet and specific goals for her behaviors.

   • Set a time frame for achievement. Because you have been talking with the CNA about restorative care over the past few weeks, the time frame for achievement of this goal may be shorter than the rest. Set up the next meeting when you can discuss progress with the CNA.

   • Determine what you can do to help the CNA achieve the goals.

   • Outline the consequences if the CNA does not meet the goals. Discuss the potential consequences with your registered nurse supervisor before you include them in the performance plan. Consequences may range from termination to progressive discipline or transfer off the unit.

REVIEW QUESTIONS

1. The nursing team consists of two RNs, one LPN, and two UAPs. Which of the following patients should the nurse on the medical-surgical unit assign to the LPN?
   1. A patient diagnosed with heart failure who is being discharged
   2. A patient admitted with a low hematocrit and hemoglobin complaining of fatigue
   3. A patient admitted with abdominal pain, weakness, and dizziness
   4. A patient with dysphasia who needs a tube feeding

2. A staff nurse has continued to show up late for her shift, despite the multiple verbal warnings she has received. What action by the nurse manager is best in this situation?
   1. Follow the facility's established disciplinary process.
   2. Pull the nurse aside in front of coworkers and remind her she has been warned about being late.
   3. Ignore the situation for now because the nurse is late and needs to get to work.
   4. Fill out a disciplinary action form and place it in the nurse's communication folder.

3. The LPN arrives at work at long-term care facility and is told that two UAPs are assigned to work with the nursing staff during the upcoming shift. In preparing to delegate assignments to the two UAPs, which action is best for the nurse to perform *first*?
   1. Check on patients to make sure that each patient is stable before getting a report.
   2. Clearly explain how each UAP is to perform each assigned task for the upcoming shift.
   3. Look up medication actions, side effects, and safe doses for each of the assigned patients.
   4. Match patient-care tasks and assignments with the abilities of each qualified UAP.

4. Which statement *most* accurately explains why a nurse would want to accept constructive criticism?
   1. Accepting criticism graciously is an effective way to impress the human resources department.
   2. A nurse who is able to accept criticism is more likely to progress and grow professionally.
   3. Criticism motivates the nurse to become a better worker.
   4. Nurses avoid formal complaints from patients and peers if they accept criticism without question.

5. The nurse is receiving a bedside report from another nurse. The nurse giving the report begins to talk about another patient who is not assigned to the reporting nurse. Which action by the nurse receiving the report is best in this situation?
   1. Ask the nurse to clarify whom the nurse is reporting on.
   2. Ask the nurse to move out into the hallway to continue the discussion.
   3. Ask the nurse not to talk so loudly.
   4. Ask the nurse to report only on the assigned patient.

References

Covey, S. (2013). *The 7 habits of highly effective people: Powerful lessons in personal change.* New York: Simon & Schuster. (Classic)

Doran, G. T. (1981). There's a S.M.A.R.T. way to write management's goals and objectives. *Management Review, 70*(11), 35–36. (Classic)

National Council of State Boards of Nursing. (2005). *Joint statement on delegation.* (Position statement, another has not been published) Retrieved from https://www.ncsbn.org/Delegation_joint_statement_NCSBN-ANA.pdf

Nugent, P., & Vitale, B. (2014). *Fundamentals of nursing: Content review plus practice questions.* Philadelphia: F.A. Davis.

Venes, D. (Ed.). (2009). *Taber's cyclopedic medical dictionary* (22nd ed.). Philadelphia: F.A. Davis.

Wilkinson, J. M., Treas, L. S., Barnett, K. L., & Smith, M. H. (2016). *Fundamentals of nursing: Theory, concepts, and applications* (Vol. 1). Philadelphia: F. A. Davis.

Web Resources

Performance Review www.chcf.org/~/media/MEDIA%20LIBRARY%20Files/PDF/PDF%20F/PDF%20FFGuidePerformanceAppraisals.pdf

Appendix

Answers to Review Questions

Chapter 19	Chapter 20	Chapter 21
1. 1	1. 1	1. 4
2. 2, 3, 4	2. 1, 2, 4, 5	2. 1
3. 3	3. 1	3. 4
4. 1	4. 2	4. 2
5. 1	5. 2	5. 4

Index

Note: Page numbers followed by "b," "f," and "t" indicate boxes, figures, and tables, respectively.

Ethical reasoning, 257
  process of, 258
Ethics, 251–258
  issues in, 255
    bioethics, 255–256
    genetics, 255
    stem-cell research, 255
  personal values and, 252–253
  principles of, 253, 254b
    autonomy, 254
    beneficence, 254
    fidelity, 254–255
    justice, 254
    nonmaleficence, 254
    veracity, 255
  theories of
    deontology, 256–257
    utilitarianism, 257
Ethnic, definition of, 176
Ethnic groups, in U.S., 186–187
Ethnicity, 47–48
Ethnocentrism, 184
Euclid, 102
European Americans, 186
Evaluation
  delegation and, 314
  of performance, 323–325
Evidence-based practice (EBP), 67, 73,
  202–203
Examinations/tests
  anxiety over, managing, 94
  developing test-taking skills, 89
  essay questions, 93–94
  multiple choice, 91–92
  reviewing for, 90
  true-or-false questions, 92–93
  words to understand when
    taking, 93b
Expert power, 273–275
Extended care facilities, 60

False imprisonment, 267
Feedback
  in communication process, 164–165
  in team management, 307–308
Fidelity, as ethical principle, 254–255
Flash cards, 89–90
Fleming, Alexander, 105
Fliedner, Theodor, 6
Forming, in team building, 306
Fraud, 266

Gender roles, 179–180
Genetics, as ethical issue, 255

Goals
  as component of performance analysis,
    324, 325
  SMART mnemonic for writing, 312b
Goodrich, Annie, 9, 10

HAIs. *See* Healthcare-associated
  infections
Hammurabi, 4
Health care, financing of, 54–55
Health-care agencies, 59
  assisted living centers, 60–61
  emergent care centers, 61
  extended care facilities, 60
  home health care, 60
  hospice, 60
  hospitals, 59
  industrial clinics, 61
  inner-city clinics, 62
  physician's office, 61
  public health departments, 61
  school health clinics, 61–62
Health-care providers, having fees administered
  by agency/negotiated with insurance
  company, 55b
Health-care systems, 54
  roles/tasks of LPN in, 56–57
Health information exchange (HIE), 70
Health information systems (HIS), 70
Health Information Technology for Economic
  and Clinical Health (HITECH) Act
  (2009), 70
Health Insurance Portability and Accountability
  Act (HIPAA, 1996), 71–72
Health literacy, 73–74
Health professionals, basic rights of, 167
Healthcare-associated infections (HAIs),
  11–12
Herzberg's two-factor theory of
  motivation, 293–295, 295t
HIE. *See* Health information exchange
Hierarchy of needs (Maslow), 21, 41f, 116,
  287–289
  motivation and, 123
  priority setting and, 215–217
High-touch nursing care, 21
  vs. high-tech nursing, 22
HIPAA. *See* Health Insurance Portability and
  Accountability Act
Hippocrates, 4
Hiring, for gender/ethnic diversity,
  188–189
HIS. *See* Health information systems
Hispanic Americans, 187